Atlas of Open Partial Horizontal Laryngectomy

Francesco Mattioli • Erika Crosetti
Michael Ghirelli • Matteo Fermi • Andy Bertolin
Editors

Atlas of Open Partial Horizontal Laryngectomy

Springer

Editors
Francesco Mattioli
Otorhinolaryngology Head and Neck Surgery
University Hospital of Modena
Modena, Italy

Michael Ghirelli
ENT Unit
AUSL Romagna, Ospedale Infermi di Rimini
Rimini, Italy

Andy Bertolin
ENT Department Laryngeal Cancer Centre
Ospedale Civile di Vittorio Veneto
Vittorio Veneto, Italy

Erika Crosetti
ENT Department Head and Neck Cancer Unit
San Giovanni Bosco Hospital
Torino, Italy

Matteo Fermi
Otorhinolaryngology Head and Neck Surgery
Azienda Ospedaliero Universitaria di
Bologna IRCCS
Bologna, Italy

ISBN 978-3-031-48022-5 ISBN 978-3-031-48023-2 (eBook)
https://doi.org/10.1007/978-3-031-48023-2

This Springer imprint is published by the registered company Springer Nature Switzerland AG
The registered company address is: Gewerbestrasse 11, 6330 Cham, Switzerland

Foreword

The treatment of tumors of the larynx represents one of the most relevant topics of Head and Neck Surgery.

Open partial horizontal laryngectomies (OPHL) have become a cornerstone in the treatment of laryngeal cancer. Nowadays, the preservation of laryngeal function is one of the primary goals in the treatment of these tumors.

During the past decades, the modular system of OPHLs has been further developed, thanks to the effort of Italian Laryngological School, providing new surgical and prognostic insights regarding the management of laryngeal cancers.

OPHLs offer a surgical strategy to deal with many different types of laryngeal cancers, even in case of locally advanced.

The book herein proposed is a comprehensive work, based on many years of shared surgical experience, displaying to the scientific community and the reader the know-how of the involved teams regarding indications, surgical steps, and postoperative management of OPHLs.

The images and the high quality of the intraoperative photographs will be an important help for the reader who wish to understand this topic to the last detail.

The editors and the co-authors involved in this opera are committed, passionate, and constantly involved in the research on this topic, and this book is the result of our effort for the International Scientific Community and the clinicians interested in this extremely relevant topic.

The aim will always be to propose the best possible therapeutic option to patients affected by laryngeal cancer in order to achieve optimal oncological and functional outcomes.

It has been a great pleasure and honor for us to have the opportunity to write a foreword to this amazing book.

ENT Dept. Laryngeal Cancer Centre
Ospedale Civile di Vittorio Veneto
Vittorio Veneto, Italy
Giuseppe Rizzotto

ENT Department Head Neck Cancer Unit
San Giovanni Bosco Hospital
Torino, Italy
Oncology Department
University of Turin
Turin, Italy
Giovanni Succo

Otorhinolaryngology Head and Neck Surgery
Azienda Ospedaliero Universitaria Di Bologna IRCCS
Bologna, Italy
Alma Mater Studiorum-Università di Bologna
Bologna, Italy
Livio Presutti

Contents

Anatomy of the Larynx

1

Ignacio Javier Fernandez, Cecilia Lotto, and Davide Dal Molin

The larynx is an uneven and median organ forming part of the upper airways. Phonation, respiration, and swallowing are its main functions. It is located in the infrahyoid region, below the hyoid bone and the tongue base. Its boundaries are anteriorly by the strap muscles, posteriorly the hypopharynx, superiorly the tongue base and valleculae and inferiorly the trachea.

The larynx is a compound organ formed by epithelium, ligaments, cartilages, muscles, and connective, neural and adipose tissues. The upper border is placed at the fourth cervical vertebra level, while the inferior one corresponds to the sixth cervical vertebra.

1.1 Laryngeal Framework

1.1.1 Cartilages (Fig. 1.1)

1. **Thyroid cartilage**

   The thyroid cartilage represents the largest cartilage of the whole laryngeal skeleton. It is constituted by two rectangular plates (or laminas) attached together by front end, forming an acute angle whose amplitude is variable depending on sex. In the upper part of the cartilage, the two laminas stay apart from each other, forming the thyroid notch. Each lamina has attached on its back end, a superior and an inferior cornua. The superior cornua is in contact with the greater horns of the hyoid bone, while the inferior cornua articulates with the cricoid cartilage forming the cricothyroid joint. This joint is a synovial joint and allows the anteroposterior sliding and rotation of the inferior thyroid cornua upon the cricoid cartilage.

   An important landmark is the superior tubercle, a cartilaginous eminence situated at the junction of the greater cornua with its respective thyroid ala. Just 1 cm below the superior tubercle, both the superior laryngeal nerve and artery pass through the thyrohyoid membrane to innervate the supraglottic region.

   On the anterior surface of the lamina stands the oblique line, a cartilage relief goes from posterior to anterior and from superior to inferior. Thyrohyoid and sternothyroid muscles anchor on this eminence [1–3].

   The vocal folds are located 0.5 cm under the superior margin of the thyroid cartilage, closer to the lower border of the cartilage than the upper [1].

2. **Cricoid cartilage**

   This signet ring-shaped cartilage is located under to the thyroid cartilage and upper to the trachea. It is formed by a posterior lamina, that is 20–30 mm in height, and an anterior arch that is only 3–4 mm in height. The posterior lamina articulates with the arytenoid cartilages in its superior surface thanks to the cricoarytenoid facets. The attachment with the thyroid cartilage is allowed by the cricothyroid joint facets that articulate with the lesser cornua of the thyroid cartilage. Cricothyroid membrane connects the superior margin of the cricoid arch with the inferior margin of the thyroid cartilage. Cricoid joins the first tracheal ring inferiorly by membranous attachment [1, 3].

   Cricoid represents the only tract of the airway completely encircle with cartilage.

3. **Arytenoid cartilages**

   The arytenoid cartilages are paired, and pyramidal cartilages located upper to the superior margin of the cricoid lamina. They both present an anterior vocal process, where vocal muscle and ligament attach, and a lateral muscular process where most of the intrinsic laryngeal muscles attach. In front of the anterior border of the vocal processes of these cartilages passes by an imaginary line that represents an important onchological breakpoint, called "Magic Line" [1–3].

I. J. Fernandez (✉) · C. Lotto
University of Bologna, Bologna, Italy

D. Dal Molin
Department of Otorhinolaryngology-Head and Neck Surgery, Azienda Ospedaliero Universitaria di Bologna IRCCS, Bologna, Italy
e-mail: davide.dalmolin@studio.unibo.it

F. Mattioli et al. (eds.), *Atlas of Open Partial Horizontal Laryngectomy*, https://doi.org/10.1007/978-3-031-48023-2_1

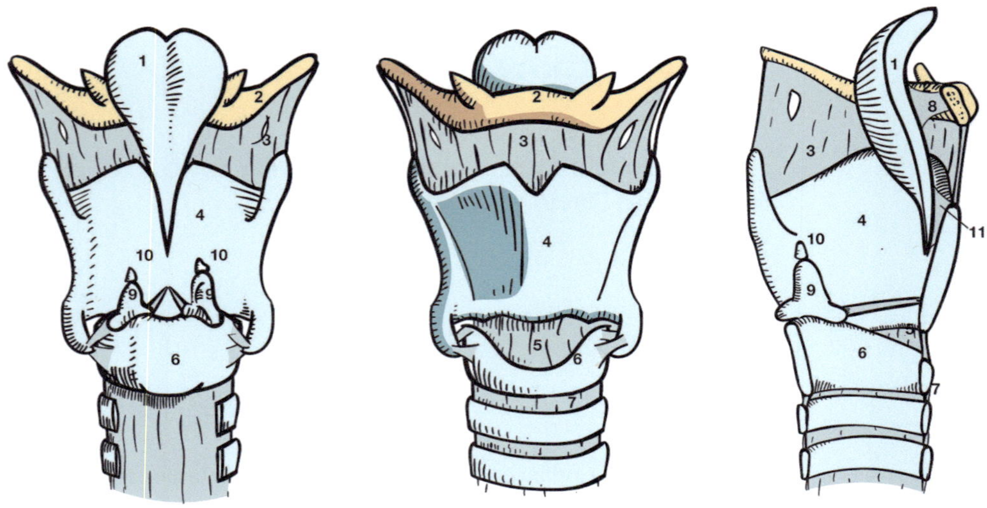

Fig. 1.1 (1) Epiglottis, (2) Hyoid bone, (3) Thyrohyoid membrane, (4) Thyroid cartilage, (5) Median cricothyroid ligament, (6) Cricoid cartilage, (7) Cricotracheal ligament, (8) Hyoepiglottic ligament, (9) Arytenoid cartilages, (10) Cuneiform and corniculate cartilages, (11) Thyroepiglottic ligament

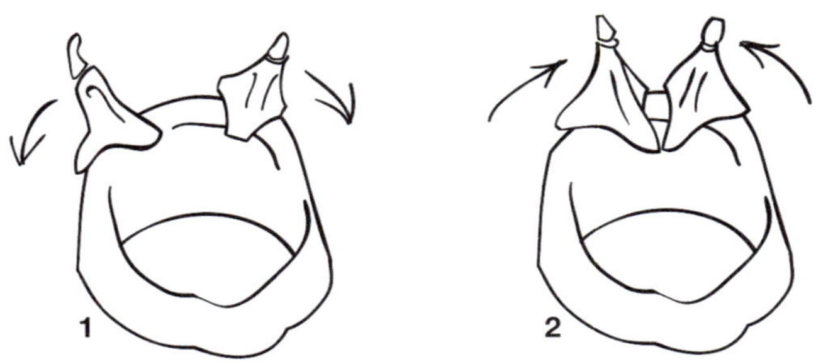

Fig. 1.2 (1) Abduction, (2) Adduction

Phonation, respiration, and swallowing happen thanks to their movements (Fig. 1.2).

4. **Cuneiform and corniculate cartilages**

   Cuneiform cartilages are two little rod-like cartilages included in both aryepiglottic folds providing additional structural support. Corniculate cartilages are two little cone-like cartilages located upper to the arytenoid apex and they are curved medially and posteriorly. They move with the corresponding arytenoid [1, 3].

5. **Epiglottis**

   Epiglottis is the only elastic cartilage of the larynx. It is oval leaf-shaped cartilage, located posterior to the hyoid bone and the thyroid cartilage. It forms a mucosal fold that separates the base of tongue by the larynx. Thanks to its posterior displacement during swallowing, it falls over the laryngeal vestibule preventing inhalation.

   The inferior part of the cartilage is attached to the inner surface of the thyroid cartilage just inferior to the thyroid notch. Its anterior surface relates to the base of tongue by three mucosal folds, the glossoepiglottic folds. It divides the anterior surface of the epiglottis in a superior part, covered by mucosa, and an inferior part, covered by adipose tissue belonging to the thyro-hyoid-epiglottic space. The posterior epiglottic surface is covered by the laryngeal mucosa [1–4].

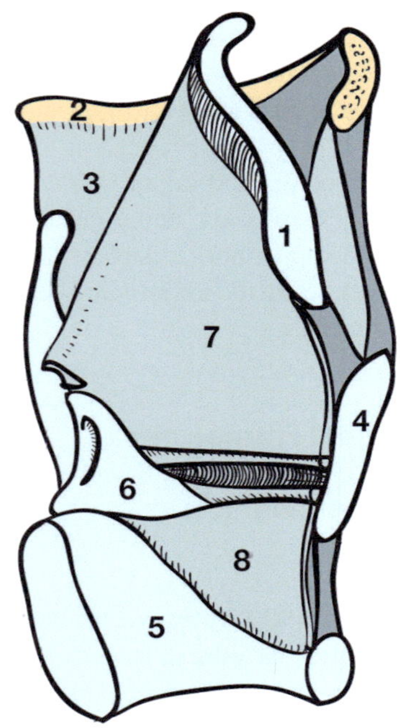

Fig. 1.3 (1) Epiglottis, (2) Hyoid bone, (3) Thyrohyoid membrane, (4) Thyroid cartilage, (5) Cricoid cartilage, (6) Arytenoid cartilages, (7) Quadrangular membrane, (8) Conus elasticus

1.1.2 Connective Membranes and Ligaments (Fig. 1.3)

1. **Quadrangular membrane**

   The quadrangular membrane is an elastic support structure of the supraglottic larynx. It extends from the lateral margin of the epiglottis to the medial surface of the arytenoid cartilages. Its superior margin is free and thickened, forming the aryepiglottic ligament. The inferior margin, also thickened, forms the vestibular ligament [1, 3].

2. **Conus Elasticus**

   Conus elasticus is a fibroelastic membrane located in the glottis and subglottic spaces. It attaches inferiorly to the superior margin of the cricoid cartilage and the inner surface of the first tracheal ring. The conus extends superiorly to the anterior commissure and the vocal process of the arytenoid cartilage. Its superior free margin represents the vocal ligament [2, 3].

1.1.3 Intrinsic Ligaments

1. Thyroepiglottic ligament joins the inferior part of the epiglottis to the inner surface of the thyroid cartilage.
2. Median cricothyroid ligament: it runs between the inferior margin of the thyroid cartilage and the superior margin of cricoid cartilage.
3. Cricocorniculate ligament arises from the superior margin of the cricoid lamina, it runs superiorly between the arytenoid cartilage to the corniculate cartilage [1–3].

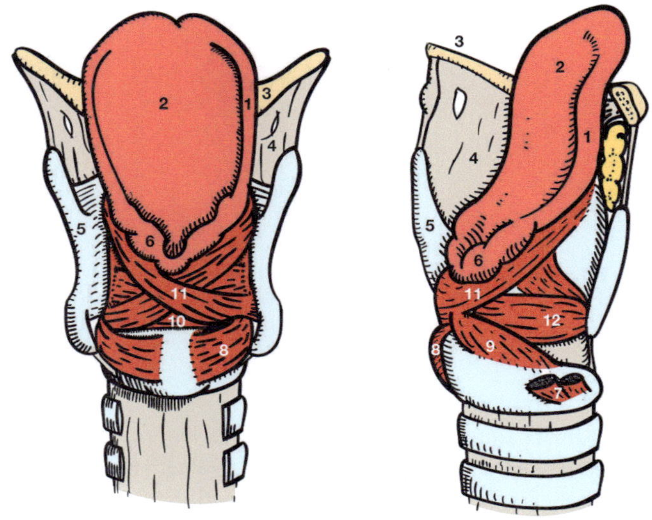

Fig. 1.4 (1) Aryepiglottic fold, (2) Epiglottis, (3) Hyoid bone, (4) Thyrohyoid membrane, (5) Thyroid cartilage, (6) Arytenoid cartilages, (7) Cricothyroid muscle, (8) Posterior cricoarytenoid muscle, (9) Lateral cricoarytenoid muscle, (10) Interarytenoid oblique muscle, (11) Interarytenoid transverse muscle, (12) Thyroarytenoid muscle

1.1.4 Extrinsic Ligaments

The extrinsic ligament connects the larynx with hyoid bone, tongue, pharynx, and first tracheal ring [1–3].

1. Thyrohyoid membrane: it extends from the inferior margin and the greater horns of the hyoid bone to the superior margin and superior cornua of the thyroid cartilage. It is laterally crossed by the internal branch of the superior laryngeal nerve and the superior laryngeal vessels.
2. Cricotracheal ligament: it runs between the inferior margin of cricoid cartilage to the superior margin of the first tracheal ring.
3. Hyoepiglottic ligament: it extends from the hyoid bone to the anterior surface of epiglottis. It helps the epiglottic replacement after swallowing.
4. Glossoepiglottic ligament: it forms the median glossoepiglottic fold and joins the tongue to the epiglottis.
5. Pharyngoepiglottic ligament: they form the lateral glossoepiglottic fold which runs between pharynx and the lateral margin of the epiglottis.

1.2 Laryngeal Muscles

1.2.1 Intrinsic Muscles (Fig. 1.4)

1. **Cricothyroid muscle**

   Cricothyroid muscle is in the antero-inferior part of the larynx. It is shaped like a triangle with its apex fixed to the cricoid arch and its base fixed to the inferior margin and the inferior cornu of the thyroid cartilage. This muscle is formed by two bellies: pars recta (medial and with vertical direction) and pars obliqua (lateral, with oblique direction from front to back). During contraction, the muscle raises the cricoid arch and pushes back the posterior cricoid lamina. The result is lengthening, tightening, and thinning the vocal folds [1–3].

   Its innervation is supplied by the external branch of the superior laryngeal nerve.
2. **Posterior cricoarytenoid muscle**

   This muscle is located posterior to the cricoid cartilage, deeper to the pharyngeal mucosa. Its belly originates through the entire height of the cricoid lamina, and it goes laterally and superiorly to the muscular process of the corresponding arytenoid cartilage. The two muscle contractions permit the abduction of the vocal folds and are principally responsible for control of the glottic airway. Its innervation is supplied by the inferior laryngeal nerve [1–3].
3. **Lateral cricoarytenoid muscle**

   This muscle is located laterally to the conus elasticus and is covered by the thyroid cartilage. It arises from the superior margin of the cricoid lamina to the muscular process of the arytenoid. Contraction displaces the muscular process laterally and anteriorly, while the vocal process moves medially. The result is vocal fold adduction and lengthening. This muscle runs lateral and in large part parallel with the thyroarytenoid muscle. Its innervation is supplied by the inferior laryngeal nerve [1–3].
4. **Interarytenoid oblique muscle**

   This muscle is superior to the posterior cricoarytenoid muscle and is covered by the pharyngeal mucosa.

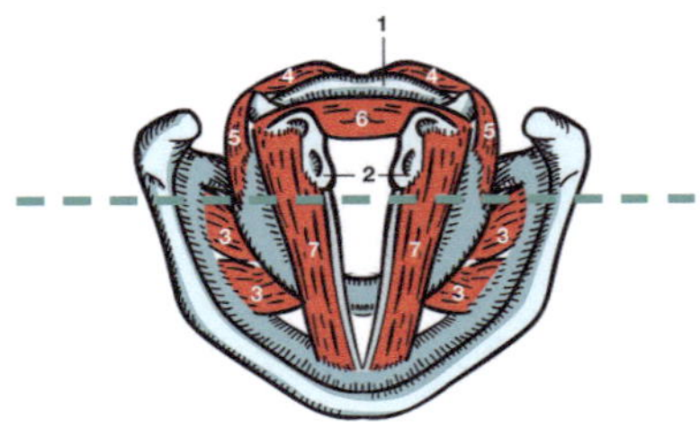

Fig. 1.5 (1) Cricoid cartilage, (2) Aryenoid cartilages, (3) Cricothyroid muscle, (4) Posterior cricoarytenoid muscle, (5) Lateral cricoarytenoid muscle, (6) Interarytenoid transverse muscle, (7) Thyroarytenoid muscle

Its fibers attach to each arytenoid apex and run obliquely (in the interarytenoid mucosal fold) to attach to the posterior face on the opposite side. Contraction of the muscles leads to arytenoid adduction, closure of the posterior glottis, and narrowing of the laryngeal inlet [1–3].

Its innervation is supplied by the inferior laryngeal nerve.

5. **Interarytenoid transverse muscle**

   This muscle is nonpaired and posteriorly covered by the interarytenoid oblique muscle. This muscle runs horizontally between the lateral margins of each arytenoid cartilage. Contraction of this muscle approaches the two cartilages and closes the posterior glottis [1–3].

   Its innervation is supplied by the inferior laryngeal nerve.

6. **Thyroarytenoid muscle** (Fig. 1.5)

   The thyroarytenoid muscle arises from the posterior face of the thyroid cartilage, where the acute angle is located. It runs posteriorly and cranially to the arytenoids. This muscle consists of two bellies: the externus and the internus. The thyroarytenoid externus inserts on the lateral surface of the arytenoid, while the internus bellies insert on the vocal process of the arytenoid. This portion of the muscle is also known as vocalis muscle. Contraction led to vocal folds shortening and thickening [1–3].

   Its innervation is supplied by the inferior laryngeal nerve.

1.2.2 Extrinsic Muscles (Fig. 1.6)

Extrinsic laryngeal muscles permit movements of elevation and depression of the larynx within the neck, connecting the laryngeal framework to the mandible, skull base, sternum, and scapula. These muscles comprise the suprahyoid group and the infrahyoid group. The suprahyoid muscles are the digastric muscle (anterior and posterior belly), mylohyoid, geniohyoid, and stylohyoid muscles. The thyropharyngeus (or inferior pharyngeal constrictor) and stylopharyngeus muscles together with suprahyoid muscles move the larynx superiorly and take part of the group of the elevators of the larynx [1, 3].

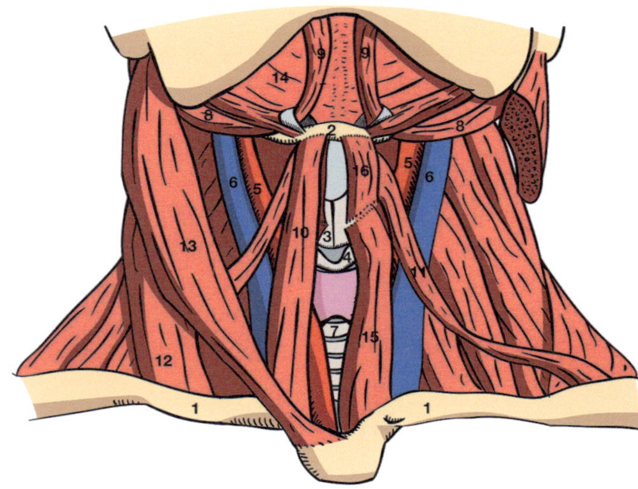

Fig. 1.6 (1) Clavicle, (2) Hyoid bone, (3) Thyroid cartilage, (4) Cricoid cartilage, (5) Carotid artery, (6) Giugular vein, (7) Trachea, (8) Posterior belly of the digastric muscle, (9) Anterior belly of the digastric muscle, (10) Sternohyoid muscle, (11) Omohyoid muscle, (12) Clavicular belly of the sternocleidomastoid muscle, (13) Sternal belly of the sternocleidomastoid muscle, (14) Mylohyoid muscle, (15) Sterno-thyroid muscle, (16) Thyro-hyoid muscle

The infrahyoid muscles are the sternothyroid, sternohyoid, and omohyoid muscles (superior and inferior belly) which act by moving inferiorly the larynx and can be grouped into the depressors of the larynx. Finally, the thyrohyoid muscle is an infrahyoid muscle which elevates the thyroid cartilage and reduces the distance between hyoid bone and thyroid cartilage.

1.3 Vocal Fold Microscopic Structure (Fig. 1.7)

Adult vocal folds have a layered structure consisting of the epithelium; the superficial, intermediate, and deep layers of the lamina propria; and the vocalis muscle. These layers can be divided into 3 sections: a cover, consisting of the epithelium and superficial layer of the lamina propria; a transition zone, consisting of the intermediate and deep layers of the lamina propria or vocal ligament; and a body, consisting of the vocalis muscle [1, 3, 5].

The most superficial layer is the squamous epithelium. Deep to the epithelium is located in the Reinke's space, the most superficial layer of the lamina propria, made up of sparse collagenous and elastic fibers within a glycoprotein matrix that vibrates markedly during phonation. The viscoelastic property of the lamina propria, especially the superficial layer, is very important for the vibratory behavior of the structure. Age-related changes in the collagenous and elastic

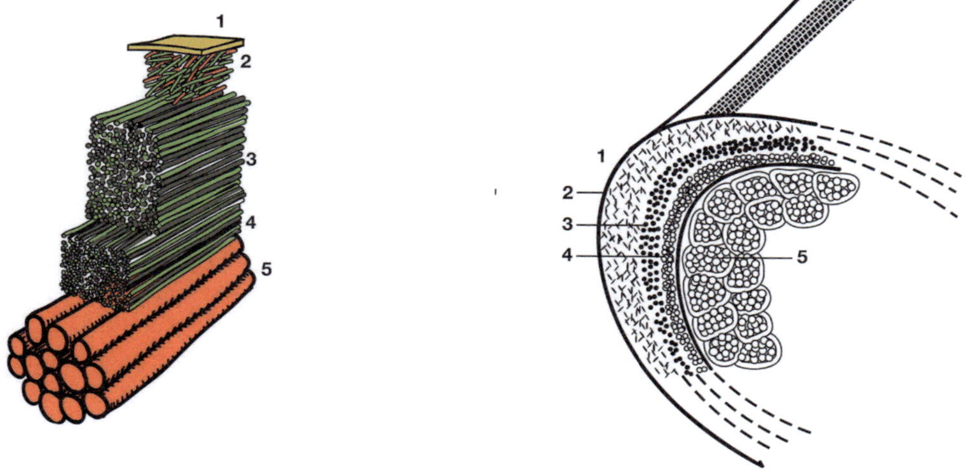

Fig. 1.7 (1) Epithelium, (2) Superficial layer of lamina propria (Reinke's space), (3) Intermediate layer of lamina propria, (4) Deep layer of lamina propria, (5) Vocalis muscle

fibers in the superficial layer of the lamina propria contribute to some extent to aging of the voice [5].

The intermediate layer is primarily made up of elastic fibers, whereas the deep layer is chiefly composed of collagen fibers. Together they form the vocal ligament which continues inferiorly with the conus elasticus.

The supraglottic larynx presents a cylindrical epithelial coating of a respiratory type with a rich supply of seromucous glands.

The subglottic larynx presents a structure similar to the trachea as regard the cylindrical coating of a respiratory type and the distribution of the seromucous glands.

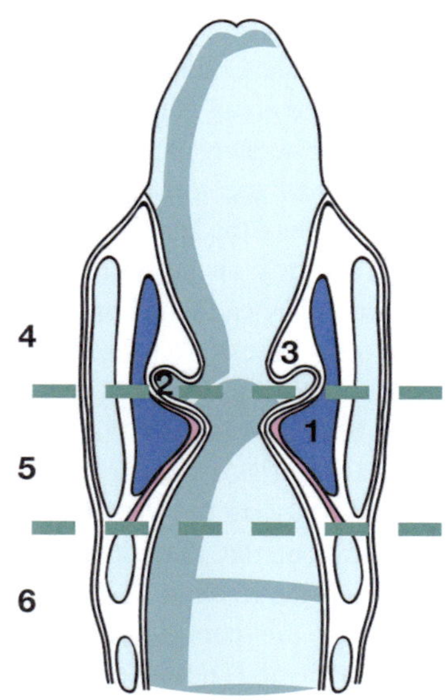

Fig. 1.8 (1) Vocal fold, (2) Ventricle, (3) Ventricular fold, (4) Supraglottic space, (5) Glottic space, (6) Subglottic space

1.4 The Laryngeal Spaces

An anatomical space is defined as any demarcated portion of the body, which can be an area of the surface, a segment of tissues, or a cavity. The main laryngeal spaces are the pre-epiglottic space and paraglottic space. Both spaces are clinically relevant (Fig. 1.8) [1, 4, 6–8].

1. **Pre-epiglottic space**

   The pre-epiglottic space, also called Boyer's space, is a triangular structure containing mostly adipose tissue, but also some elastic fibers, collagen fibers, and lots of lymphatic ducts. The pre-epiglottic space is surrounded by the hyoepiglottic membrane superiorly. This ligament is formed by collagen fibers lying in an anteroposterior direction, stretching from the periosteum of the superior edge of the hyoid bone to the anterior perichondrium of the free part of the epiglottis. The central part of the membrane is thicker where it forms the median hyoepiglottic ligament which extends caudally to the lingual surface of the epiglottis. Anteriorly the pre-epiglottic space is bounded by the thyrohyoid membrane and thyroid cartilage. The thyrohyoid membrane runs between the inferior margin of the hyoid bone and the superior margin of the thyroid cartilage. At this level, the median thyrohyoid ligament constitutes a median thickening of the membrane, and it is anchored to the superior margin of the hyoid bone, connecting with the fibers of the hyoepiglottic ligament. Posteroinferiorly the pre-epiglottic space is limited by the thyroepiglottic ligament and the ventral face of epiglottic cartilage. The most lateral fibers of the thyroepiglottic ligament continue with the fibers of the quadrangular membrane. The posterior end of the pre-epiglottic space is located near the anteroposterior midpoint of the thyroid lamina. The pre-epiglottic is adjacent to the paraglottic spaces in their lateral limit located posteroinferiorly and it is separated from them by a layer of fiber tissue (the so-called thyroglottic ligament), whereas the two spaces are not clearly delineated from each other postero superiorly. Therefore, at this level, the pre-epiglottic space continues from the lateral margins of the epiglottis toward the ary-epiglottic folds without anatomical boundaries [9].

2. **Paraglottic space**

   The paraglottic space is a laryngeal space filled by loose connective tissue, adipose tissue, lymphatic and blood vessels, and finally the Morgagni's ventricle.

   The paraglottic space is delimited by the thyroid cartilage laterally, by the piriform recess dorsally, and by the quadrangular membrane, vocal muscle, and conus elasticus medially.

   More specifically in its inferior part, the paraglottic space is bordered by the median cricothyroid ligament anteriorly, by the vocal muscle and conus elasticus medially and by the cricoarytenoid joint posteriorly. Both regions, the cricoarytenoid joint and the paraglottic space, are separated only by a small area of apposition of the lateral and posterior cricoarytenoid muscle. Anteriorly at the level of the cricothyroid ligament, there aren't any cartilage borders. This could represent a possible route for extra-laryngeal cancer spread.

   At the level of subglottic region, the conus elasticus divides into two bands, a lateral one, of more dense connective tissue, that inserts on the superior edge of the cricoid cartilage and bounds the cricothyroid space from below, and a medial one that continues inferiorly with the elastic membrane of the trachea.

   Supero-medially, the paraglottic space is in direct communication with the adipose tissue of the pre-epiglottic space. It should be underlined, that in some cases, the paraglottic space is separated from the pre-epiglottic by a collagenous fiber septum. Small projections of the paraglottic adipose tissue extend between the caudal fibers of the thyroarytenoid muscle.

   The vessels in this anatomical area have a cranio-caudal orientation, and this factor is crucial for the spreading of cancer.

1.5 Anterior Commissure

The larynx is divided into three main areas as supraglottic, glottic, and subglottic spaces. The vocal folds form the glottis. The right and left vocal cords join together anteriorly to form the anterior commissure, which adheres to the inner surface of the thyroid cartilage. The vocal ligament of each side continues anteriorly into the Broyles' ligament that inserts directly into the thyroid cartilage, within a small area with absent perichondrial layer. This area represents a crucial point for the possible spreading of cancer involving the anterior commissure.

Olofsson's description considers the anterior commissure, an area of mucosa located between the vocal cords, bounded superiorly by a line joining the angle of the ventricles and extending inferiorly for not more than 3 mm. The AJCC and Ogura consider the glottis, and therefore also the anterior commissure, as being included between the horizontal plane passing through the free margin of the vocal cord and a virtual plane located 1 cm more caudally [10].

Assessment of the anterior commissure is an important component of the radiologists' evaluation of many primary lesions of the true and false vocal cords to ascertain whether disease has spread across the midline.

1.6 Vascularization (Fig. 1.9)

The larynx is vascularized by two main arteries: the superior and the inferior laryngeal arteries.

- The **superior laryngeal artery** originates near the upper margin of the thyroid cartilage from the superior thyroid

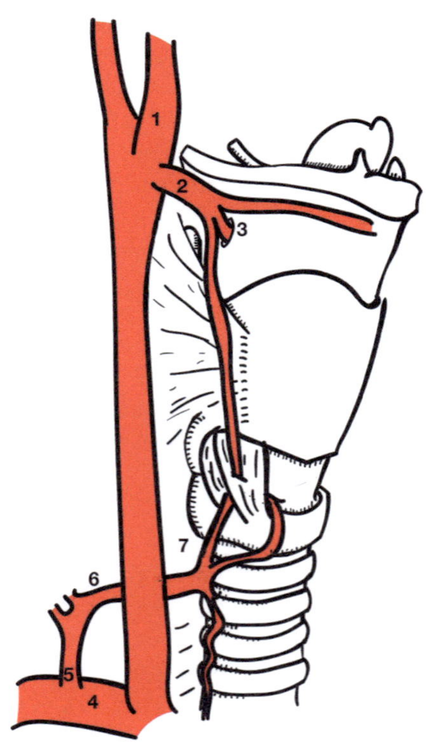

Fig. 1.9 (1) External carotid artery, (2) Superior thyroid artery, (3) Superior laryngeal artery, (4) Subclavian artery, (5) Thyrocervical trunk, (6) Inferior thyroid artery, (7) Inferior laryngeal artery

artery, branch of the external carotid artery, and accompanies the internal branch of the superior laryngeal nerve. They pass through the thyrohyoid membrane to reach the larynx.

- The **inferior laryngeal artery** originates from the inferior thyroid artery, branch of the thyrocervical trunk. It enters the larynx by passing deep to the inferior margin of the inferior constrictor muscle of the pharynx. Together with the recurrent laryngeal nerve, ascends in the groove between the esophagus and the trachea.

Veins draining the larynx accompany the arteries.

- **Superior laryngeal veins** drain into superior thyroid veins which, in turn, drain into the internal jugular veins.
- **Inferior laryngeal veins** drain into inferior thyroid veins, which drain into the left brachiocephalic vein.

1.7 Lymphatics

The lymphatics drain the region above and below the vocal folds, as lymphatic vessels are very densely represented in the supraglottis and subglottis. Those above the glottic space follow the superior laryngeal artery and terminate in deep cervical nodes, at the level of carotid bifurcations (Robbins level IIa and III). Those below the glottic space drain into deep nodes associated with the inferior thyroid artery or with nodes associated with the upper trachea (Robbins levels III, IV, and VI). Lymphatic vascularization is poor at glottic level, more evident at the level of anterior commissure and very rich at the level of posterior commissure, where lymphatics cross the midline, giving a bilateral drainage (Robbins level II and III) [11].

1.8 Innervation (Fig. 1.10)

Sensory and motor innervation of the larynx is supplied two branches of the vagus nerve:

1. **Superior laryngeal nerve**. It originates from the inferior vagal ganglia and descends medial to the internal carotid artery and divides into internal and external branches just above the level of the greater cornua of the hyoid bone. The external branch descends along the lateral wall of the pharynx, penetrates toward the inferior constrictor of the pharynx, and ends into the fiber of the cricothyroid muscle. The internal branch passes antero-inferiorly to penetrate the thyrohyoid membrane, together with the superior laryngeal artery. It is mainly sensory and supplies the laryngeal and hypopharyngeal mucosa. It divides commonly into a medial branch supplying the sensory innervation of the epiglottis, hyo-thyro-epiglottic space and supraglottis, and a lateral branch supplying the vocal cords, subglottic space, and mucosa of the pyriform sinus [1, 3].

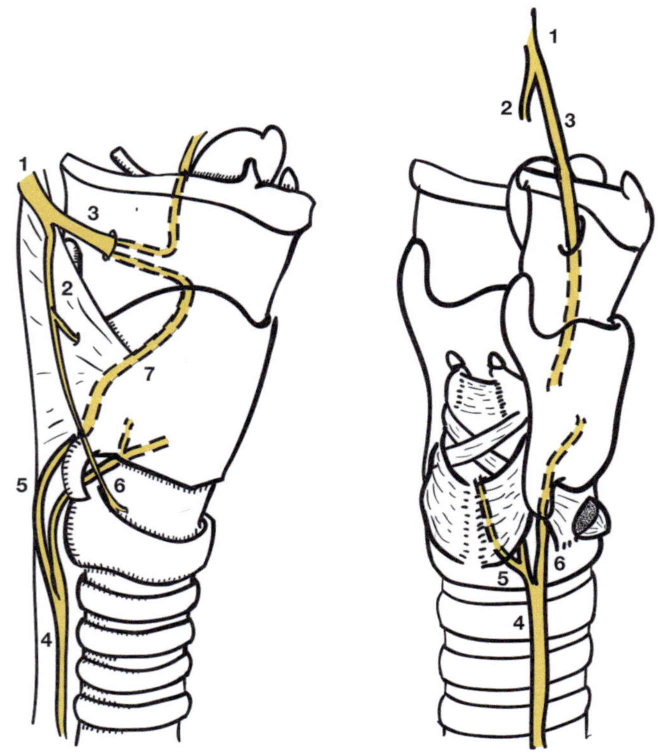

Fig. 1.10 (1) Superior laryngeal nerve, (2) External branch, (3) Internal branch, (4) Inferior or recurrent laryngeal nerve, (5) Posterior branch, (6) Anterior branch, (7) Galen's loop

2. **Inferior or recurrent laryngeal nerve**. Recurrent laryngeal nerves have a distinct course on the right and left side. The left recurrent laryngeal nerve is longer than the right one, as it originates from the vagus nerve in the mediastinum, surrounds the aortic arch, and runs upwards into the lateral groove between trachea and esophagus and behind the left thyroid lobe. The right one originates from the right vagus nerve, in the thoracic inlet and surrounds the right subclavian artery. The right recurrent nerve ascends into the neck following an oblique (superior-medial) direction, eventually joining the right groove formed by the esophagus and trachea. Both nerves penetrate the larynx deep to the margin of inferior constrictor of the pharynx and posterior to the joint between the inferior cornu of the thyroid cartilage and cricoid cartilage. In the internal part of the larynx, they divide in an anterior and in a posterior branch. The posterior branch connects with the internal branch of the superior laryngeal nerve, forming the "Galen's loop." The recurrent laryngeal nerves are motor to all intrinsic muscles of the larynx except for the cricothyroid muscle [1, 3].

References

1. Lucioni M. Practical guide to neck dissection. 2nd ed. Springer Verlag; 2013.
2. Rosen CA, Simpsons CB. Operative techniques in laryngology. Springer Verlag; 2008.
3. Gray H. Gray's anatomy. The anatomical basis of clinical practice. 41st ed. Elsevier; 2015.
4. Reidenbach MM. The periepiglottic space: topographic relations and histological organization. J Anat. 1996;188(Pt 1):173–82.
5. Sato K. Reticular fibers in the vocal fold mucosa. Ann Otol Rhinol Laryngol. 1998;107(12):1023–8.
6. Reidenbach MM. Borders and topographic relationships of the paraglottic space. Eur Arch Otorrinolaringol. 1997;254(4):193–5.
7. Reidenbach MM. The paraglottic space and transglottic cancer: anatomical considerations. Clin Anat. 1996;9(4):244–51.
8. Sato K, Kurita S, Hirano M. Location of the preepiglottic space and its relationship to the paraglottic space. Ann Otol Rhinol Laryngol. 1993;102(12):930–4.
9. Dayal VS, Bahri H, Stone PC. Preepiglottic space: an anatomic study. Arch Otolaryngol Head Neck Surg. 1972;95(2):130–3.
10. Ortug G, Liman Z, Ortug A. A dissectional study of the level of anterior commissure of the larynx. Ear Nose Throat J. 2021;100(10S):983S–8S.
11. Robbins KT, Clayman G, Levine PA, et al. Neck dissection classification update: revision proposed by the American Head and Neck Society and the American academy of otolaryngology—head and neck surgery. Arch Otolaryngol Head and Neck Surg. 2002;128(7):751–8.

Diagnostic Work-Up in Laryngeal Oncology

2

Erika Crosetti, Andy Bertolin, Ilaria Bertotto, Daniele Regge, and Giovanni Succo

In the current scenario where "precision surgery" of laryngeal cancer is taking hold, with the implementation of organ and functional preservation strategies, an equally precise diagnostic work-up is highly warranted.

The selection of laryngeal cancer (LC), still manageable by open partial horizontal laryngectomy (OPHL), requires a very precise endoscopic and radiological work-up.

2.1 Endoscopic Work-Up

The endoscopic evaluation for the diagnosis and staging of malignant laryngeal neoplasms has been enriched in recent years with new tools, to plan a "custom tailored" therapeutic choice, aimed at safeguarding the organ and functions.

Given the large number of tools available today, it is undoubtedly difficult to identify the gold standard for the endoscopic staging of laryngeal tumors. Every exam provides a contingent of information, each of which is useful for reducing the rate of up- and downstaged patients in the pre-treatment phase.

Indirect videolaryngoscopy, with rigid telescopes (angled 70° and 90°) or flexible instruments and the white light source (WL) or stroboscopic one (STROBO-L), is the standard diagnostic approach in the diagnosis of laryngeal tumors.

The image quality has been greatly improved with the introduction of high-definition cameras (HDTV) and flexible videoendoscopes with high-quality distal microchips, respectively.

The breakthrough in terms of additional information obtainable in indirect laryngoscopy was then possible thanks to the development of further endoscopic tools, such as autofluorescence (AF), narrow band imaging (NBI), and coherent optical tomography.

Lastly, the most recent endoscopic methods on the market were ECE (Enhanced Contact Endoscopy) [1] and HD SPIES technology (Storz Professional Image Enhancement System) (KARLSTORZ GmbH & Co., Tuttlingen, Germany).

These new endoscopic tools provide important biological information and are useful to improve pre- and intraoperative assessment of the superficial extent of the lesion and to identify new areas of malignant transformation, that are distinct from the primary lesion.

This new interpretation of endoscopy, that is, associating the two-dimensional and macroscopic assessment of a lesion with a study aimed at understanding its biology and assuming its histology, is defined as "biological endoscopy."

The *Narrow Band Imaging (NBI) endoscopy*, recently introduced and borrowed from gastroenterological experiences, is an innovative system of optical technology that, by

Supplementary Information The online version contains supplementary material available at https://doi.org/10.1007/978-3-031-48023-2_2. The videos can be accessed individually by clicking the DOI link in the accompanying figure caption or by scanning this link with the SN More Media App.

E. Crosetti (✉)
ENT Department Head and Neck Cancer Unit, San Giovanni Bosco Hospital, Torino, Italy

A. Bertolin
ENT Department Laryngeal Cancer Centre, Ospedale Civile di Vittorio Veneto, Vittorio Veneto, Italy

I. Bertotto
Radiology Unit, FPO IRCCS Candiolo Cancer Institute, Candiolo, Turin, Italy
e-mail: ilaria.bertotto@ircc.it

D. Regge
Radiology Unit, FPO IRCCS Candiolo Cancer Institute, Candiolo, Turin, Italy

Department of Surgical Sciences, University of Turin, Turin, Italy
e-mail: daniele.regge@ircc.it

G. Succo
ENT Department Head Neck Cancer Unit, San Giovanni Bosco Hospital, Torino, Italy

Oncology Department, University of Turin, Turin, Italy

F. Mattioli et al. (eds.), *Atlas of Open Partial Horizontal Laryngectomy*, https://doi.org/10.1007/978-3-031-48023-2_2

means of a double filter, exclusively selects two wavelengths of 415 and 540 mm (corresponding to blue and green light). In this way, the vascular architecture of the mucosal surface is emphasized, ensuring the detection of precancerous and neoplastic lesions, thanks to their characteristic neoangiogenic hypervascularization.

Vascular morphological alterations include capillary intrapapillary vascular loops (IPCL) that hypertrophy and increase in density in inflammatory lesions, up to becoming tortuous in dysplastic lesions and highly irregular in neoplastic ones; well-demarcated dark area in the context of a normal mucosa, with the presence of dark punctiform lesions, increase in vascular density or presence of tortuous and irregular vessels, with densely represented capillary loops; an hypertrophic vessel afferent to the lesion, which comes from the periphery, branching irregularly into vascular loops in the context of the lesion and surrounding tissues.

Many recent publications have demonstrated the degree of reliability of NBI in the early diagnosis and staging of tumors of the upper aero-digestive tracts, showing high values of sensitivity (SE), specificity (SP), positive predictive value (VPP), negative predictive value (NPV), and diagnostic accuracy.

Moreover, the NBI technology, combined with HDTV, proved to be extremely advantageous in intraoperative upstaging and in the best definition of surgical margins in transoral laryngeal surgery [2–5].

One of the most interesting features of the NBI is also its high specificity, when compared, for example, to the autofluorescence endoscopy, with the possibility of distinguishing the NBI patterns characteristic of inflammatory and neoplastic lesions.

The ability to discriminate "true positive" endoscopic pictures from "false positives" is certainly strongly conditioned by the clinician's experience, which can be acquired with a relatively short learning process (about 6 months).

The "false positives" are generally represented by pictures of chronic inflammation and mucositis following previous radiotherapy, in which there is a widespread increase in density and hyperplasia of the capillaries, without the characteristic clear demarcation toward the surrounding mucosa. In this clinical setting, the NBI confirms an additional value with an SE, SP, VPP, VPN, and AC of 100%, 98%, 92%, 100%, and 98%, respectively.

Autofluorescence (AF) of normal and pathological laryngeal tissues has been studied since 1980. In 1984, Alfano [6], using the principle that the biochemical composition and histomorphological architecture of the tissue profile determine their spectral characteristics of fluorescence, demonstrated that the AF technique could effectively differentiate normal tissue from pre-neoplastic and tumor pathological tissue.

The autofluorescence endoscopy (AF) has found application in the diagnosis of superior aero-digestive tract pathology, with particular interest in the evaluation of laryngeal lesions of the larynx. Recent studies reported sensitivity (SE) and specificity (SP) values varying between 97% and 87%, and 87% and 78%, respectively [7].

The use of AF in direct microlaryngoscopy has been considered by many authors to be the gold standard, with an increase in SE (92–87% vs 71–75%) and an increase in accuracy diagnostic (AC) by 12%. Furthermore, the combination of the two diagnostic procedures (direct microlaryngoscopy + AF) results in a statistically significant increase in SE to 97–100%, if compared with the SE of direct microlaryngoscopy alone or of AF only.

In a recent article [8], the systematic application of AF endoscopy during microlaryngoscopy has allowed a better definition of the superficial extension of the lesion, in particular of its margins, even in the presence of abundant superficial keratosis. A prospective evaluation of the diagnostic accuracy of surficial extension and TNM staging was conducted in 73 patients with glottic cancer, undergoing transoral laser surgery. The use of direct AF resulted in disease-free surface margins in 97.2% of cases and small surface margins in 2.8%. An improvement in diagnostic accuracy occurred in 16.4% while in 8.2% of cases there was an up-staging of the TNM classification. The sensitivity of direct AF was 96.5% and the specificity was 98.5%.

The AF endoscopy enriched the pre- and intraoperative work-up of multistep endoscopy, providing information on the biological characteristics of the disease. In a recent paper [9] on a cohort of 140 patients with suspected laryngeal cancer, who underwent a series of indirect laryngeal endoscopic examinations (WL endoscopy with HDTV camera, laryngostroboscopy, and AF endoscopy) and subsequently undergoing direct microlaryngoscopy (MLD) (WL endoscopy with HDTV camera and AF endoscopy), higher sensitivity (97.9%) and specificity (90.5%) values were obtained compared to the single methods, allowing a better therapeutic planning of superficial lesions and a more accurate orientation of the mapping biopsies of widespread lesions.

The most recently introduced bio-endoscopic tool is the *SPIES endoscopy*, a technology that allows to evaluate a lesion through the chromatic representation of the different wavelengths of the visible light spectrum mediated by a high-definition camera. SPIES technology allows to appreciate and evaluate the mucosal surface and subepithelial vascularization depending on the selected wavelength (Clara, Clara + Chroma, Chromz, Spectra A, Spectra B). The main target of this new endoscopic device is neoangiogenesis, a prerequisite for the progression of precancerous lesions in frankly neoplastic lesions. Similarly to NBI technology, SPIES technology also requires a certain degree of experience in order to minimize the percentage of false positives.

It is important to emphasize that the assessment of the real limits of surficial extension of a laryngeal lesion can only be performed during direct laryngoscopy. The diagnostic work-up performed in indirect laryngoscopy is burdened by a considerable number of downstaged patients, even with the best technologies and good expertise of clinicians (especially in the case of lesions that extend toward the bottom of the ventricle, lesions of the anterior commissure or characterized by an important hypertrophy of the false cords or dyskeratosis, etc.)

Indirect endoscopic staging allows to "approach" the patient more correctly and to raise the degree of suspicion toward the more frankly borderline lesions.

The significant elements of this evaluation are the quality of the image in terms of definition and chromatic fidelity, the possibility of reaching the proximity of the lesion and of exploring the blindest parts (ventricles, anterior commissure, commissure of the false cords, hypoglottic cone); angled vision; optical and digital enhancement techniques (autofluorescence, NBI, HD SPIES) focusing on the peripheral extremes and angles of the lesions, especially if hyperkeratotic; the ability to record the exam and review it by freezing the image on the most significant frames.

First of all, the use of flexible instruments and rigid telescopes determines a first dichotomy: the videolaryngoscopy is increasingly orienting itself toward a philosophy of "single exam," conducted in an cabinet, with compliant patient (prepared with pre-anesthetic drug) in order to enhance the versatility and angular vision of the instruments, which at the same time allow the static and dynamic examination of all laryngeal structures (vocal cords and arytenoids), the use of the digital optical enhancement of the NBI, the continuation of the endoscopic investigation of the entire airway and digestive tract, and finally the completion of the exam with a microbiopsy.

The endoscopy with rigid telescopes determines a more orthodox and less versatile diagnostic liturgy, providing an image quality still unattainable for videolaryngoscopes and, when coupled to the HDTV camera, even superior to microscopic vision.

In this case, the diagnostic strategy involves two distinct phases. The indirect examination with the dynamic assessment of the patient prepared with local anesthesia. A second phase, which involves the direct evaluation of the larynx, with the patient in narcosis, completes the diagnosis on the "less visible" parts such as the ventricle, the commissure of the true and false vocal cords, the hypoglottic cone, using telescopes with different angles (0° –70° –120°), with the possibility of equal use of HD SPIES endoscopy, completion of the examination on the airways and digestive system, and biopsy assessment of the lesion.

To maximize the potential of this diagnostic strategy, it is advisable to use special laryngoscopes, with a "large" proximal section, which do not require the direct engagement of the tip of the instrument in the laryngeal vestibule. In our experience, the Lindholm laryngoscope is optimal for this purpose.

The final evaluation of the real extent of the lesion must only be the product of information from the imaging with the information of the complete endoscopic work-up ("dynamic" exams in indirect laryngoscopy + "static" exams in direct laryngoscopy).

2.2 Imaging

In the patient's work-up, the endoscopic assessment provides an accurate definition of the superficial tumoral extension and functional data on the motility of the vocal cords and arytenoids. Based on this preliminary information, head and neck surgeons query the radiologist with specific questions on the extent of submucosal neoplastic involvement. In this context, the introduction in clinical practice of a structured checklist that includes all the key anatomical structures to be assessed by the radiologist allows a more meticulous and systematic imaging assessment. Furthermore, this tool facilitates a cooperative attitude between the radiologist and the surgeon, especially in cases of equivocal radiological findings, allowing the best possible surgical planning.

In the staging of laryngeal cancer, "*precision imaging*" translates into the accurate evaluation of very small anatomical critical subsites and adequate characterization of tissues, focusing on the distinction between tumor and peritumoral inflammatory changes. The overall aim of imaging is therefore to reduce the risk of overstaging of the disease and consequently of overtreatment.

Contrast-enhanced multidetector computed tomography (CECT) is the first-line imaging technique for laryngeal cancer assessment [10]. The short acquisition time needed to cover a large body volume reduces motion artifacts. In addition, multiplanar reconstructions allow the assessment of tumor spread on the other planes (i.e., coronal or sagittal). Finally, reconstructions on an axial plane parallel to the glottis must be obtained to avoid misinterpretation [11].

The main limitation of CT in laryngeal cancer staging is the low sensitivity. In particular, the CT-scan inaccuracy in the assessment of neoplastic invasion of the cartilages and of extralaryngeal spread is well known [12, 13]. The poor representation of adipose tissue in the paraglottic space at the glottic level makes the evaluation of tumor spread, especially in the posterior compartment, difficult [14].

Magnetic resonance imaging (MRI) is a second-level technique in the assessment of laryngeal cancer. MRI is characterized by a high intrinsic tissue contrast resolution, enhanced by the multiparametric approach that combines information from different sequences (morphological T1 and T2 weighted, diffusion weighted imaging (DWI), and post Gadolinium administration acquisition). Consequently, it has a greater potential than CT to characterize different tissues. However, long acquisition times and motion artifacts still represent two challenging technical aspects of larynx MRI. Diagnostic accuracy of MRI and its potential advantage over CT in the local staging of laryngeal cancer are strictly dependent on the quality of MR images. High-quality examinations can be obtained by adopting state-of-the-art MR techniques as reported in literature guidelines [1, 10, 11, 14].

Precise assessment of submucosal tumoral spread and accurate report of critical areas are key issues for optimal partial surgical planning. The small size of the laryngeal subsites requires high spatial resolution. Moreover, slice thickness should not exceed 3 mm to avoid "partial volume effect" artifacts. The use of local surface coils, alone or combined with head coils, is strongly advocated. Surface coils have a small field of view but sufficient to cover the larynx and hypopharynx and provide an increased signal-to-noise ratio [10, 13, 14].

Ensuring adequate patient cooperation is challenging during MR scanning. Motion artifacts, mainly related to frequent swallowing, especially in cases of bulky laryngeal tumor in non-compliant subjects, may drastically reduce image quality. Correct coil positioning by a trained technician and adequate instructions to the patient on breathing and swallowing during image acquisition contribute to quality of MR examination. Furthermore, MRI technological improvements have reduced acquisition time, minimizing the effects of patient voluntary and physiologic movements, without an increase in scanning time.

Proper MRI scanning, i.e., orientation of the axial plane parallel to the true vocal folds plane, and of the coronal plane orthogonal to it, is crucial for a correct interpretation of radiological findings.

DWI, e.g., molecular diffusion, is a functional technique that represents the Brownian motion of water protons in a tissue. In high cellular density tissues, such as solid tumors, molecular diffusion is restricted. At the qualitative visual assessment, this phenomenon translates into a high signal intensity of the tumor on images acquired at high *b*-values and a low signal intensity on the corresponding ADC map. Due to tissue heterogeneity and the geometrical features of head and neck region, the acquisition of good quality DW images is challenging [15]. Indeed, DW images could present with a low spatial resolution and geometric distortions that reduce its quality [13].

A multiparametric approach integrating signal intensity information from morphological sequences, DWI, and contrast-enhanced acquisitions, allows MRI to distinguish tumoral tissue from edema and peritumoral inflammation. By using a multiparametric approach in the evaluation of primary laryngeal cancer, MRI provides a more accurate assessment of the paraglottic space and cartilages than CT, thus improving specificity values [10, 13, 16]. Ravanelli et al. [12], in a retrospective analysis of 17 patients affected by cT3 glottic SCC with arytenoid fixation demonstrated that MR, performed with a state-of-the-art technique, was able to predict tumoral invasion of posterior laryngeal compartment/cricoarytenoid unit distinguishing it form inflammatory involvement [14]. Furthermore, MR reliably detects extralaryngeal spread, providing more accurate information than CT. Finally, state-of-the-art multiparametric MRI is preferable to CT in the preoperative work-up to evaluate submucosal disease spread in patients scheduled for OPHL [17].

In patients previously treated with (chemo)radiotherapy or surgery and with suspicion of tumor persistence or recurrence, MRI may play a role in the differential diagnosis between tumoral tissue and post-treatment changes (e.g., fibrosis, scar, inflammation, and edema) [10].

In the assessment of nodal staging, the presence of neck metastatic nodes or suspected ones, the involved levels, unilaterality or bilaterality, and signs of extra-nodal extension should be evaluated and reported by the radiologist as well as the presence of Delphian node and of its metastatic invasion. Ultrasonography has a complementary role in the characterization of nodes and is the preferred method for percutaneous imaged-guided biopsy, bearing in mind that imaging cannot detect microscopic disease within a node [18].

On the basis of endoscopic and radiological aspects, it was possible to propose a laryngeal compartmentalization, using a vertical virtual plane tangential to the arytenoid vocal process and perpendicular to the ipsilateral thyroid lamina (the so-called magic plane) [17].

Therefore, an adequate preoperative endoscopic and imaging work-up able to reliably distinguish among such different causes of arytenoid fixation are strongly warranted and might greatly help in subclassifying these lesions according to more detailed etiologies in the future.

2.3 Case Example 1

A 59 year old male affected by a right glottic-transglottic squamous cell carcinoma (SCC) G3.

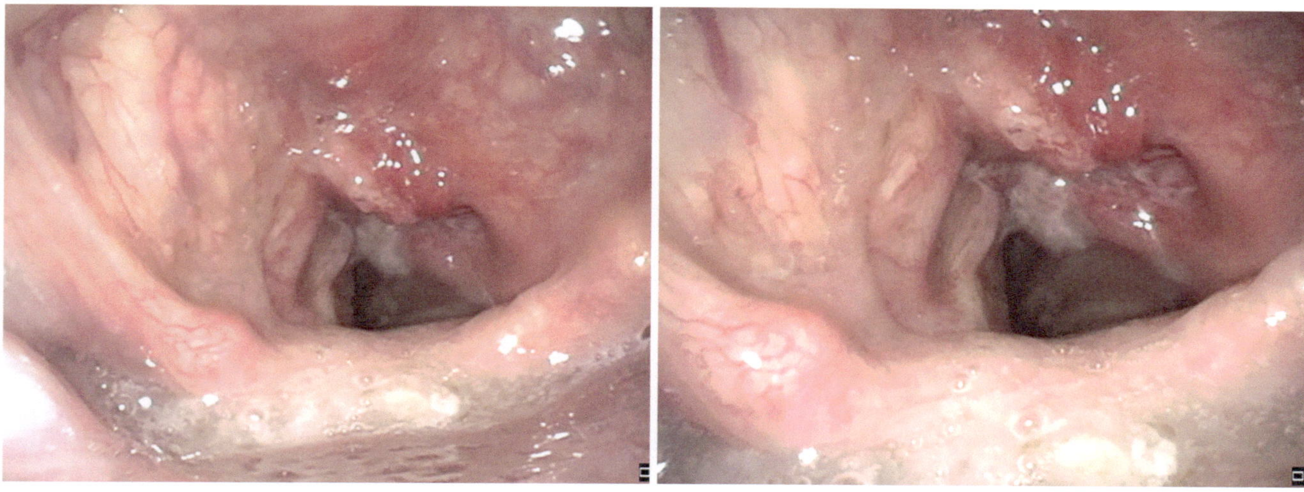

Pre-operative endoscopy. The tumor involves the right vocal cord and extends to the right false cord and the petiolus of epiglottis, showing a clear transglottic spreading
The motility of right vocal cord is absent
The motility of the right arytenoid is preserved (Video 2.1)

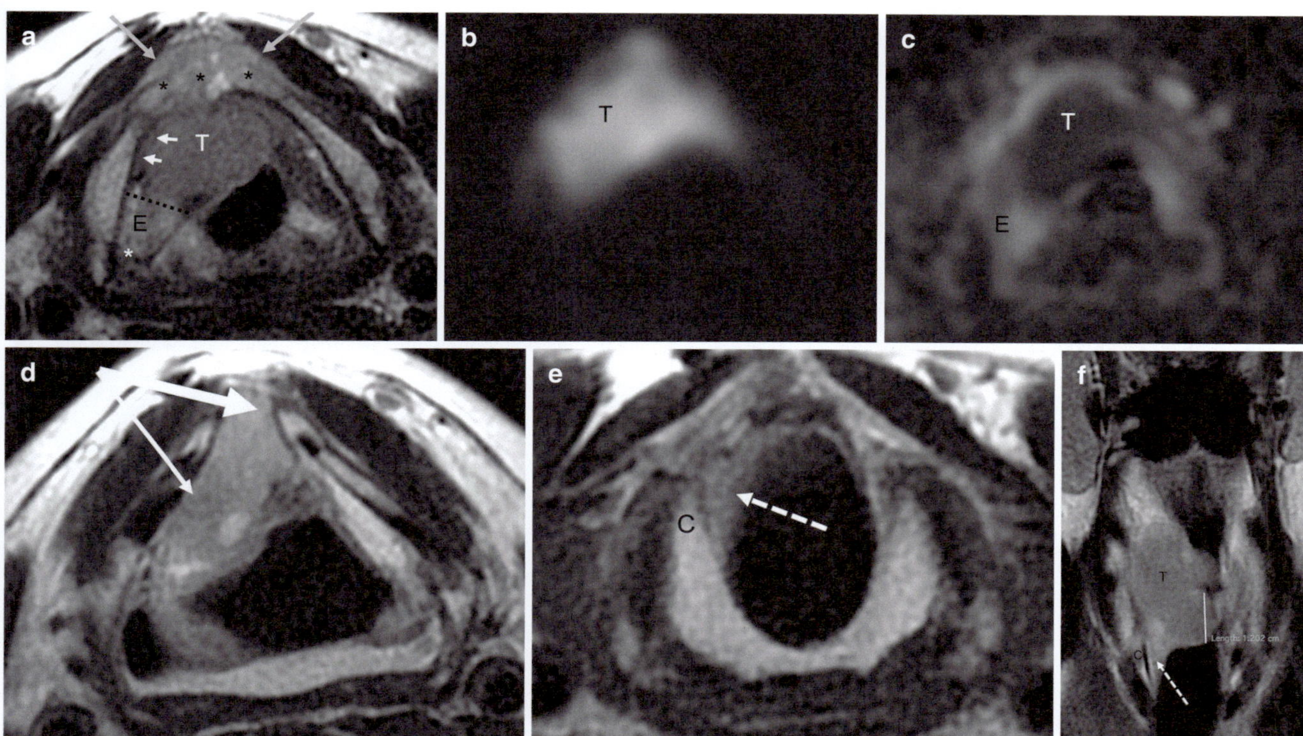

The glottic level demonstrated by FSE T2-weighted (**a**) DWI b1000 (**b**), ADC map (**c**). A large tumor (T) with intermediate signal intensity on T2 (**a**), high signal intensity on DWI b1000 (**b**), and restriction on the ADC map (**c**) invades the anterior laryngeal compartment. In the T2-weighted image, (**a**) the lesion infiltrates the right true vocal cord and extends to the contralateral side, it invades the right anterior paraglottic space (short white arrows) and involves massively the thyroid cartilage (asterisks) spreading into the extralaryngeal soft tissue (gray arrows). Behind the "magic plane" (**a**) (black dotted line), alterations brighter than the tumor on T2 (**a**) and without restriction on the ADC map (**c**) indicative of peritumoral edema (**e**) involve the posterior paraglottic space, expanding the thyrocricoarytenoid space (**a**) (white asterisk)
The lesion has a transglottic spreading as demonstrated in the axial FSE T2-weighted (**d**) and coronal FSE T1-weighted postcontrast images (**f**). At the supraglottic level (**d**) the fat tissue of the right superior paraglottic space (thin white arrow) and of the pre-epiglottic space (thick white arrow) is replaced by the tumor. The lesion has minimal subglottic extension (**f**). In the FSE T2-weighted sequence at the subglottic level (**e**) the dashed white arrow points at a submucosal thickening brighter than the tumor and characterized by enhancement (**f**) indicative of peritumoral edema adjacent to the inner cortex of the cricoid (**c**) without tumoral involvement of the cartilage itself (**e, f**). *FSE* fast spin echo, *DWI* diffusion-weighted imaging, *ADC* apparent diffusion coefficient

2.4 Case Example 2

A 68 year old male affected by a left glottic SCC

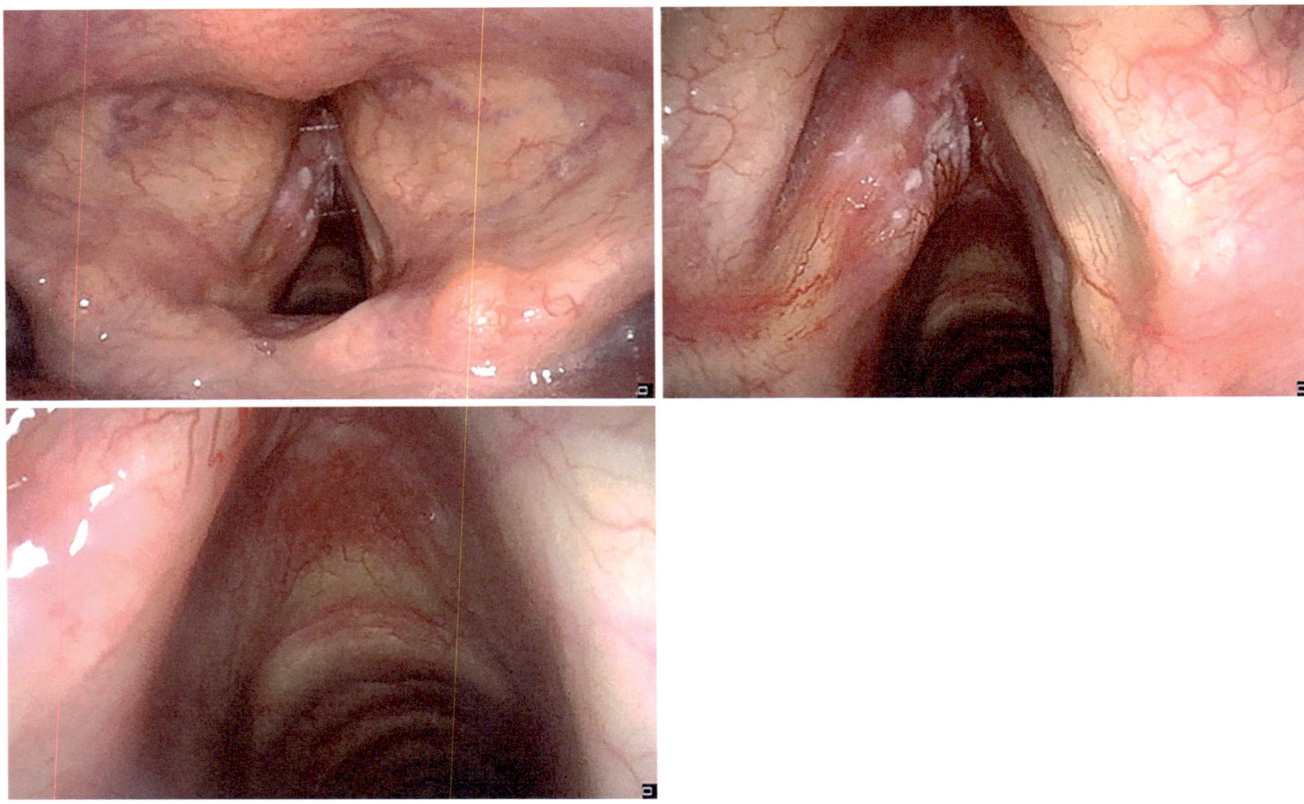

Pre-operative videoendoscopy: the tumor involves the left vocal cord reaching the anterior commissure. Minimal submucosal swelling at the level of conus elasticus on the left side
The motility of both vocal cords and arytenoids is preserved (Video 2.2)

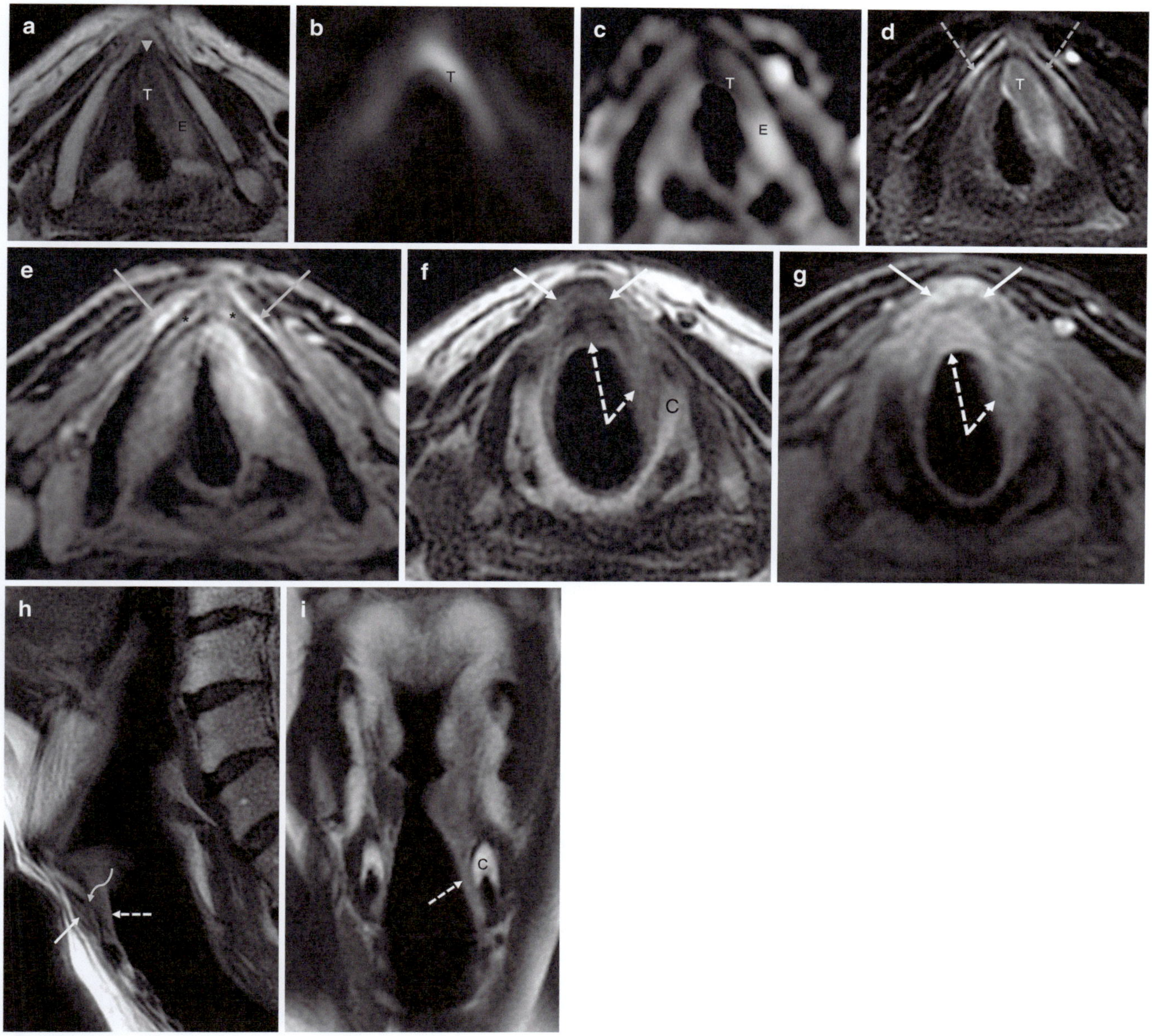

The glottic level is depicted on different MRI sequences FSE T2-weighted (**a**), DWI b1000 (**b**), ADC map (**c**), fat sat T2-weighted (**d**), and 3D gradient echo fat sat T1 postcontrast injection (**e**)
MRI demonstrates a left glottic neoplastic lesion (T) with an intermediate signal intensity on T2-weighted (**a**), high intensity on the DWI b 1000 sequence (**b**) and low signal on the ADC map, indicative of restriction (**c**). The tumor infiltrates the anterior two thirds of the left true vocal cord (**a**) up to the anterior commissure (gray arrowhead). Bright alteration on T2-weighted (**a**) without restriction (**c**), due to edema (**e**) surrounds the tumor
The lesion is adjacent to the inner cortex of the left thyroid lamina (**d**); the bone marrow of the thyroid cartilage shows a brighter signal intensity than the tumor (dashed gray arrows) and enhancement (**e**) (black asterisks) indicative of inflammatory changes. In the T1-weighted postcontrast image (**e**) a linear enhanced alteration is detected outside the larynx (gray arrows). Subglottic level on axial FSE T2-weighted (**f**) and 3D gradient echo fat sat T1 postcontrast (**g**); FSE T2 weighted on sagittal (**h**) and coronal (**i**) planes
T2-weighted images in the three planes show a neoplastic submucosal thickening (white dashed arrows) with enhancement (**g**) in the anterior and left side of subglottic level. At the same level extralaryngeal spread (**f, g, h**) (white arrows) through the cricothyroid membrane (**h**) (curved arrow) is present. The cricoid cartilage (**f, i**) (**c**) does not show abnormal alterations suspicious of invasion. *FSE* fast spin echo, *DWI* diffusion-weighted imaging, *ADC* apparent diffusion coefficient

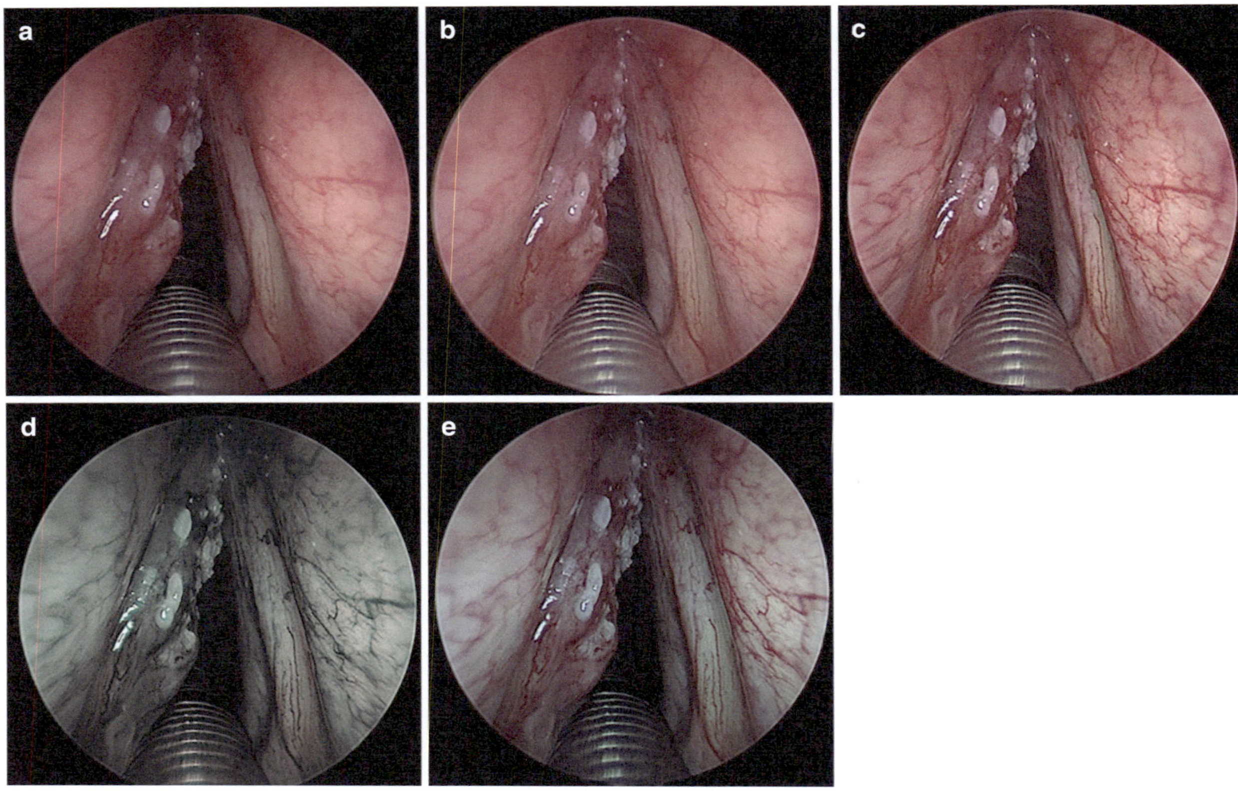

Intraoperative work-up (0° rigid telescope HD SPIES): the tumor infiltrates the left vocal cord and extends to the anterior commissure (**a**: white light; **b**: Clara; **c**: clara + chroma; **d**: spectra A; e: spectra B)

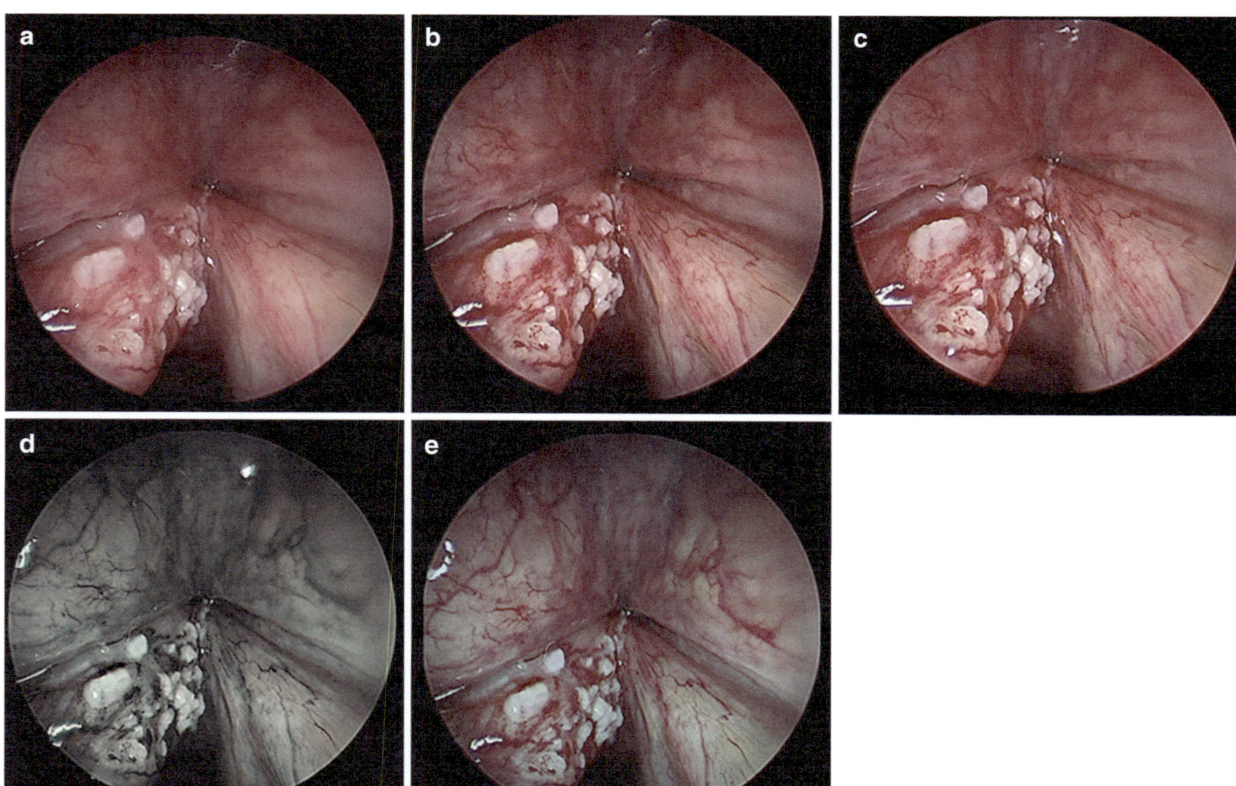

Intraoperative work-up (70° rigid telescope HD SPIES): the tumor infiltrates the left vocal cord and extends to the anterior commissure (**a**: white light; **b**: Clara; **c**: clara + chroma; **d**: spectra A; **e**: spectra B)

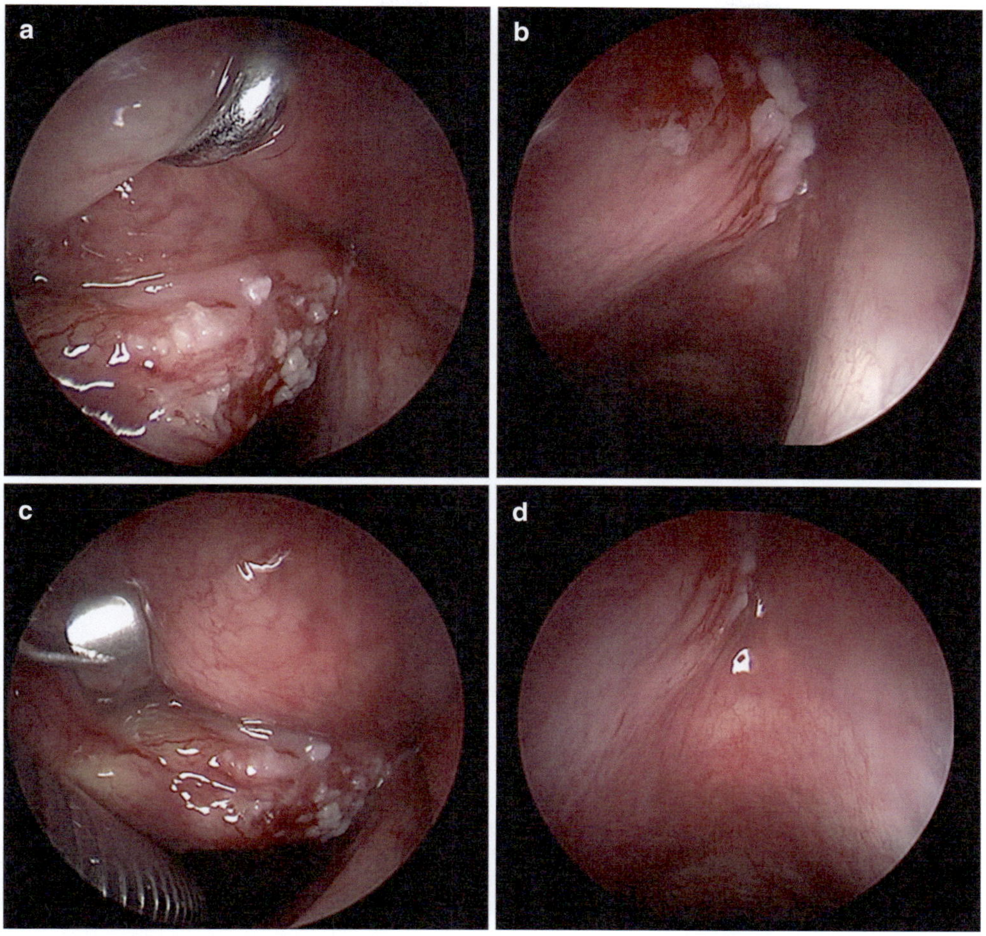

Intraoperative work-up (70° rigid telescope HD SPIES): the tumor infiltrates the left ventricle and extends to the subglottic region. Posteriorly, the tumor reaches the vocal process of left arytenoid

2.5 Case Example 3

A 62-year-old female affected by supraglottic SCC

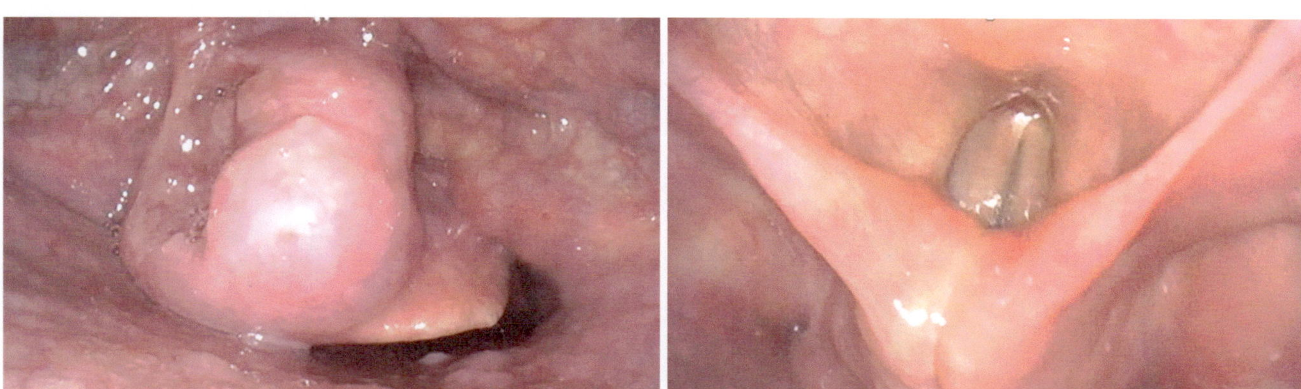

Pre-operative work-up. The tumor involves the left lingual aspect of epiglottis and left glosso-epiglottic vallecula
The motility of both vocal cords and arytenoids is preserved (Video 2.3)

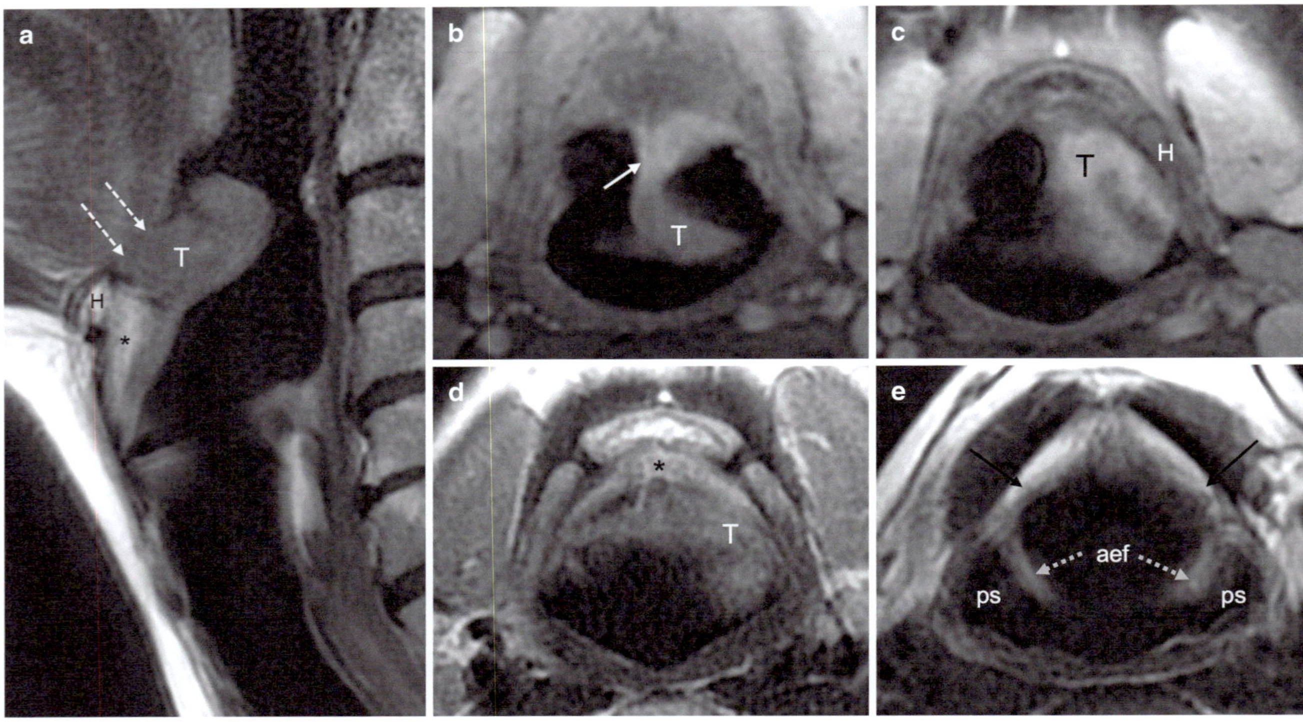

MRI FSE T2-weighted sequence on sagittal plane (**a**), 3D gradient echo fat sat T1 postcontrast injection on axial plane (**b**, **c**) and FSE T2 weighted on axial plane (**d**, **e**)
At supraglottic level, the neoplastic tissue (T) with intermediate signal intensity on T2 weighted (**a**) and enhancement (**b**, **c**) involves the left side of lingual surface of the suprahyoid epiglottis cartilage extending to the glossoepiglottic fold (**b**) (white arrow). The lesion is adjacent to the base of the tongue (**a**) (dashed white arrows) and close to the hyoid bone (H) that does not show any abnormalities suspicious of invasion (**a**, **c**). The pre-epiglottic space (black asterisk) is normal in both sagittal (**a**) and axial planes (**d**). In the T2-weighted axial image (**e**), black arrows indicate the high signal intensity of non-invaded superior paraglottic spaces and gray dashed arrows point at normal aryepiglottic folds. Piriform sinuses (ps) appear regular
A left level II neck node (**c**) (N) smaller than 1 cm in short axis diameter is detected

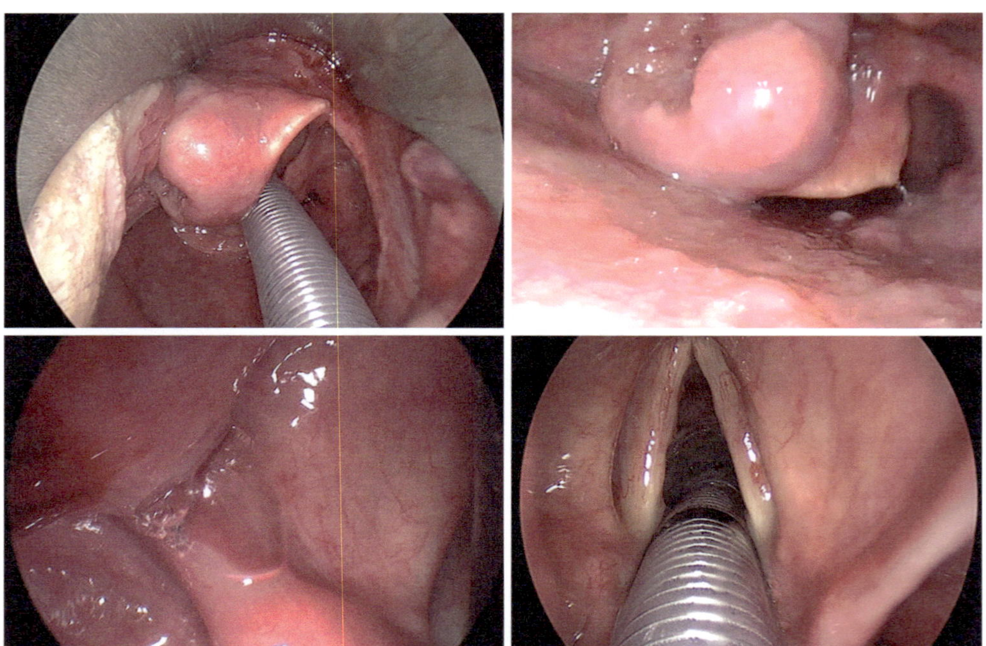

Intraoperative work-up (0° rigid telescope). The tumor infiltrates the left lingual aspect of epiglottis and left glosso-epiglottic vallecula. The glottis plane is not involved

2.6 Case Example 4

A 54 year old male affected by persistence of left glottic SCC after radiotherapy

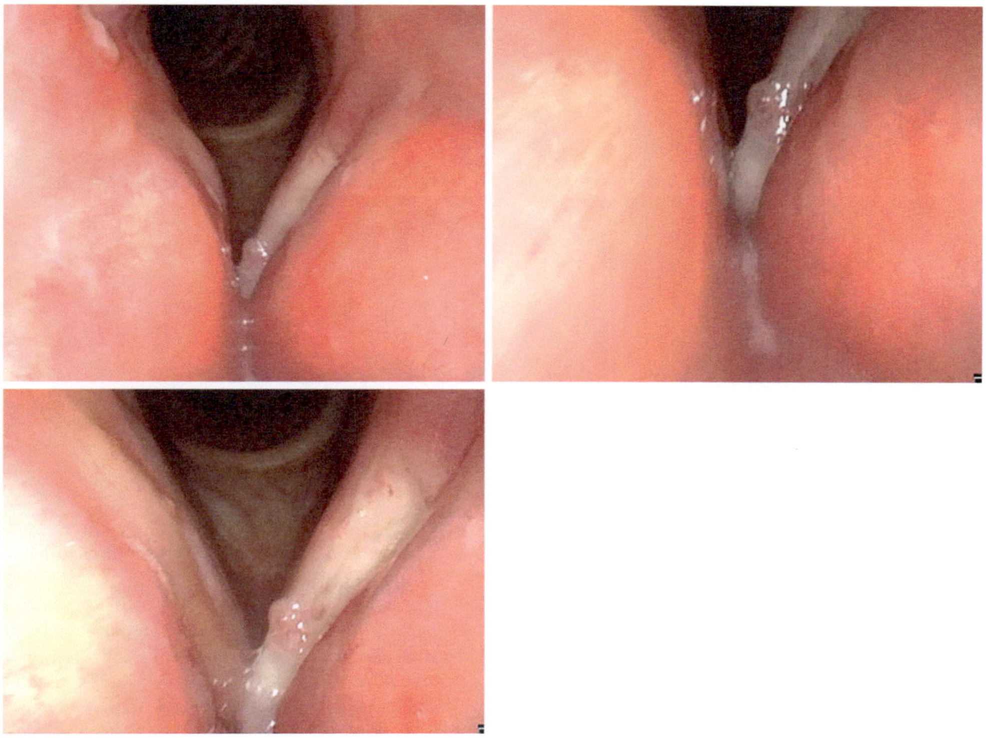

Pre-operative work-up. The tumor involves the left vocal cord reaching the anterior commissure
The motility of both vocal cords and arytenoids is preserved (Video 2.4)

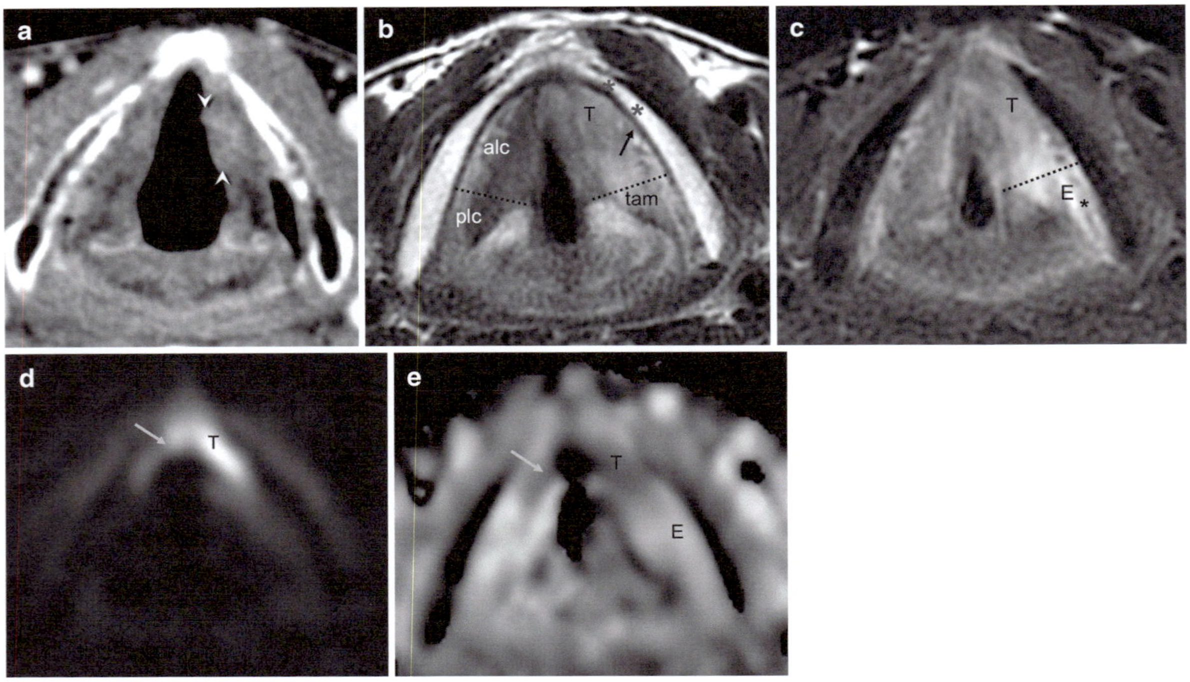

CT axial scan after radiation therapy for left glottic SCC (**a**). At the glottic level arrowheads delimit an area with moderate contrast enhancement in the left true vocal cord, suspected of tumor persistence
Glottic level detected by different MR sequences FSE T2-weighted (**b**), FSE fat sat T2 weighted (**c**), DWI b1000 (**d**), ADC map (**e**). The black dotted lines (**b**, **c**) indicate the "magic plane" (described by Succo et al.) that separates the anterior laryngeal compartment (alc) form the posterior laryngeal compartment (plc). In the anterior third of the left true vocal cord MR images show a tumoral tissue (T) with intermediate signal intensity on T2 (**b**, **c**), high signal on DWI b1000 (**d**) and low signal on ADC map indicative of restricted diffusion (**e**). A small alteration (grey arrow) suspected of tumoral spread to the anterior third of the right true vocal cord is depicted on DWI b1000 (**d**) and ADC map (**e**). On the left side the tumor invades the anterior paraglottic space (**b**) (black arrow) without any abnormalities within the thyroid cartilage (grey asterisks). High signal intensity alterations on T2 (**b**), better depicted on fat sat T2 (**c**) without restriction of diffusion (**d**, **e**) correspond to post-treatment inflammatory edema (E) and involve the posterior part of the thyroarytenoid muscle (tam) (**b**) and the posterior paraglottic space (**c**) (black asterisk)
FSE fast spin echo, *DWI* diffusion-weighted imaging, *ADC* apparent diffusion coefficient

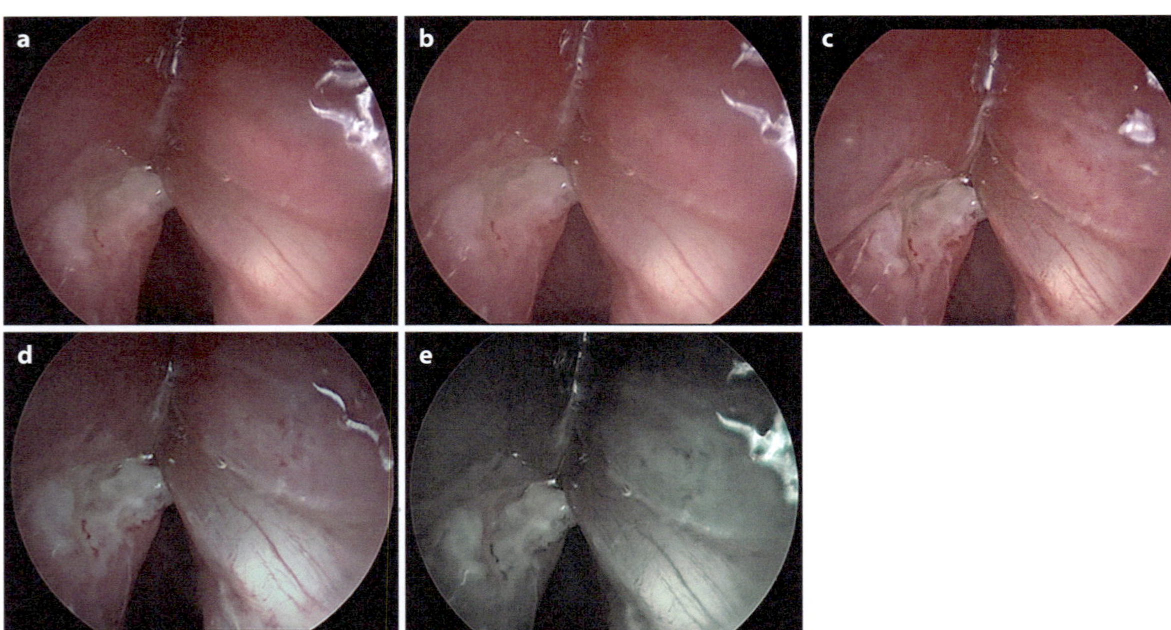

Intra-operative work-up (70° rigid telescope HD SPIES): the tumour involves the left vocal cord and the anterior commessure (**a**: white light; **b**: Clara; **c**: clara + chroma; **d**: spectra B; **e**: spectra A)

2.7 Case Example 5

A 69 year old male affected by left glottic SCC

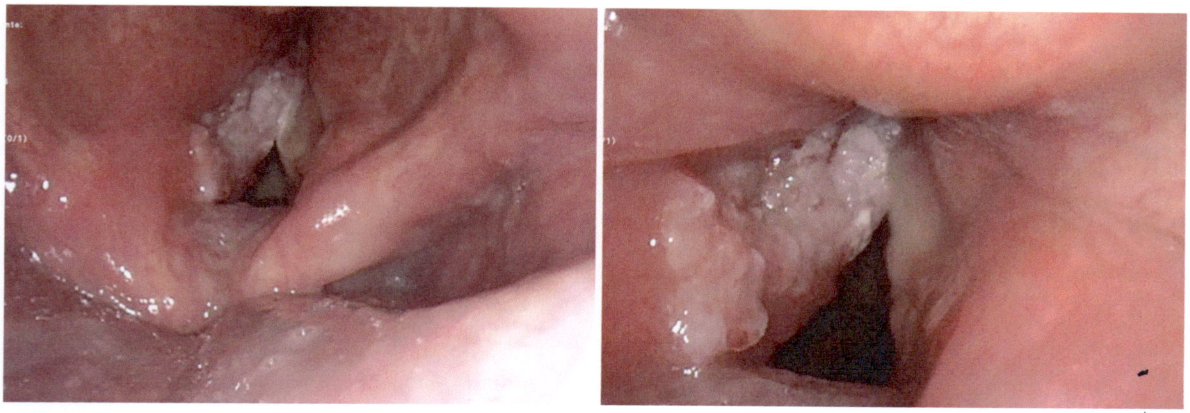

Pre-operative work-up. The tumor involves the left vocal cord, the left false cord, reaching the vocal process of arytenoid and showing a transglottic extension
The motility of left vocal cord is absent
The motility of left arytenoid is preserved (Video 2.5)

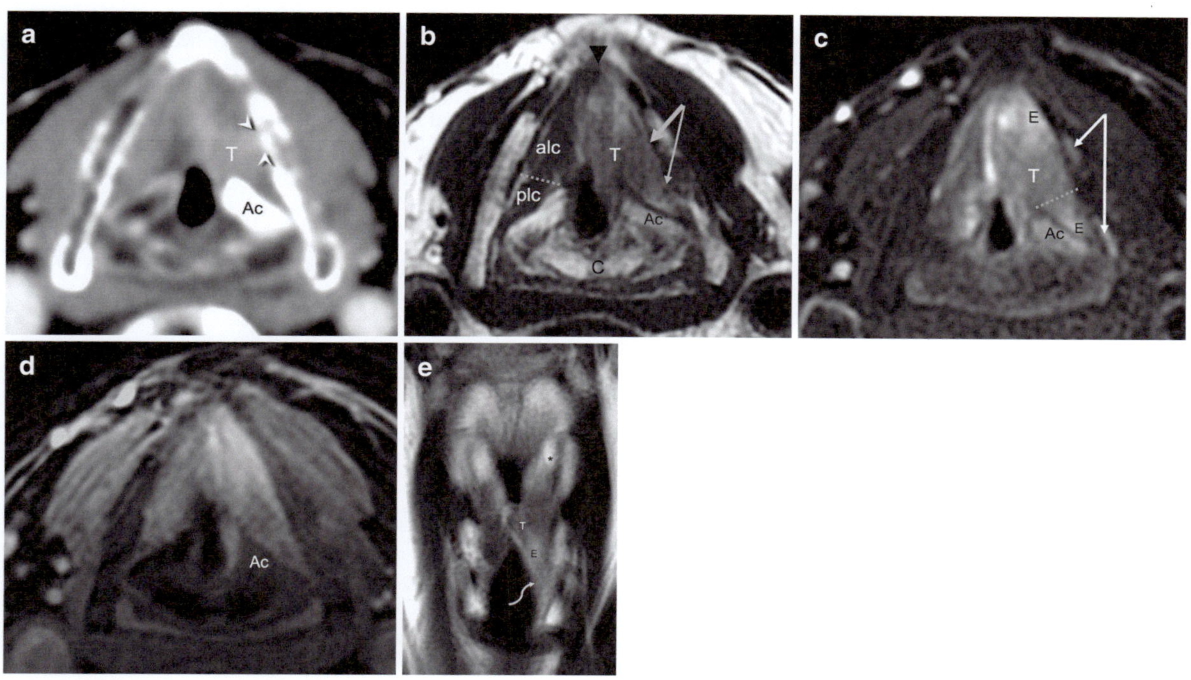

Contrast-enhanced CT scan on axial plane (a) demonstrates a tumor (T) that infiltrates the left true vocal cord, the paraglottic space and contacts the inner cortex of the thyroid cartilage (arrowheads). The left arytenoid cartilage (Ac) shows marked sclerosis that may be due to both the cartilage inflammatory changes for tumor vicinity and neoplastic infiltration
MR sequences FSE T2-weighted (**b**), FSE fat sat T2-weighted (**c**), 3D gradient echo fat sat T1 postcontrast injection (**d**) at the glottic level. The "magic plane" (**b**, **c**) (gray dotted lines) defines the anterior laryngeal compartment (alc) and posterior laryngeal compartment (plc). On the T2-weighted sequences (**b**, **c**) the tumor (T) shows intermediate signal intensity, infiltrates the left true vocal cord in both the compartments (**c**) and reaches the anterior commissure (**b**) (arrowhead). The lesion (**b**) invades both the anterior paraglottic space (thick gray arrow) and posterior paraglottic space (thin gray arrow). High signal intensity alterations indicating edema (E) better demonstrated on fat sat T2-weighted sequence (**c**) surround the tumor. The left arytenoid cartilage (**c**) (Ac) shows diffuse alteration brighter than the adjacent tumor, indicating bone marrow edema, without significant enhancement (**d**). White arrows (**c**) point at bright alterations inside the left thyroid lamina due to edema for the tumor vicinity. The cricoid lamina (C) appears normal (**b**)
On the coronal FSE T2-weighted image (**e**) edema (E) surrounding the tumor (T) extends to the subglottic level where hyperintense submucosal thickening is demonstrated (curved arrow), without signs of tumor involvement. The left superior paraglottic space (asterisk) shows normal fat tissue signal intensity. *FSE* fast spin echo

References

1. Puxeddu R, Sionis S, Gerosa C, Carta F. Enhanced contact endoscopy for the detection of neoangiogenesis in tumors of larynx and hypopharynx. Laryngoscope. 2015;125(7):1600–6.
2. Sumiyama K, Kaise M, Nakayoshi T, et al. Combined use of a magnifying endoscope with a narrow band imaging system and a multibending endoscope for en bloc EMR of early stage gastric cancer. Gastrointest Endosc. 2004;60:79–84.
3. Uedo N, Ishihara R, Iishi H, et al. A new method of diagnosing gastric intestinal metaplasia: narrow-band imaging with magnifying endoscopy. Endoscopy. 2006;38:819–24.
4. Watanabe A, Taniguchi M, Tsujie H, et al. The value of narrow band imaging endoscope for early head and neck cancers. Otolaryngol Head Neck Surg. 2008;138:446–51.
5. Piazza C, Cocco D, De Benedetto L, Del Bon F, Nicolai P, Peretti G. Narrow band imaging and high definition television in the assessment of laryngeal cancer: a prospective study on 279 patients. Eur Arch Otorhinolaryngol. 2010;267:409–14.
6. Alfano RR, Tata DB, Cordero JJ, et al. Laser induced fluorescence spectroscopy from native cancerous and normal tissue. IEEE J Quantum Electron. 1984;20:284–91.
7. Arens C, Dreyer T, Glanz H, Malzahn K. Indirect autofluorescence laryngoscopy in the diagnosis of laryngeal cancer and its precursor lesions. Eur Arch Otorhinolaryngol. 2004;261:71–6.
8. Succo G, Garofalo P, Fantini M, Monticone V, Abbona GC, E. Crosetti Direct autofluorescence during CO_2 laser surgery of the larynx: can it really help the surgeon? Acta Otorhinolaryngol Ital. 2014;34(3):174–83.
9. Crosetti E, Pilolli F, Succo G. A new strategy for endoscopic staging of laryngeal carcinoma: multistep endoscopy. Acta Otorhinolaryngol Ital. 2012;32(3):175–81.
10. Maroldi R, Ravanelli M, Farina D. Magnetic resonance for laryngeal cancer. Curr Opin Otolaryngol Head Neck Surg. 2014;22(2):131–9. https://doi.org/10.1097/MOO.0000000000000036.
11. Chiesa-Estomba CM, Ravanelli M, Farina D. Imaging checklist for preoperative evaluation of laryngeal tumors to be treated by transoral microsurgery: guidelines from the European Laryngological Society. Eur Arch Otorhinolaryngol. 2020;277(6):1707–14. https://doi.org/10.1007/s00405-020-05869-0.
12. Ravanelli M, Agazzi GM, Farina D, et al. New developments in imaging of laryngeal cancer. Curr Otorhinolaryngol Rep. 2017;5:49–55. https://doi.org/10.1007/s40136-017-0145-5.
13. Becker M, Monnier Y, de Vito C. MR imaging of laryngeal and hypopharyngeal cancer. Magn Reson Imaging Clin N Am. 2022;30(1):53–72. https://doi.org/10.1016/j.mric.2021.08.002.
14. Ravanelli M, Paderno A, Del Bon F, et al. Prediction of posterior paraglottic space and cricoarytenoid unit involvement in endoscopically T3 glottic cancer with arytenoid fixation by magnetic resonance with surface coils. Cancers (Basel). 2019;11(1):67. https://doi.org/10.3390/cancers11010067.
15. Thoeny HC, De Keyzer F, King AD. Diffusion-weighted MR imaging in the head and neck. Radiology. 2012;263(1):19–32. https://doi.org/10.1148/radiol.11101821.
16. Becker M, Zbären P, Casselman JW, et al. Neoplastic invasion of laryngeal cartilage: reassessment of criteria for diagnosis at MR imaging. Radiology. 2008;249(2):551–9. https://doi.org/10.1148/radiol.2492072183.
17. Succo G, Cirillo S, Bertotto I, Maldi E, Balmativola D, Petracchini M, Gned D, Fornari A, Motatto GM, Sprio AE, Manca A, Crosetti E. Arytenoid fixation in laryngeal cancer: radiological pictures and clinical correlations with respect to conservative treatments. Cancers (Basel). 2019;11(3):360. https://doi.org/10.3390/cancers11030360.
18. Stoeckli SJ, Haerle SK, Strobel K, et al. Initial staging of the neck in head and neck squamous cell carcinoma: a comparison of CT, PET/CT, and ultrasound-guided fine-needle aspiration cytology. Head Neck. 2012;34(4):469–76. https://doi.org/10.1002/hed.21764.

TNM Staging and Its Surgical Implications

3

Andy Bertolin, Marco Lionello, and Fabio Canal

3.1 Introduction

A correct oncological staging represents the prerequisite for an adequate treatment of the laryngeal cancer. The TNM, now in its eighth edition [1], is still the most widely used staging system worldwide for laryngeal squamous cell carcinoma (LSCC).

The clinical staging of LSCC includes the endoscopic analysis of the local extent of the disease and laryngeal motility and the radiological study of the involved structures.

A comprehensive preoperative endoscopic examination of the larynx requires a rigid or flexible high-definition laryngoscope in white light (WL) and narrow-band imaging (NBI) to adequately define the extent of the disease (Fig. 3.1). A panendoscopy of the upper aero-digestive tract is also necessary to rule out a second synchronous tumor. In the case of intermediate-advanced stage lesions, a preoperative endoscopy under general anesthesia with rigid angled telescopes (0°, 30°, 70°) in WL and NBI or autofluorescence with eventual mapping biopsies of the lesion represents a fundamental diagnostic tool [2].

In the study of laryngeal motility, it is essential to define whether the motility is normal, impaired, or absent, but also to distinguish between vocal cord and arytenoid motility. In the case of an early superficial lesion of the vocal cord with normal motility, an infiltration of the thyroarytenoid muscle or paraglottic spaces can be reasonably ruled out and a simple laryngoscopy may be diagnostic. In the event of impaired vocal cord motility, a radiological study is mandatory to evaluate the state of the paraglottic spaces and of the intrinsic laryngeal muscles. The involvement of these structures may determine the shift from an endoscopic to an open surgical approach. An impaired motility or fixation of an arytenoid, on the other hand, might be associated with a posterior

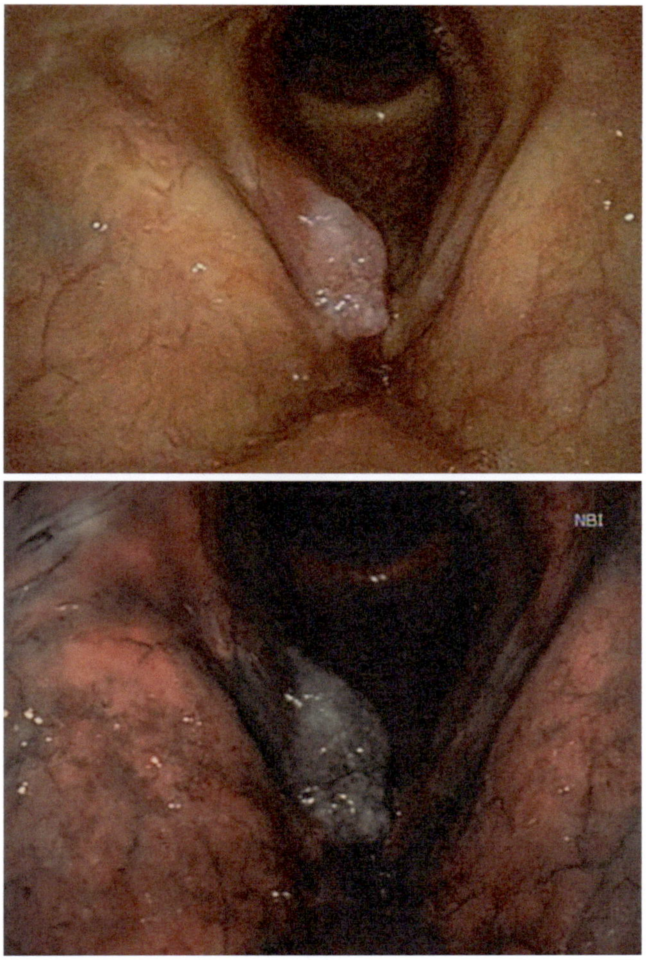

Fig. 3.1 Preoperative endoscopy in white light (WL) and narrow-band imaging (NBI)

A. Bertolin
ENT Department Laryngeal Cancer Centre, Ospedale Civile di Vittorio Veneto, Vittorio Veneto, Italy
e-mail: andy.bertolin@aulss2.veneto.it

M. Lionello (✉)
Otorhinolaryngology Unit, Ospedale Civile di Vittorio Veneto, Vittorio Veneto, Italy
e-mail: marco.lionello@auls2.veneto.it

F. Canal
Pathology Unit, Santa Maria Degli Angeli Hospital, Pordenone, Italy
e-mail: fabio.canal@asfo.sanita.fvg.it

F. Mattioli et al. (eds.), *Atlas of Open Partial Horizontal Laryngectomy*, https://doi.org/10.1007/978-3-031-48023-2_3

spreading of a glottic lesion, a negative prognostic factor that often leads to perform a more aggressive surgery such as supratracheal laryngectomy (OPHL III) [3].

As concerns for radiological examination, the contrast-enhanced computerized tomography (CT) scan of the neck is today the most widespread examination for the initial staging of laryngeal cancer. If available, however, the contrast-enhanced magnetic resonance (MR) should be considered the first choice, in consideration of the best anatomical detail achieved by modern acquisition techniques, also aided using surface coils. Actually, these techniques allow us to obtain fundamental information on the staging of the disease, including: (1) the involvement of the different laryngeal sites and subsites; (2) the involvement of the paraglottic spaces and/or the pre-epiglottic space; (3) erosion, infiltration, overcoming of the laryngeal cartilages; exteriorization to prelaryngeal tissues or infiltration of adjacent organs (base of the tongue, hypopharynx, trachea, esophagus); (4) the presence of lymph node or distant metastases.

At diagnosis, the PET-CT is indicated in advanced cases to rule out distant metastases or in defining the state of suspicious enlarged neck nodes. It is also useful in the follow-up and restaging.

The importance of TNM lies in its detailed classification of LSCC that is homogeneous by prognostic stages, reproducible and comparable, therefore able to compare the effectiveness of the different treatments and the experiences of the different centers.

Considering the current literature on the subject, radiotherapy alone or in combination with chemotherapy finds wide space in the integrated treatment of laryngeal cancer. However, the non-surgical area is beyond the scope of this discussion, so we will analyze in detail the indications for the different types of surgical treatment based on TNM staging.

3.2 Early Stages (cT1–T2, N0, and M0)

For these locally spread laryngeal tumors, a laryngeal function-preserving option is preferable. For early-stage LSCCs, transoral laser microsurgery (TLM) and radiotherapy (RT) provide comparable oncological outcomes in terms of local control and survival, with a trend in favor of RT for functional vocal outcomes [4].

Considering surgical options, in most cases, LSCC at early stages (cTis–T1–T2) can be endoscopically managed, while open surgery is considered in cases with bad laryngeal exposure for recurrences.

For early glottic lesions, the CO_2 laser-assisted TLM represents the mainstay of treatment, given the high precision of the laser free beam, low morbidity and hospitalization time, and good oncological and functional outcomes.

Local control, laryngeal preservation rate, and disease-specific survival with TLM are reported of 85–87%, 94–98%, and 99%, respectively, for glottic pT1, and 66–82%, 79–86%, and 98%, respectively, for glottic pT2 [5, 6].

For early glottic lesions (cT1a), the first-choice treatment is TLM if laryngeal exposure is satisfactory. It has been reported that glottic cT1a squamous cell carcinoma invades the thyroarytenoid muscle in <10% of cases at diagnosis [7, 8]. Therefore, a type III cordectomy (transmuscular) is oncologically safe in the majority of glottic cT1a (Fig. 3.2).

Primary lesions of the anterior commissure can be endoscopically managed in most cases with a cordectomy type VI, in case of adequate laryngeal exposure [9]. However, these cases need to be carefully evaluated, even with contrast-enhanced CT scan or MR. A tumor of the anterior commissure that anteriorly spreads through the thyroid cartilage into prelaryngeal tissues (cT4a) may be erroneously under-staged with endoscopic assessment alone (Fig. 3.3).

Glottic carcinoma is classified as cT1b when it involves both vocal cords without impairing vocal cord mobility or extending to other laryngeal subsites. Treatments for cT1b glottic SCC include TLM, radiation therapy, and open surgery. The two-stage bilateral cordectomy for cT1b glottic carcinoma consists of TLM performed in two steps to reduce the risk of anterior synechiae, without affecting oncological radicality. Bertolin et al. reported that cT1b patients treated with two-stage bilateral cordectomy achieved local control in 96% of cases, with 95% disease-specific, and a 95% organ preservation rate. They developed anterior synechiae less frequently after two-stage bilateral cordectomy and experienced no higher recurrence rate or shorter disease-free survival than patients treated with a single-stage procedure. In selected cases (no suspect of paraglottic space invasion and no primary tumor of the anterior commissure), two-stage bilateral cordectomy could be considered the primary approach for the treatment of early glottic cT1b carcinomas [10] (Fig. 3.4).

When considering glottic cT2 lesions, we should distinguish between neoplasms with normal vocal cord motility and those with impaired vocal cord motility. It was reported that the latter have got a worse prognosis than the former [11]. When approaching these lesions through TLM, this should be kept in mind to perform wider resections.

Moreover, we should consider clinical understaging. Peretti et al. reported that glottic cT2 lesions that became pT3 at pathological examination (because unexpected involvement of the inferior paraglottic space) showed dramatically higher recurrence rate and worse survival [12].

Although TLM for cT2 laryngeal cancer with unimpaired vocal cord mobility still represents a sound option, open partial horizontal laryngectomy (OPHL) offers higher local control and laryngeal preservation rates for selected patients with impaired mobility of vocal cords and suspected involvement of the paraglottic space. Five-year overall survival (OS), disease-specific survival (DFS), locoregional control, local control, laryngeal function preservation, and

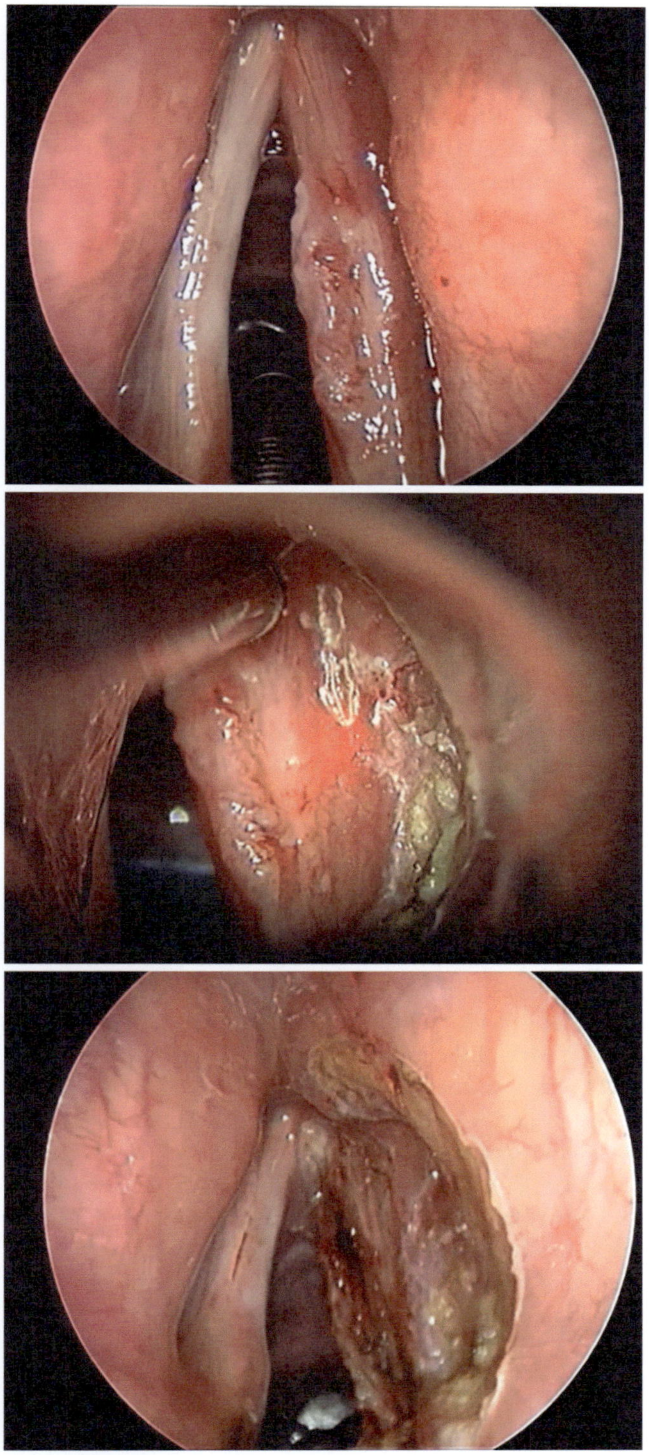

Fig. 3.2 Right cordectomy type III (transmuscular) for cT1a glottic carcinoma

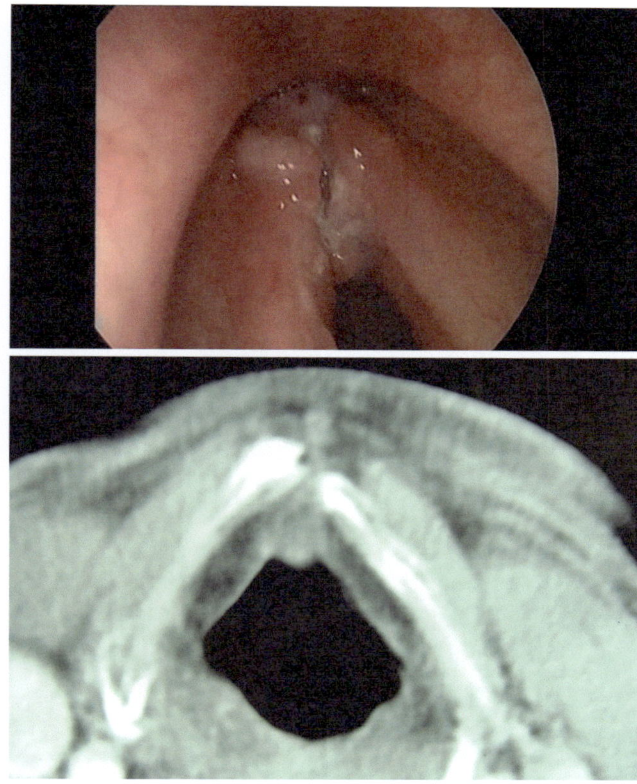

Fig. 3.3 Primary tumor of the anterior commissure spreading through the thyroid cartilage into prelaryngeal tissues (cT4a)

laryngectomy-free survival rates were reported of 93.1%, 98.0%, 97.1%, 97.5%, 97.8%, and 98.5%, respectively [13].

The results achieved with TLM in early supraglottic carcinoma are comparable to those of open supraglottic laryngectomy in terms of local control and survival. Ambrosch et al reported the outcome of 48 patients with early supraglottic carcinoma treated with TLM. The 5-year local control rate was 100% for T1 cases and 89% for T2 cases [14].

At supraglottis, the transoral robotic surgery (TORS) can find indication, in particular in cases of bad laryngeal exposure with conventional TLM. Ansarin and coworkers compared 10 patients submitted to TLM and TORS, respectively, for cT1–3 cN0–cN2c supraglottic cancer and concluded that TORS seems as safe and effective as TLM. Shorter TORS operating times are probably attributable to prior experience with TLM. For laryngeal exposure, length of feeding tube placement and margin evaluability, TLM was superior [15].

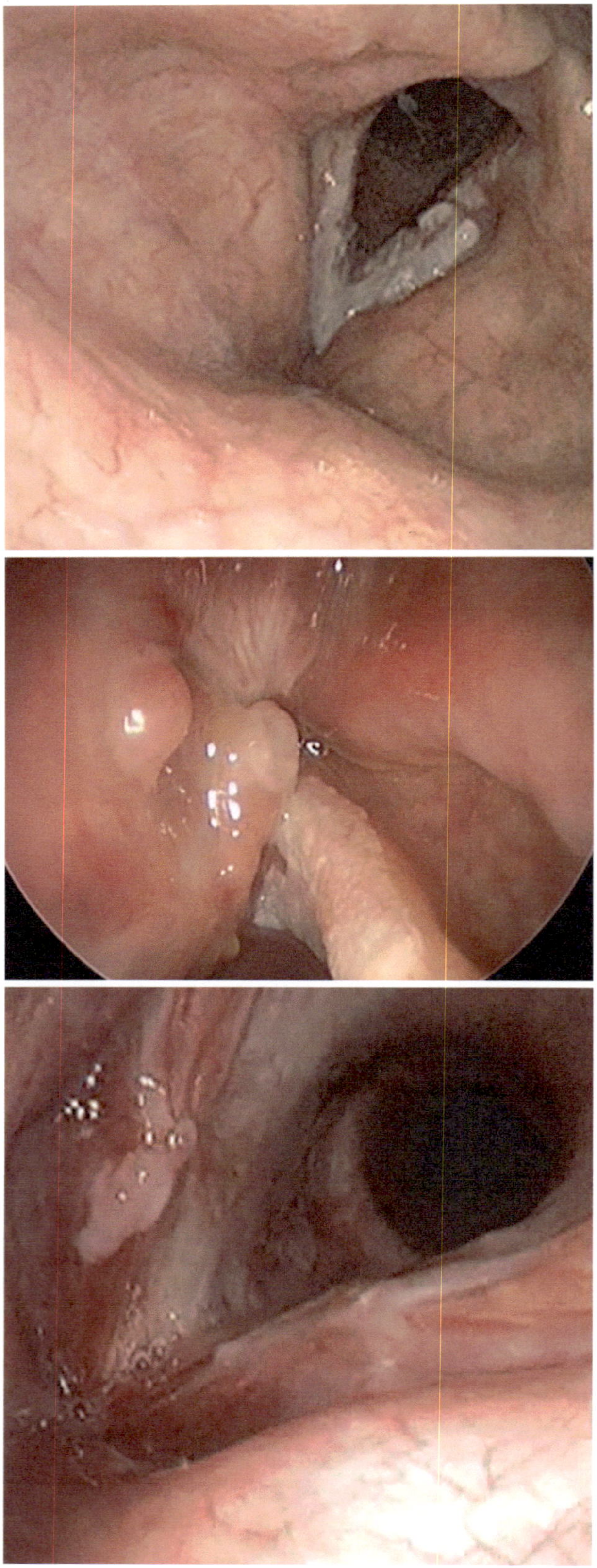

Fig. 3.4 Two-stage bilateral cordectomy: (1) preoperative endoscopy; (2) intraoperative endoscopy before the second procedure; (3) postoperative endoscopy

3.3 Locally Intermediate: Advanced Stages (cT3–T4)

TLM and TORS are not considered a standard treatment for locally advanced laryngeal tumors although, in appropriately selected patients, the outcomes published in the literature sound encouraging [15–18].

Locally intermediate LSCC (cT2–T3) represents the classic indication for OPHL. For selected intermediate LSCC, OPHLs provide oncological outcomes comparable with total laryngectomy (TL) [19].

The TL remains the first choice for cT4a LSCC, however, reserving non-surgical organ preservation treatment for patients who refuse the destructive surgical option. For locally advanced LSCC, the indication to OPHL has to be carefully evaluated and considered only in very selected cases (anterior cT4a, with minimal invasion of prelaryngeal tissues).

Absolute contraindications to OPHL are represented by (I) lesions spreading through the tongue base and pyriform sinus, (II) lesions with significant infiltration of the pre-epiglottic space affecting the hyoid bone, lesions affecting the interarytenoid space, the posterior commissure, and both the arytenoid cartilages, (III) extensive extralaryngeal extension involving the thyroid gland, infrahyoid muscles, cervical skin, jugular vein, or common carotid artery, (IV) lesions extending to the first tracheal ring.

Succo and coworkers recently analyzed the oncological outcomes of cT3–T4a LSCC patients treated with OPHL and recognized a different prognostic meaning of the anterior vs posterior localization of the tumor. They found that the anterior lesions (with referral to a coronal plane situated at the anterior edge of the arytenoid cartilages) had a significantly better prognosis than posterior ones [20].

The posterior spreading of the tumor, through the inferior paraglottic space, was related to worsening of the prognosis. Lucioni et al. hypothesized an anatomical explanation while the thyroid lamina is an excellent barrier to the tumor anterior spreading, posteriorly it can proceed toward the pyriform sinus, retrocricoid region, and through the thyro-cricoid membrane toward the paralaryngeal spaces [3]. Therefore, posterior pT3 glottic lesions oncologically behave as pT4a lesions.

Moreover, the posterior spreading of the lesion toward the thyro-cricoarytenoid space (TCAS) and the cricoarytenoid joint (condition that endoscopically results in ipsilateral arytenoid fixation) determines the impossibility to approach posterior cT3 lesions with supracricoid laryngectomy (OPHL II) and the need for shifting to supratracheal laryngectomy (OPHL III) or TL.

Therefore, anterior glottic cT3 lesions (impaired/absent vocal cord motility and normal arytenoid motility) can be safely approached with OPHL type II in most cases and are related to

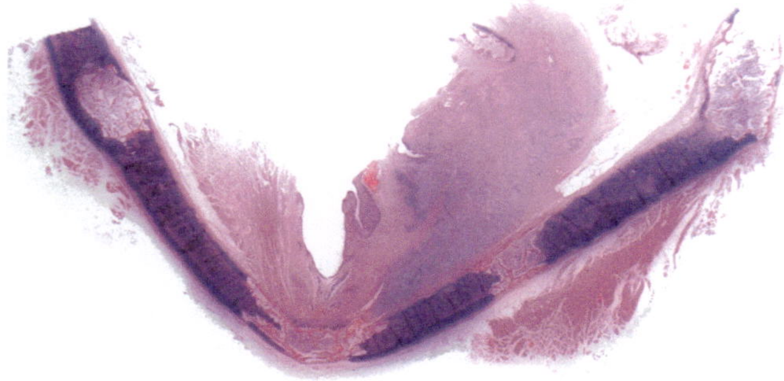

Fig. 3.5 Glottic pT3 carcinoma treated with OPHL: involvement of the inferior paraglottic space

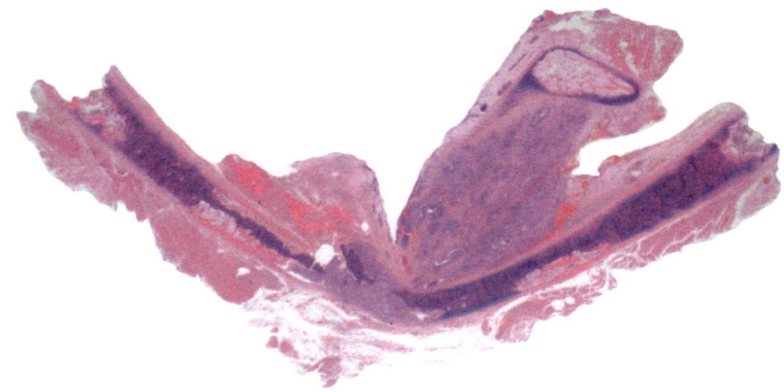

Fig. 3.7 Glottic pT4a carcinoma treated with OPHL. The lesion spreads through the thyroid cartilage, with initial invasion of prelaryngeal tissues

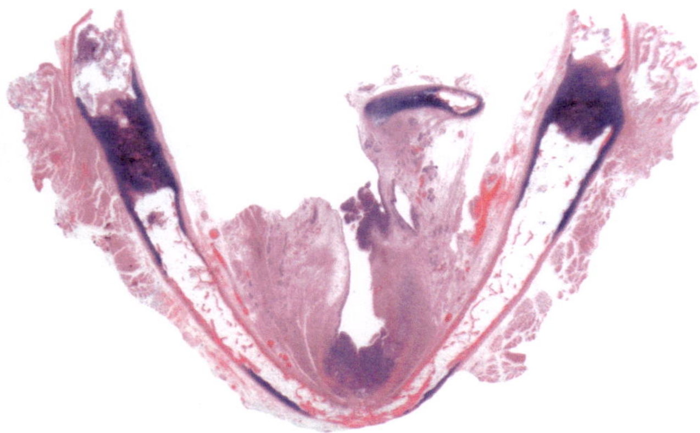

Fig. 3.6 Glottic pT3 carcinoma treated with OPHL: erosion of the inner cortical of the thyroid cartilage

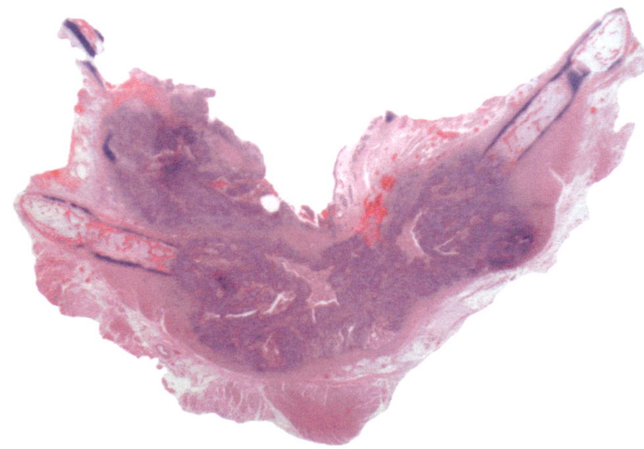

Fig. 3.8 Glottic pT4a carcinoma treated with TL. The lesion spreads through the thyroid cartilage, with massive invasion of prelaryngeal tissues. Safe margins

the absolute best prognosis (Fig. 3.5). In cases with anterior subglottic extension, an OPHL type III may be considered and the shift (OPHL II > III) can even be intraoperative with a modular approach [21]. For anterior cT3 treated with OPHL, the disease-specific survival (DSS) and local control were reported of 97% and 96%, respectively [19] (Fig. 3.6). In these cases, OPHL warrants a better oncological outcome than TLM (whose local control ranges between 44% and 72% for glottic tumor and 70–87% for supraglottic carcinoma) [16, 22, 23].

For selected anterior neoplasms that present initial spreading to prelaryngeal tissues through the thyroid cartilage (cT4a), OPHL could be reasonably considered as a conservative alternative to total laryngectomy (Figs. 3.7 and 3.8). In these cases, DSS and local control were reported as 93% and 78%, respectively [20].

On the other hand, posterior cT3 lesions (absent arytenoid motility) need for more radical surgery (OPHL III vs total laryngectomy). Here the reported DSS and local control after OPHL were 90% and 89%, respectively [20].

For posterior pT4a, OPHL provides dismal oncological results (DSS and local control of 86% and 81%, respectively) [20]. In these cases, total laryngectomy should be preferred.

3.4 Recurrences

Recurrent LSCC must be correctly restaged, to evaluate the local extension of the relapse, the nodal status, but also distant metastases or second tumors. A contrast enhanced MR may be necessary to distinguish between tumor and post-attinic changes. A restaging PET-CT has got a role in evaluating regional and distant metastases. The treatment of recurrent laryngeal cancer depends on the stage of the relapsing disease (rTNM), the type of previous treatment, and the general conditions of the patient.

An early recurrence after TLM (rcT1a) can be approached with further laser resection with good oncological outcomes, while for intermediate-advanced relapses (rcT2–T3–T4a), an open surgery approach should be preferred. In choosing the best treatment, the age of the patient should also be considered, since younger patients present higher risk of further recurrence [24, 25]. The possibility of a salvage conservative approach depends on the previously mentioned issues.

On the other hand, a recurrence after OPHL generally needs radical total laryngectomy for salvage.

The recurrence rates after primary non-surgical treatment for LSCC have been reported to range between 9% and 21% in tumor T1 and 28% and 37% in T2 glottic carcinomas [26, 27], whereas for supraglottic cancer, the failure rates are 24–30% and 25–45% for T1 and T2 lesions, respectively. The first choice for treatment in these cases is a conservative surgery. On the other hand, many patients with LSCC relapse after failed RT present with advanced tumors. The reason could be the chronic laryngeal inflammation that makes challenging an early identification of both symptoms and endoscopic signs of local recurrence. Moreover, the patterns of local relapse after irradiation lead to difficulties in correct restaging of the neoplasm [28].

For these reasons, TLM resection of laryngeal relapses after RT is at high risk of failure although promising results have been reported [29].

TL represents the standard of care for surgical salvage of radiation failure in laryngeal cancer. Salvage TL for stage T1 and T2 squamous cell carcinoma of the larynx has been reported to ensure cancer control in 75% of patients [30] and, considering all stages combined, a 5-year OS rate of 43–55% [31].

In selected patients (rcT1–T2–T3), when proper selection criteria for conservation laryngeal surgery are adopted, OPHL can be considered for salvage after RT failure. LC rates after salvage partial laryngectomy range between 67% and 100%, OS between 56% and 95%, and DSS between 81% and 100%, respectively. Moreover, the incidence of major postoperative complications seems comparable with that of salvage TL (41.2% for previous chemoradiotherapy, 29.4% for previous RT) [32].

3.5 The Neck Status

The occurrence of neck node metastases dramatically worsens the laryngeal cancer prognosis. Therefore, it must be carefully investigated in the diagnostic staging work up. Furthermore, the presence of regional metastases significantly influences the kind of treatment due to the probability of need for adjuvant radiotherapy or chemoradiotherapy (in case of extranodal extension). The suspicion of node metastasis (>cN1) is not an absolute contraindication to open partial laryngectomies. On the other hand, an extensive extralaryngeal extension involving the thyroid gland, infrahyoid muscles, cervical skin, and internal jugular vein are considered contraindications to conservative surgery.

The supraglottic region is richly supplied with lymphatics. Invasive supraglottic LSCC presents with node metastases at diagnosis in 25–75% of cases when all stages are considered [33]. Furthermore, considering the embryological derivation, bilateral metastases are not unusual [34]. In case of supraglottic lesions, a bilateral neck dissection must be considered in particular for neoplasms crossing the midline.

Early-stage glottic carcinoma (cT1–T2) is accepted to have a low incidence of lymph node metastasis (0–10%), while the reported incidence with more advanced stage disease (cT3–T4) varies between 10% and 35% [35]. Therefore, for intermediate-advanced stage disease, an elective ipsilateral neck dissection is mandatory in cN0 patients, while it can be omitted in case of early glottic cancer.

Moreover, it was reported that, in posterior T3 and T4a lesions, the risk of lymph node metastases with extracapsular extension (ENE +) is 2.5 times greater than in anterior lesions [20]. Considering this, OPHLs must be reserved for carefully selected cases of posterior cT3 (and contraindicated for posterior cT4a) given the high risk of poor functional outcome following adjuvant treatment. In these cases, total laryngectomy with neck dissection ± adjuvant treatment remains the gold standard treatment.

Neoplasms with subglottic extension spread initially to the paratracheal and recurrent lymph nodes [36]. Therefore, in these cases, a dissection of the anterior compartment (VI level) should be carried out.

3.6 Conclusions

The TNM staging system allows us to properly stage the laryngeal cancer and offer to the patient the best surgical options. On the other hand, the modern management of LSCC is multidisciplinary and organ sparing protocols should be offered to the patient, when appropriate, as long as surgery. Anyway, when deciding to carry out an organ conservative intervention, the first goal is to not carry out other adjuvant treatments.

Besides the tumor features, when choosing the best treatment, other patient-related variables have necessarily to be considered, such as the patient's age, general conditions, compliance to postoperative rehabilitation, and suitability for any adjuvant treatment.

The age of the patient must be carefully considered, since the biological behavior of LSCC seems to be more aggressive in young people, who may benefit from more radical surgeries.

Laryngeal surgery is a patient-tailored surgery, and, after a meticulous selection of fitting patients, different surgical options can be proposed.

References

1. Brierley JD, Gospodarowicz MK, Wittekind C. TNM classification of malignant tumours. 8th ed. Chichester, UK: John Wiley and Sons; 2017.

2. Crosetti E, Pilolli F, Succo G. A new strategy for endoscopic staging of laryngeal carcinoma: multistep endoscopy. Acta Otorhinolaryngol Ital. 2012;32(3):175–81.
3. Lucioni M, Lionello M, Guida F, Sovran F, Canal F, Rizzotto G, Bertolin A. The thyro-cricoarytenoid space (TCAS): clinical and prognostic implications in laryngeal cancer. Acta Otorhinolaryngol Ital. 2020;40(2):106–12.
4. Guimarães AV, Dedivitis RA, Matos LL, Aires FT, Cernea CR. Comparison between transoral laser surgery and radiotherapy in the treatment of early glottic cancer: a systematic review and meta-analysis. Sci Rep. 2018;8(1):11900.
5. Sjögren EV. Transoral laser microsurgery in early glottic lesions. Curr Otorhinolaryngol Rep. 2017;5(1):56–68.
6. Lucioni M, Marioni G, Bertolin A, Giacomelli L, Rizzotto G. Glottic laser surgery: outcomes according to 2007 ELS classification. Eur Arch Otorhinolaryngol. 2011;268(12):1771–8.
7. Lionello M, Bertolin A, Nardello E, Giacomelli L, Canal F, Rizzotto G, Marioni G, Lucioni M. Could the infiltration of the thyroarytenoid muscle define the pT2 glottic carcinoma? Head Neck. 2019;41(10):3639–46.
8. Pittore B, Ismail-Koch H, Davis A, Parodo G, Ledda GP, Brennan PA, Puxeddu R. Thyroarytenoid muscle invasion in T1 glottic carcinoma. Eur Arch Otorhinolaryngol. 2009;266(11):1787–91.
9. Remacle M, Van Haverbeke C, Eckel H, et al. Proposal for revision of the European Laryngological Society classification of endoscopic cordectomies. Eur Arch Otorhinolaryngol. 2007;264(5):499–504.
10. Bertolin A, Lionello M, Salis G, Rizzotto G, Lucioni M. Two-stage CO_2-laser-assisted bilateral cordectomy for cT1b glottic carcinoma. Am J Otol. 2017;38:183–7.
11. Canis M, Martin A, Ihler F, et al. Transoral laser microsurgery in treatment of pT2 and pT3 glottic laryngeal squamous cell carcinoma—results of 391 patients. Head Neck. 2014;36:859–66.
12. Peretti G, Piazza C, Mensi MC, Magnoni L, Bolzoni A. Endoscopic treatment of cT2 glottic carcinoma: prognostic impact of different pT subcategories. Ann Otol Rhinol Laryngol. 2005;114:579–86.
13. Succo G, Crosetti E, Bertolin A, Lucioni M, Caracciolo A, Panetta V, Sprio AE, Berta GN, Rizzotto G. Benefits and drawbacks of open partial horizontal laryngectomies, Part A: Early- to intermediate-stage glottic carcinoma. Head Neck. 2016;38(Suppl. 1):E333–40.
14. Ambrosch P, Kron M, Steiner W. Carbon dioxide laser microsurgery for early supraglottic carcinoma. Ann Otol Rhinol Laryngol. 1998;107:680–8.
15. Ansarin M, Zorzi S, Massaro MA, et al. Transoral robotic surgery vs transoral laser microsurgery for resection of supraglottic cancer: a pilot surgery. Int J Med Robot. 2014;10(1):107–12.
16. Vilaseca I, Bernal-Sprekelsen M. Transoral laser microsurgery for locally advanced laryngeal cancer. Acta Otorrinolaringol Esp. 2013;64(2):140–9.
17. Canis M, Ihler F, Martin A, Wolff HA, Matthias C, Steiner W. Organ preservation in T4a laryngeal cancer: is transoral laser microsurgery an option? Eur Arch Otorhinolaryngol. 2013;270(10):2719–27.
18. Ozer E, Alvarez B, Kakarala K, Durmus K, Teknos TN, Carrau RL. Clinical outcomes of transoral robotic supraglottic laryngectomy. Head Neck. 2013;35(8):1158–61.
19. Succo G, Crosetti E, Bertolin A, et al. Benefits and drawbacks of open partial horizontal laryngectomies, Part B: Intermediate and selected advanced stage laryngeal carcinoma. Head Neck. 2016;38(Suppl. 1):E649–57.
20. Succo G, Crosetti E, Bertolin A, et al. Treatment for T3 to T4a laryngeal cancer by open partial horizontal laryngectomies: prognostic impact of different pathologic tumor subcategories. Head Neck. 2018;40(9):1897–908.
21. Bertolin A, Lionello M, Ghizzo M, et al. Modular approach in OPHL: are there preoperative predictors? Acta Otorhinolaryngol Ital. 2020;40(5):352–9.
22. Canis M, Ihler F, Martin A, Wolff HA, Matthias C, Steiner W. Results of 226 patients with T3 laryngeal carcinoma after treatment with transoral laser microsurgery. Head Neck. 2014;36(5):652–9.
23. Peretti G, Piazza C, Ansarin M, et al. Transoral CO_2 laser microsurgery for Tis-T3 supraglottic squamous cell carcinomas. Eur Arch Otorhinolaryngol. 2010;267:1735–42.
24. Lucioni M, Bertolin A, Lionello M, Giacomelli L, Rizzotto G, Marioni G. Salvage transoral laser microsurgery for recurrent glottic carcinoma after primary laser-assisted treatment: analysis of prognostic factors. Head Neck. 2016;38(7):1043–9.
25. Lucioni M, Bertolin A, Lionello M, Giacomelli L, Rizzotto G, Marioni G. Open partial horizontal laryngectomy for salvage after failure of CO_2 laser-assisted surgery for glottic carcinoma. Eur Arch Otorhinolaryngol. 2016;273(1):169–75.
26. DeSchyver A. Radiotherapy of laryngeal cancer. General principles and results in T1 and T2 cases. Acta Otolrhinolaryngol Belg. 1992;46:187–95.
27. Bataini JP, Brumin F. Early and moderately advanced cancers of supraglottic larynx and their management by radiotherapy. In: Kagan AR, Miles J, editors. Head and neck oncology: clinical management. New York, NY: Pergamon; 1989. p. 69–82.
28. Brandenburg JH, Condon KG, Frank TW. Coronal sections of larynges from radiation-therapy failures: a clinical-pathologic study. Otolaryngol Head Neck Surg. 1986;95:213–8.
29. Ramakrishnan Y, Drinnan M, Kwong FN, et al. Oncologic outcomes of transoral laser microsurgery for radiorecurrent laryngeal carcinoma: a systematic review and meta-analysis of English-language literature. Head Neck. 2014;36(2):280–5.
30. Schwaab G, Mamelle G, Lartigau E, et al. Surgical salvage treatment of T1/T2 glottic carcinoma after failure of radiotherapy. Am J Surg. 1994;168:474–5.
31. Philippe Y, Espitalier F, Durand N, Ferron C, Bardet E, Malard O. Partial laryngectomy as salvage surgery after radiotherapy: oncological and functional outcomes and impact on quality of life. A retrospective study of 20 cases. Eur Ann Otorhinolaryngol Head Neck Dis. 2014;131:15–9.
32. Bertolin A, Lionello M, Ghizzo M, et al. Salvage open partial horizontal laryngectomy after failed radiotherapy: a multicentric study. Laryngoscope. 2020;130(2):431–6.
33. Sinard RJ, Netterville JL, Garrett CG, Ossoff RH. Cancer of the larynx. In: Myers EN, Suen JY, editors. Cancer of the head and neck. 3rd ed. Philadelphia: Saunders; 1996. p. 381–421.
34. Marks JE, Devineni VR, Harvey J, Sessions DG. The risk of contralateral lymphatic metastases for cancers of the larynx and pharynx. Am J Otolaryngol. 1992;13:34–9.
35. Yang CY, Andersen PE, Everts EC, Cohen JI. Nodal disease in purely glottic carcinoma: is elective neck treatment worthwhile? Laryngoscope. 1998;108:1006–8.
36. Lucioni M, D'Ascanio L, De Nardi E, Lionello M, Bertolin A, Rizzotto G. Management of paratracheal lymph nodes in laryngeal cancer with subglottic involvement. Head Neck. 2018;40(1):24–33.

Patients' Selection Criteria

4

Erika Crosetti, Marco Fantini, Alessandro Pagliassotto, and Giovanni Succo

Open Partial Horizontal Laryngectomies (OPHLs) represent oncologically safe procedures but can be challenging for the neolarynx rehabilitation process. Therefore, an accurate patient selection is crucial in the pre-operative setting. Several Authors investigated laryngeal functional outcomes after OPHLs, suggesting that overall functional recovery is generally satisfactory concerning the main neolarynx functions (voice, breathing, and swallowing) even if a great variability can be observed [1, 2]. Voice quality is usually well preserved after Type I OPHLs, since vocal folds are spared, while is highly and similarly deteriorated after Type II and Type III OPHLs [3–5]. Nevertheless, a satisfactory level of oral communication is generally achieved through a substitution voice after a proper rehabilitation [6]. Swallowing recovery after open partial laryngectomies is a challenging process and has been widely investigated [7–11]. Swallowing is always severely impaired immediately after surgery, but generally recovers in about 6 months, with patients finally reaching a free oral diet [1, 8]. Nevertheless, chronic aspirations and post-swallowing residues can remain as long-term findings in some patients, increasing the risk of aspiration pneumonia and death [1, 2, 12].

Concerning tracheal cannula removal, naso-gastric tube (NGT) feeding, and length of hospital stay, a review by Schindler et al. reported great literature variability regarding supracricoid partial laryngectomy, with mean decannulation time ranging from 8 to 105 days, mean NGT removal time ranging from 10 to 88 days, and mean length of hospital stay ranging from 5 to 104 days, as reported by different authors [1]. Succo et al. reported that good Laryngeal Function Preservation (LFP), meaning no need for NGT, decannulation, no need for PEG positioning, intelligible speech, and no need for total laryngectomy, is generally achieved after OPHLs, with LFP rates at 5 years ranging from 91.2% to 98.5%, according to the extent of disease [13, 14]. Given that functional recovery after open partial laryngectomy can be challenging and is affected by great heterogeneity, determining prognostic factors for difficult functional recovery is crucial for an optimal patient selection in the pre-operative setting.

Gallo et al. investigated factors associated with post-operative morbidity after OPHLs. The Authors analyzed by logistic regression the associations of patients-related factors, disease-related factors, and type of surgery with post-operative acute complications (airway complications, dysphagia, bleeding, surgical site infection, dehiscence of pexy, emphysema, and pharyngocutaneous fistulas), finding that older age, alcohol consuming, advanced cT status, and more extended partial laryngectomies were related to higher rates of overall and airway complications (pneumonia, emphysema, fistula, and dysphagia). Nomograms were developed for prediction of postsurgical complications to reach a better patient selection in the surgical planning process [15].

Apart from post-operative acute morbidity, the process of functional recovery after OPHL is crucial for the patient's survival and quality of life. We recently investigated in a cohort of 131 consecutive patients who underwent Type I, Type II, or Type III OPHL, a series of patient-related variables to define pre-operative prognostic factors for functional and clinical outcomes after OPHLs [16]. We found that age > 70 years, female sex, smoking habits, BMIs > 25 at diagnosis, presence of cervical spine osteophytosis, comorbidities, and cT3–cT4 staging were significantly associated with poorer functional and clinical outcomes. The multivariate analysis showed that cT3–cT4 staging and BMI < 25 were independent risk factors for sequelae, PEG positioning;

E. Crosetti (✉)
ENT Department Head and Neck Cancer Unit, San Giovanni Bosco Hospital, Torino, Italy

M. Fantini
Otorhinolaryngology Department—Head Neck Cancer Unit, San Giovanni Bosco Hospital, Turin, Italy

A. Pagliassotto
Otorhinolaryngology Unit, Martini Hospital, Turin, Italy
e-mail: alessandro.pagliassotto@aslcittaditorino.it

G. Succo
ENT Department Head Neck Cancer Unit, San Giovanni Bosco Hospital, Torino, Italy

Oncology Department, University of Turin, Turin, Italy

F. Mattioli et al. (eds.), *Atlas of Open Partial Horizontal Laryngectomy*, https://doi.org/10.1007/978-3-031-48023-2_4

late tracheal cannula removal. Smoking habits and age > 70 years were independent risk factors for late NGT removal.

It is not surprising that age may impact as an independent risk factor for late tracheal cannula and NGT removal, since elderly patients have a slower functional recovery. Despite that, our data confirm that age itself may not represent a risk factor for late sequelae or need for PEG positioning, as previously reported by other Authors [17, 18].

Cervical spine osteophytosis may also represent a risk factor for sequelae and need for PEG positioning. It is well known that cervical spine osteophytosis can lead to swallowing disorders because of extrinsic compression of the pharynx and esophagus, disturbances of normal epiglottic tilt, and induction of cricopharyngeal spasm [19]. Such condition may determine severe dysphagia after OPHL, requiring gastrostomy and prolonged rehabilitation. In patients, undergoing open partial laryngeal surgery is therefore mandatory to investigate the presence of such condition and considering a surgical osteophytectomy before proceeding with the open partial laryngectomy [20] (Fig. 4.1a, b).

Considering cT status, an intermediate-advanced cT staging at diagnosis requires larger surgical resection, explaining the associations with higher incidence of PEG positioning and sequelae for cT3 and cT4 laryngeal tumors. As previously reported by Succo et al., intermediate and selected advanced stage laryngeal carcinomas undergoing OPHL have higher rates of sequelae when compared to early-to intermediate stage diseases (15.3% vs. 12%, respectively). Similarly, 5 years LFP is higher for patients who had an early-to-intermediate stage carcinoma when compared to patients with intermediate and selected advanced stage laryngeal tumors (97.8% vs. 92.6%, respectively) [13, 14].

BMI-related findings must be considered carefully as well, as significant associations were found between lower BMIs and sequelae or PEG positioning, both in the univariate and in the multivariate analysis. It has to be considered that there were not obese patients among our study population, but slightly underweight, normal weight, and overweight patients. In the first days after an OPHL procedure, even if enteral and parenteral feeding is provided, patients usually experience a considerable loss of weight, ranging—in our experience—from 8 to 10 kg. In terms of functional recovery and swallowing rehabilitation, when the process requires longer than normal, having a higher BMI may be an advantage, as fat tissue represents a fundamental energy reservoir. On the contrary, normal weight and underweight patients experiencing troubles with the swallowing recovery process may suffer from malnutrition and, consequently, they may develop higher risk of persisting dysphagia and need for PEG positioning. To our knowledge, no data exist in Literature about the influence of preoperative BMI and functional recovery after OPHLs. Previous studies underlined the association between malnutrition, sarcopenia and swallowing impairment in dysphagic patients, determining higher risk of aspiration [21–23]. Some Authors studied the effect of BMI on dysphagia recovery in stroke units, concluding that higher BMIs correlate with a complete swallowing recovery [24]. These findings could suggest possible similarities with patients undergoing partial laryngeal surgery.

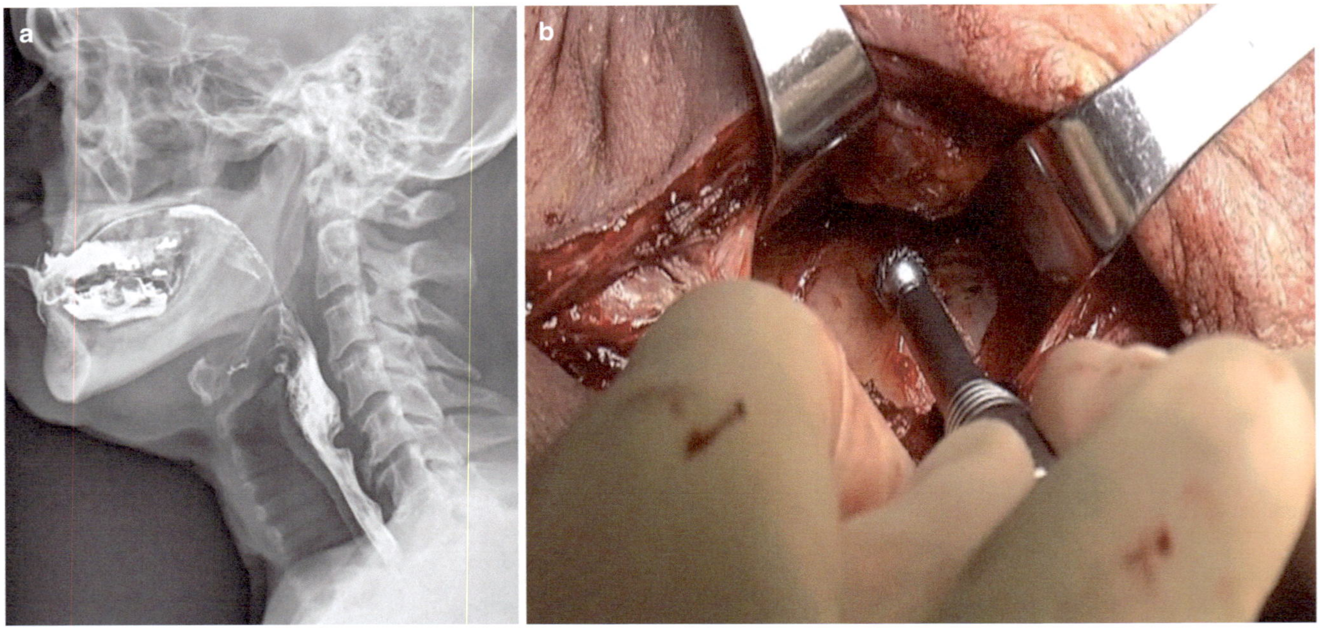

Fig. 4.1 C5–C6 cervical spine osteophytosis in a patient who underwent OPHL and developed dysphagia (**a**). Surgical removal's osteophytosis (**b**)

Age, BMI, smoking habits, and cT status should be therefore taken carefully into account when planning an OPHL. Even if not emerging as independent risk factors in our analysis, we believe that cervical spine osteophytosis and comorbidities should be considered carefully as well, since in our experience they strongly impact on the patient's clinical and functional recovery after surgery. In conclusion, knowing prognostic factors associated with higher risk for poorer functional outcomes after Open Partial Horizontal Laryngectomies (OPHLs) is crucial for clinicians and surgeons. The identification of the most relevant prognostic factors associated with worse functional and clinical recovery outcomes may help defining the best surgical option for each patient, not only from an oncological perspective, but also considering post-operative morbidity and quality of life.

References

1. Schindler A, Pizzorni N, Mozzanica F, et al. Functional outcomes after supracricoid laryngectomy: what do we not know and what do we need to know? Eur Arch Otorhinolaryngol. 2016;273(11):3459–75. https://doi.org/10.1007/s00405-015-3822-3.
2. Schindler A, Fantini M, Pizzorni N, et al. Swallowing, voice, and quality of life after supratracheal laryngectomy: preliminary long-term results. Head Neck. 2015;37(4):557–66. https://doi.org/10.1002/hed.23636.
3. Estomba CC, Reinoso FB, Lorenzo AL, Conde JF, Nores JA, Hidalgo CS. Functional outcomes of supraglottic squamous cell carcinoma treated by transoral laser microsurgery compared with horizontal supraglottic laryngectomy in patients younger and older than 65 years. Acta Otorhinolaryngol Ital. 2016;36(6):450–8. https://doi.org/10.14639/0392-100X-864.
4. Peretti G, Piazza C, Cattaneo A, De Benedetto L, Martin E, Nicolai P. Comparison of functional outcomes after endoscopic versus open-neck supraglottic laryngectomies. Ann Otol Rhinol Laryngol. 2006;115(11):827–32. https://doi.org/10.1177/000348940611501106.
5. Schindler A, Pizzorni N, Fantini M, et al. Long-term functional results after open partial horizontal laryngectomy type IIa and type IIIa: a comparison study. Head Neck. 2016;38(Suppl. 1):E1427–35. https://doi.org/10.1002/hed.24254.
6. Fantini M, Gallia M, Borrelli G, et al. Substitution voice rehabilitation after open partial horizontal laryngectomy through the proprioceptive elastic method (PROEL): a preliminary study. J Voice. 2020; https://doi.org/10.1016/j.jvoice.2020.04.025.
7. Di Santo D, Bondi S, Giordano L, et al. Long-term swallowing function, pulmonary complications and quality of life after supracricoid laryngectomy. Otolaryngol Head Neck Surg. 2019;161(2):307–14. https://doi.org/10.1177/0194599819835189.
8. Breunig C, Benter P, Seidl RO, Coordes A. Predictable swallowing function after open horizontal supraglottic partial laryngectomy. Auris Nasus Larynx. 2016;43(6):658–65. https://doi.org/10.1016/j.anl.2016.01.003.
9. Pizzorni N, Schindler A, Castellari M, Fantini M, Crosetti E, Succo G. Swallowing safety and efficiency after open partial horizontal laryngectomy: a videofluoroscopic study. Cancers. 2019;11(4):549. https://doi.org/10.3390/cancers11040549.
10. Lips M, Speyer R, Zumach A, Kross KW, Kremer B. Supracricoid laryngectomy and dysphagia: a systematic literature review. Laryngoscope. 2015;125:2143–56. https://doi.org/10.1002/lary.25341.
11. Zica GM, de Freitas AS, Silva ACAE, et al. Swallowing, voice and quality of life of patients submitted to extended supratracheal laryngectomy. Einstein. 2020;18:eAO5390. https://doi.org/10.31744/einstein_journal/2020ao5390.
12. Gallo O, Deganello A, Gitti G, et al. Prognostic role of pneumonia in supracricoid and supraglottic laryngectomies. Oral Oncol. 2009;45(1):30–8. https://doi.org/10.1016/j.oraloncology.2008.03.013.
13. Succo G, Crosetti E, Bertolin A, et al. Benefits and drawbacks of open partial horizontal laryngectomies, part A: early- to intermediate-stage glottic carcinoma. Head Neck. 2016;38(Suppl. 1):E333–40. https://doi.org/10.1002/hed.23997.
14. Succo G, Crosetti E, Bertolin A, et al. Benefits and drawbacks of open partial horizontal laryngectomies, part B: intermediate and selected advanced stage laryngeal carcinoma. Head Neck. 2016;38(Suppl. 1):E649–57. https://doi.org/10.1002/hed.24064.
15. Gallo O, Cannavicci A, Bruno C, Maggiore G, Locatello LG. Survival outcomes and prognostic factors of open partial laryngeal surgery: a thirty years' experience. Ann Otol Rhinol Laryngol. 2020;129(7):669–76. https://doi.org/10.1177/0003489420905616.
16. Fantini M, Crosetti E, Affaniti R, Sprio AE, Bertotto I, Succo G. Preoperative prognostic factors for functional and clinical outcomes after open partial horizontal laryngectomies. Head Neck. 2021; https://doi.org/10.1002/hed.26845. Epub ahead of print
17. Crosetti E, Caracciolo A, Molteni G, et al. Unravelling the risk factors that underlie laryngeal surgery in elderly. Acta Otorhinolaryngol Ital. 2016;36(3):185–93. https://doi.org/10.14639/0392-100X-817.
18. Schindler A, Favero E, Capaccio P, Albera R, Cavalot AL, Ottaviani F. Supracricoid laryngectomy: age influence on long term functional results. Laryngoscope. 2009;119(6):1218–25. https://doi.org/10.1002/lary.20172.
19. Abdel-Aziz M, Azab N, El-Badrawy A. Cervical osteophytosis and spine posture: contribution to swallow disorders and symptoms. Curr Opin Otolaryngol Head Neck Surg. 2018;26(6):375–81. https://doi.org/10.1097/MOO.0000000000000488.
20. Yoshimatsu Y, Tobino K, Maeda K, et al. Management of airway obstruction due to diffuse idiopathic skeletal hyperostosis in the cervical spine: a case report and literature review. Intern Med. 2019;58(2):271–6. https://doi.org/10.2169/internalmedicine.1071-18.
21. Veldee MS, Peth LD. Can protein-calorie malnutrition cause dysphagia? Dysphagia. 1992;7(2):86–101. https://doi.org/10.1007/BF02493439.
22. Kuroda Y, Kuroda R. Relationship between thinness and swallowing function in Japanese older adults: implications for sarcopenic dysphagia [published correction appears in J Am Geriatr Soc. 2012 Dec;60(12):2385]. J Am Geriatr Soc. 2012;60(9):1785–6. https://doi.org/10.1111/j.1532-5415.2012.04123.x.
23. Smithard D, Hansjee D, Henry D, et al. Inter-relationships between frailty, sarcopenia, undernutrition and dysphagia in older people who are admitted to acute frailty and medical wards: is there an older adult quartet? Geriatrics. 2020;5(3):E41. https://doi.org/10.3390/geriatrics5030041.
24. Ikenaga Y, Nakayama S, Taniguchi H, et al. Factors predicting recovery of oral intake in stroke survivors with dysphagia in a convalescent rehabilitation ward. J Stroke Cerebrovasc Dis. 2017;26(5):1013–9. https://doi.org/10.1016/j.jstrokecerebrovasdis.2016.12.005.

5 Open Partial Horizontal Laryngectomy Type I (OPHL 1)

Gabriele Molteni, Davide Dal Molin, Edoardo Serafini, and Valerio Arietti

5.1 Introduction

Treatment of cancer of the supraglottic larynx is constantly evolving to provide patients with the best functional outcome regarding speech, swallowing, and breathing while ensuring oncological radicality. Open partial supraglottic laryngectomy was first described by Alonso in 1947 [1]. Although time has passed since its description, it continues to play an important role in the conservative management of supraglottic laryngeal cancer [2], together with transoral laser supraglottic laryngectomies [3] and nonsurgical organ preservation strategies. When properly indicated, supraglottic laryngectomy offers cure rates similar to those of total laryngectomy with high local control rates [4, 5]. Furthermore, open partial horizontal laryngectomies (OPHLs) can also play a role in the treatment of recurrent radioresistant laryngeal carcinoma in selected cases [6, 7].

Indications for OPHL type I include tumors of the supraglottic larynx, with at least one unaffected arytenoid cartilage [8], with or without extension to the mucosa of valleculae, base of tongue, one arytenoid cartilage until the medial wall of one piriform sinus. Furthermore, even primary tumors of base of tongue or valleculae limited to these sites or extended to supraglottic larynx in young and relatively fit patients can be managed through this surgical approach.

Adequate patient selection is mandatory to achieve satisfactory oncological and functional outcomes. Vocal folds preservation allows very good phonatory function, however, the epiglottis removal might hamper adequate swallowing function recovery if patients are not able to attend adequate rehabilitation. Most patients undergoing OPHL 1 an achieve a complete oral diet with all consistencies by 10–14 days after surgery. However, the risk of aspiration pneumonia is significant in patients with inadequate laryngeal sensibility and low pulmonary reserve. This surgical option is therefore not suitable for patients with cardiopulmonary impairment so severe that they cannot temporarily tolerate moderate amounts of aspiration. This group of patients should not be addressed to this surgical procedure.

5.2 Classifications

OPHL type I, also known as supraglottic laryngectomy [9], provides resection of the entire supraglottis, including the pre-epiglottic space and the upper half of the thyroid cartilage. Inferiorly, the resection includes the petiole of the epiglottis down to the anterior commissure and the ventricular folds. Posteriorly, the resection border passes anterior to the arytenoids and transects the ventricular fold and the aryepiglottic fold. Superiorly, the incision cuts through the valleculae along the posterior aspect of the hyoid bone (Fig. 5.1). Reconstruction of the larynx is accomplished by performing a thyrohyoidopexy.

In selected cases, the procedure may be extended to [9, 10]:

- One arytenoid (OPHL I + ARY): represents an extension of the earlier procedure to one arytenoid. To prevent aspiration and improve phonatory outcome, the separated vocal fold might be fixed postero-medially to the cricoid plate.

G. Molteni (✉) · E. Serafini
Department of Otorhinolaryngology-Head and Neck Surgery, Azienda Ospedaliero Universitaria di Bologna IRCCS, Bologna, Italy

Alma Mater Studiorum—Università di Bologna, Bologna, Italy
e-mail: g.molteni@unibo.it; edoardo.serafini3@unibo.it

D. Dal Molin
Department of Otorhinolaryngology-Head and Neck Surgery, Azienda Ospedaliero Universitaria di Bologna IRCCS, Bologna, Italy
e-mail: davide.dalmolin@studio.unibo.it

V. Arietti
Division of Otorhinolaryngology-Head and Neck Surgery, University Hospital of Verona Borgo Trento, Verona, Italy

F. Mattioli et al. (eds.), *Atlas of Open Partial Horizontal Laryngectomy*, https://doi.org/10.1007/978-3-031-48023-2_5

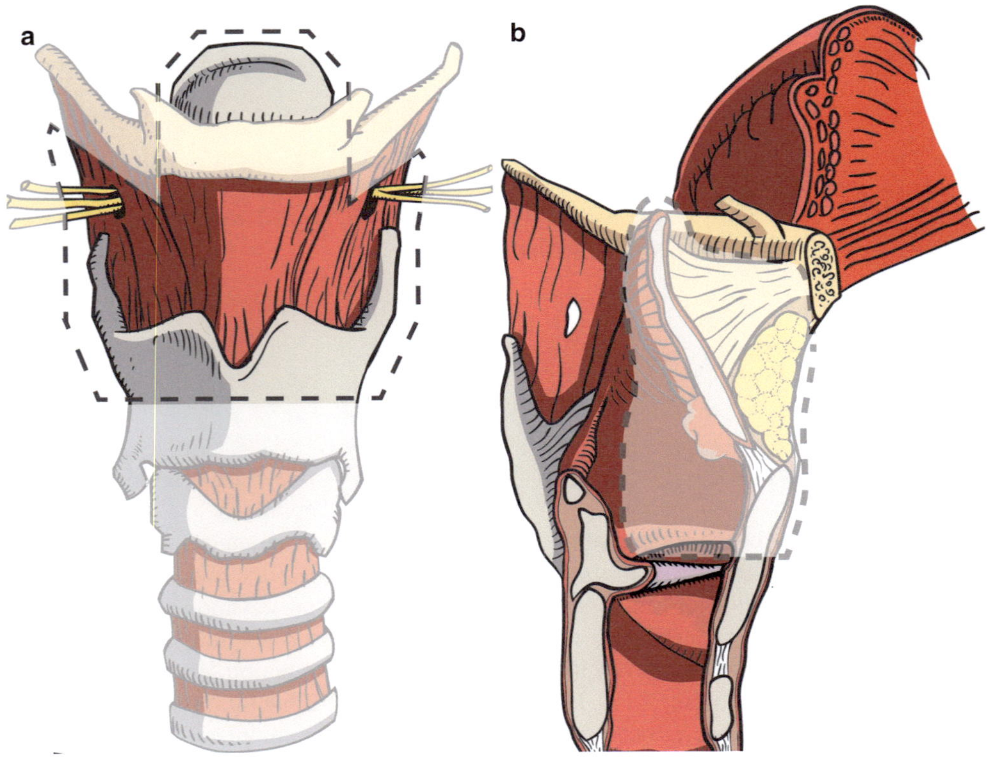

Fig. 5.1 Schematic drawing. (**a**) Coronal view; (**b**) sagittal view. The dotted line shows the supraglottic laryngeal resection

- Base of tongue (OPHL type I + BOT): represents an extension of the classic OPHL type I to a limited portion of the base of the tongue not overcoming the circumvallate papillae.
- Pyriform sinus (OPHL Type I + PYR): represents an extension of OPHL type I to the medial aspect of the pyriform sinus. Extension to the fundus or lateral wall of pyriform sinus prevents enough mucosal sparing to perform its reconstruction during the next phase.

5.3 Indications and Contraindications

Main Indications for OPHL Type I Are as Follows:

1. T1 tumors of the suprahyoid of infrahyoid epiglottis.
2. T2 supraglottic cancers involving epiglottis, valleculae, mucosa of the base of tongue, aryepiglottic folds, or medial aspect of pyriform sinus [11, 12].
3. Selected T3 supraglottic carcinomas, with normal cord mobility, involving the pre-epiglottic space and/or the thyroid cartilage limited only to its supraglottic aspect without glottic involvement.
4. Selected supraglottic T4a tumors due to extension to deep/extrinsic muscle of base of tongue or with extralaryngeal extension only to strap muscles.
5. Limited primary base of tongue or valleculae tumors with or without extension to supraglottic larynx and without hyoid bone involvement.

Main Contraindications Are as Follows:

1. Transglottic extension involving the true vocal folds or paraglottic space.
2. Extensive involvement of the base of the tongue <1 cm below the papillae circumvallate or sufficient involvement to require bilateral resection of the hypoglossal or lingual nerve.
3. Involvement of the pyriform sinus more extensive than its superior medial wall.
4. Postcricoid space or interarytenoid region involvement.
5. Severe comorbidities, poor performance status, old age, or caregiver absence.

Although it is generally believed that supraglottic laryngectomy can safely include an arytenoid, swallowing is usually significantly affected when this structure is removed via the conventional open approach. Another problem is when the tumor extends to the vallecula and base of the tongue. Surgery is still feasible, however, this type of tumor involvement requires partial resection of the base of the tongue, which might compromise functional outcomes. Furthermore, involvement of the base of the tongue from supraglottic cancer is usually advocated as T4a tumor, thus requiring postoperative radiation therapy, which might further worsen functional swallowing results [4].

Poor performance status is a contraindication to supraglottic laryngectomy that must be evaluated on an individual basis. Inadequate pulmonary reserve to tolerate the anticipated aspiration is a contraindication as well. Age and pulmonary function were used as rigid selection criteria in the past, today, however, a more pragmatic approach is proposed focusing on biological age rather than chronological one. Although most patients are heavy smokers and have chronic bronchitis, this condition can sometimes be improved before surgery. Considering that some degree of aspiration is likely in the early postoperative period [13], the degree of pulmonary impairment remains controversial in the decision to perform conservative laryngectomy. Some authors advocate routine pulmonary function testing in all patients, while others suggest the use of a clinical assessment, such as the ability to walk up two flights of stairs without showing respiratory distress [14]. Neurologic disease with swallowing problems and esophageal strictures disqualifies the patient for supraglottic laryngectomy. Although supraglottic laryngectomy may be feasible, total laryngectomy may be required if free surgical margins are not likely to be achieved without an irrecoverable functional outcome. The main aim of surgery is in every case the complete resection of the tumor. Preservation of laryngeal function is a secondary but of paramount importance goal of the procedure and patient selection must be carefully considered. Both the patient and the family must be highly motivated and demonstrate a willingness to comply with postoperative rehabilitation instructions. The possibility of conversion to total laryngectomy should always be discussed preoperatively and put in a preoperative signed modular consent.

5.4 Surgical Steps

When performing a function-preserving laryngectomy, the surgeon must strictly adhere to several important principles. Local control is the most important principle; the patient's survival is at great risk if the tumor is not properly removed. Extensive knowledge of the anatomy and function of the larynx is required to possibly predict the extent of the tumor with confidence. A basic concept to keep in mind is that the cricoarytenoid unit is the fundamental functional unit of the larynx: laryngeal preservation surgery is not feasible unless at least one cricoarytenoid unit can be preserved. In this subheading, the surgical steps of OPHL 1 are described.

5.4.1 Patient Positioning and Surgical Setting

The procedure is performed under general anesthesia with endotracheal intubation. A prophylactic antibiotic is generally administered during anesthesia induction (e.g., cefazolin and metronidazole I.V.). The patient lies supine with the neck slightly extended and a roller under the shoulders to elevate them. Whenever possible, orotracheal intubation is preferred to avoid preoperative tracheostomy. The nasogastric feeding tube is placed.

5.4.2 Skin Incision and Subplatysmal Flap Creation

A U-shaped (Leroux-Robert) bimastoid apron flap (Fig. 5.2) is planned (in the rare cases when neck dissection is not performed, lateral extension of this incision can be more medial,

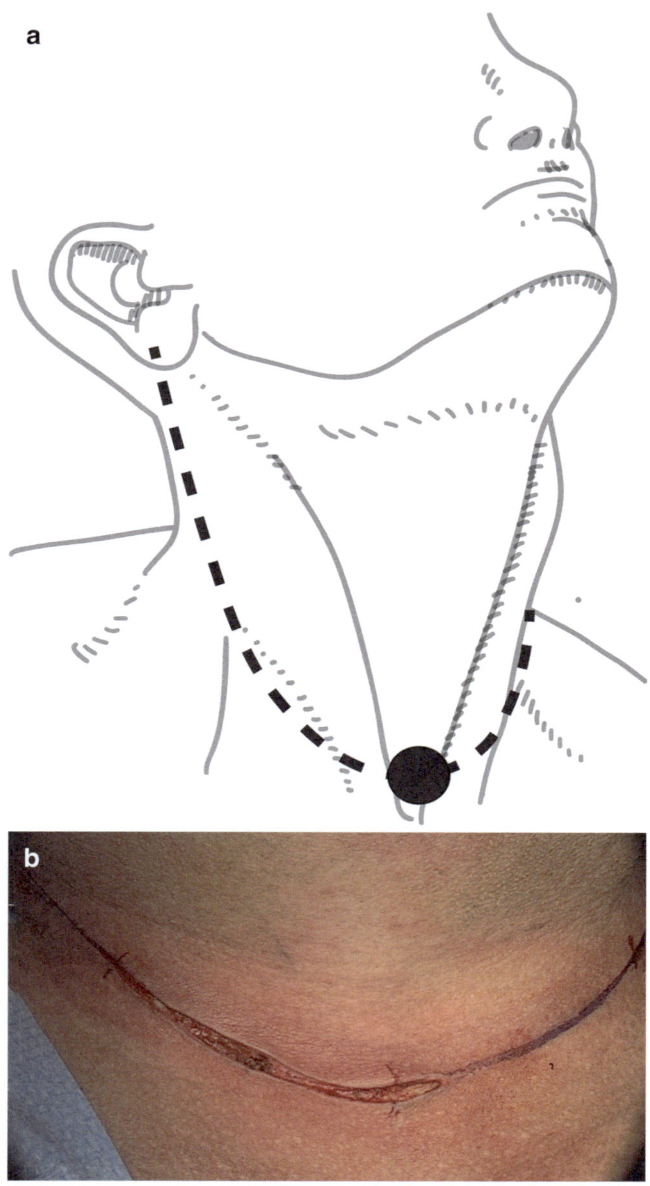

Fig. 5.2 (**a**) Schematic drawing showing the U-shaped bimastoid apron flap. (**b**) Intraoperative image showing a U-shaped bimastoid apron flap

anteriorly to the sternocleidomastoid muscles), so that the horizontal part of the incision lies at the level of cricoid cartilage. The apron flap is elevated just below the platysma muscle. A subplatysmal flap is elevated so that the external jugular vein and the greater auricular nerve remain intact. The superior flap is elevated about 1 cm above the level of the hyoid bone. If there is involvement of the thyrohyoid membrane or massive infiltration of the pre-epiglottic space, the strap muscles must be removed with the specimen.

5.4.3 Bilateral Neck Dissection

Bilateral selective neck dissection is performed in almost all patients with at least cT2 tumor. If no pathologic adenopathy (cN0) is evident during clinic-radiological evaluation, selective neck dissection of Robbins level II–IV is performed [15]. The accessory spinal nerve, jugular veins, and sternocleidomastoid muscles are preserved. Rare cases of superficial squamous cell carcinoma affecting the suprahyoid epiglottis staged cT1 can be treated without performing neck dissection.

5.4.4 Laryngotracheal Framework Skeletonization

The strap muscles are detached from the lower border of the hyoid bone and reflected downward to expose the upper half of the thyroid cartilage (Fig. 5.3). The hyoid bone is preserved. The attachments of the inferior constrictor muscle at the lateral border of the thyroid cartilage are transected (Fig. 5.4) together with muscle fibers standing along the superior border of the thyroid cartilage. Turning the larynx to the opposite side with a hook could facilitate this step. This maneuver exposes the superior horn of the hyoid bone and the upper half of the thyroid cartilage from the lateral margin to the midline (Fig. 5.5). Take care to identify and avoid any carcinoma pushing forward in the pre-epiglottic space under the thyrohyoid membrane. Once posterolateral and superior margins of thyroid cartilage are freed from muscle fibers, complete mobilization of thyroid cartilage is still limited by the lateral thyrohyoid ligament and tissues attached around and lateral to the superior horn of thyroid cartilage. These tissues together with the lateral thyrohyoid ligament should be cut. During this maneuver, attention must be paid not to damage superior laryngeal pedicle, in particular its internal branch that passes just below the great horn of the thyroid cartilage. Grabbing the larynx with a hook from the superior thyroid horn and rotating it to the opposite site while moving upward with a gauze all tissue around the superior horn prevent damaging the pedicle. When only the lateral thyroid ligament is left, it is cut with monopolar or scissors staying attached to the superior horn and paying attention not to damage the pyriform sinus mucosa.

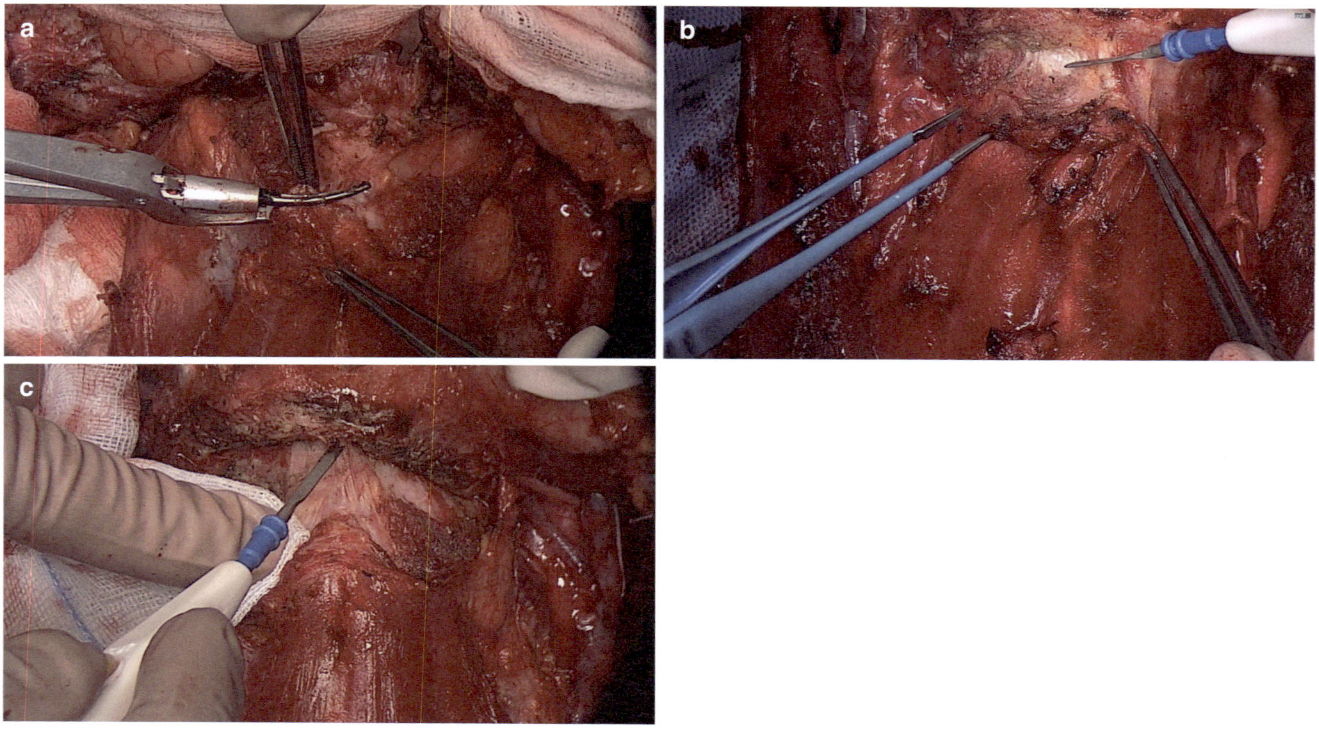

Fig. 5.3 (**a–c**) The hyoid bone is skeletonized by detaching the infrahyoid strap muscles by means of an electrocautery

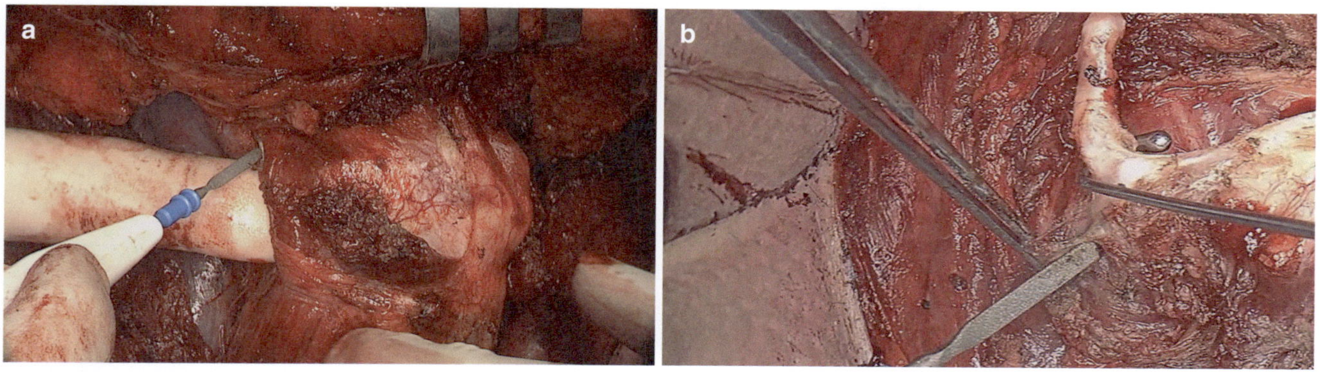

Fig. 5.4 (**a** and **b**) The inferior constrictor muscle is sectioned bilaterally along its lateral thyroid cartilage attachment. Thyrohyoid ligament should not be sectioned from the superior thyroid horn until thyroid cartilage lateral border is completely freed from muscle in order to avoid superior laryngeal nerve damage

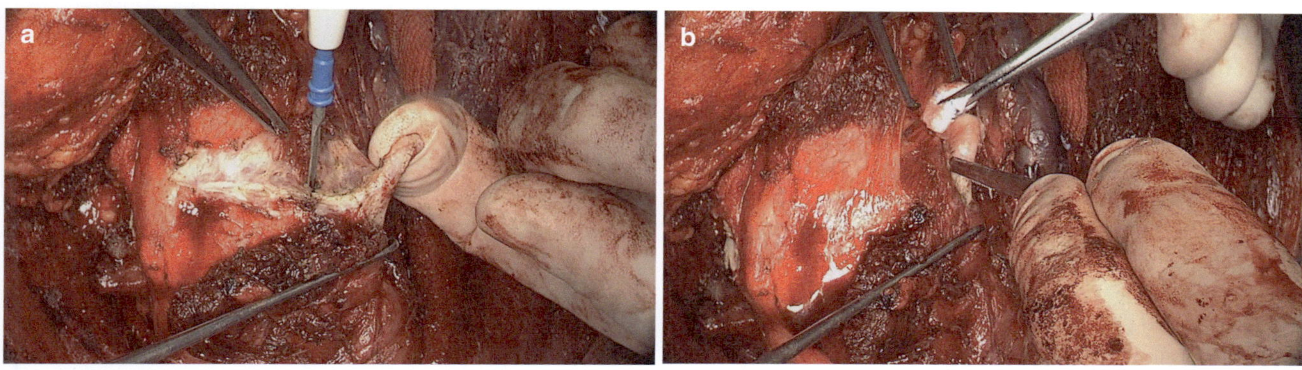

Fig. 5.5 (**a** and **b**) Right side. The greater horn of the thyroid cartilage is first freed with an electrocautery and then carefully dissected with gauze detaching pharyngeal mucosa from the upper part of thyroid cartilage in a subperichondral plane

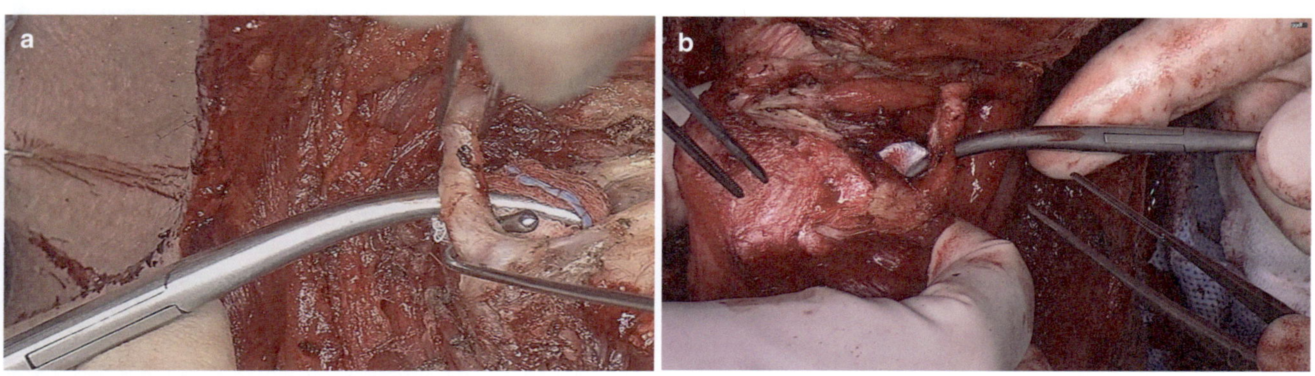

Fig. 5.6 (**a** and **b**) Left side. After thyrohyoid ligament is sectioned from the superior cornu of thyroid cartilage, mucosa of the upper part of pyriform sinus is detached from the upper part of thyroid cartilage in a sunperichondral plane with gauze or Freer (a) The same surgical step is performed on the contralateral side (b)

5.4.5 Detachment of pyriform sinus and superior thyrotomy

Inner portion of lateral and superior edge of thyroid cartilage is still attached to piriform sinus mucosa. A subperichondrial dissection of pyriform sinuses is achieved using Freer dissector or a small gauze (Fig. 5.6). During this surgical step, care must be taken to avoid entering the paraglottic space. At this time, superior laryngeal vascular pedicle can be tied and sectioned paying attention to preserve superior laryngeal nerve (which usually runs in a deeper plane) (Fig. 5.7). Some authors prefer not to section superior laryngeal artery and

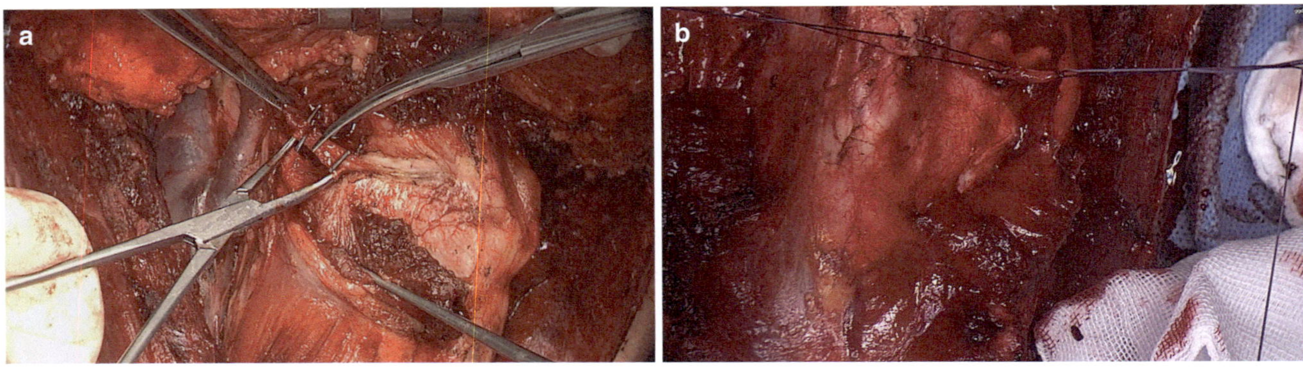

Fig. 5.7 (**a** and **b**) The laryngeal vessels are identified and sectioned. Superior laryngeal nerve runs in a deeper plane and must be preserved

vein and identifying the superior laryngeal nerve to not damage it.

Superior thyrotomy should be done just above the level of the vocal folds. The incision is made approximately midway between the thyroid notch and the inferior border of the thyroid cartilage (some authors suggest 5 mm below the superior thyroid notch), so that the larynx can be resected through the ventricle (Fig. 5.8). Section of the cartilage starts from midline and goes laterally toward the lateral portion previously divided from inner perichondrium and pyriform sinus mucosa. Alternatively, some authors suggest making this incision laterally and obliquely toward the anterior aspect of the superior horn on the less affected side, so that the attachment of the constrictor muscles may be preserved and the superior laryngeal nerve may be more easily preserved. This incision should not be made too low so as not to injure the attachment of the anterior commissure to the thyroid cartilage. We prefer a horizontal linear thyroid cartilage incision to guarantee a better match with the hyoid bone when performing thyrohyoidopexy (Fig. 5.9).

5.4.6 Pre-epiglottic Space Removal

The pre-epiglottic space is a triangular fat-containing space between the epiglottis, the hyoid bone, and the thyrohyoid membrane. Considering its frequent involvement by supraglottic tumors, this space must be removed. To completely remove this space in a hyoid-preserving approach, a subperiosteal dissection is performed along the inferior and posterior margins of the hyoid bone. Pre-epiglottic space is grab with forceps and gently pulled upward and downward while deepening subperiosteal dissection with cautery to better identify the submucosa of valleculae that is the deep plane where the pre-epiglottic fibrofatty tissue lies. Once this plane is reached, dissection is carried on downward along it to the level of the superior border of thyroid cartilage. Content of the pre-epiglottic space is reflected downward to ensure en bloc resection with the rest of the specimen (Figs. 5.10 and 5.11). To ensure that submucosa of valleculae has been reached, it is useful to pull anteriorly the pre-epiglottic tissue once it has been dissected and observe the epiglottis "pushing" against the mucosa and appearing in transparency.

5.4.7 Pharyngotomy and Laryngotomy

If not done previously, superior laryngeal artery and vein are identified, ligated, and transected. If the tumor is confined to the supraglottic larynx, the pharyngotomy incision is made through the uninvolved vallecula. This allows the subsequent mucosal incisions to be made under direct vision (Fig. 5.12). The epiglottis is grasped outside the larynx, and ventricular folds are put in direct view to confirm the extension of the tumor (Fig. 5.13).

Mucosal incision is then continued laterally along the uninvolved aryepiglottic fold and then across the anterior surface of the arytenoid muscular process to detach aryepiglottic fold and ventricular fold from it. The lower incision is made horizontally through the laryngeal ventricles to join the mucosal incisions with the cartilage incision (Fig. 5.14). The specimen is now laterally pedicled on the affected side and allows the surgeon to directly observe the extension of the tumor inside the larynx (Fig. 5.15). Final excision of the specimen is performed also on the contralateral side, under direct visualization, with adequate macroscopic margin from the tumor, preserving as much tissue and structures as possible (from the whole arytenoid to only the lateral wall of the pyriform sinus) (Fig. 5.16).

The resected specimen and surgical field are carefully evaluated, and frozen sections are sent to ensure clear margins (Fig. 5.17).

5.4.8 Focus on Resection of Supraglottis

The larynx must be opened as far as possible from the neoplastic lesion to get a safe access to the endolarynx and achieve en bloc resection with a direct vision on the tumor

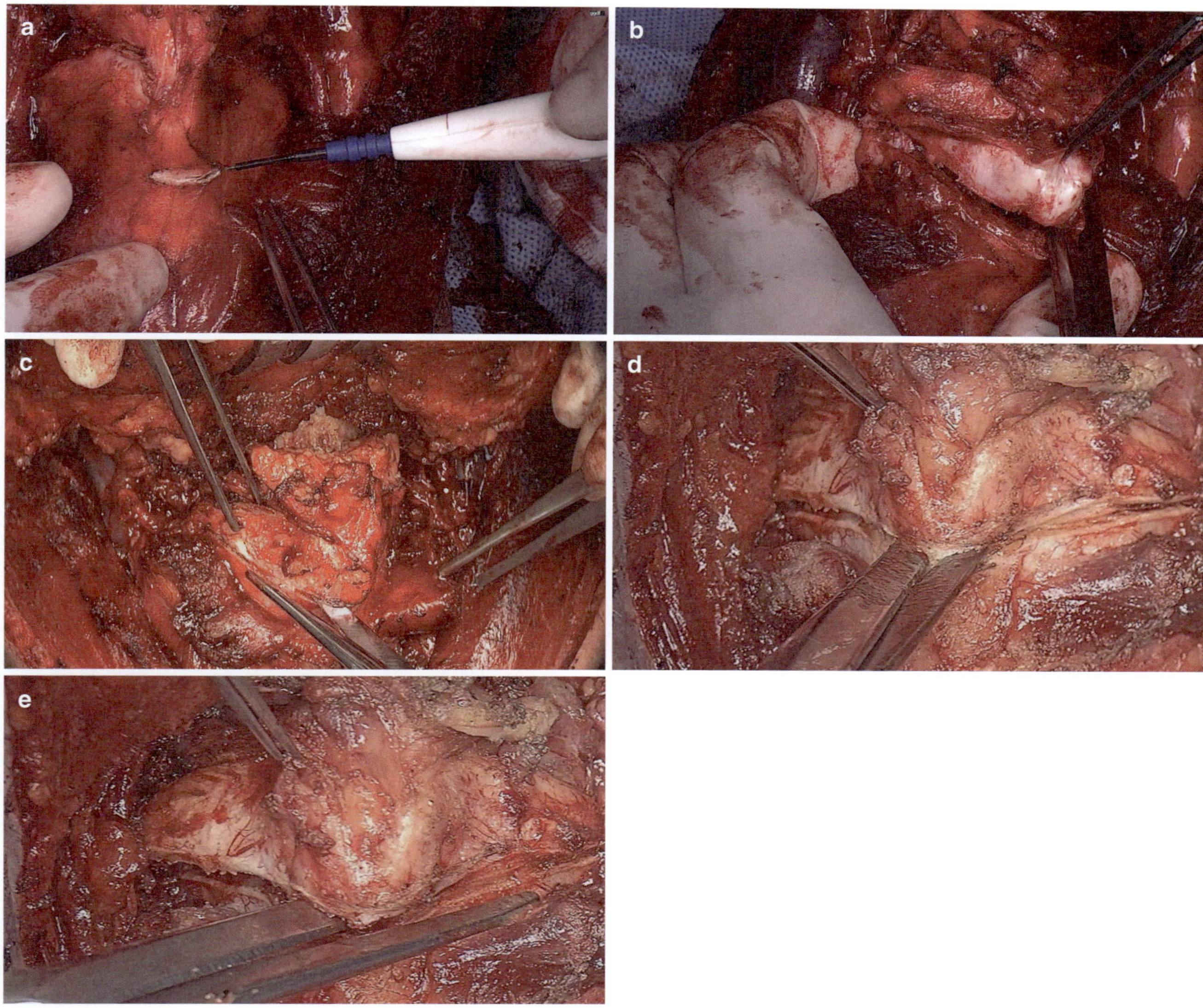

Fig. 5.8 (**a**) A median cut is performed 0.5–1 cm below the thyroid notch to assess for the proper plane above the true vocal folds; (**b–e**) The transcartilaginous bilateral cuts are performed to complete the thyrotomy

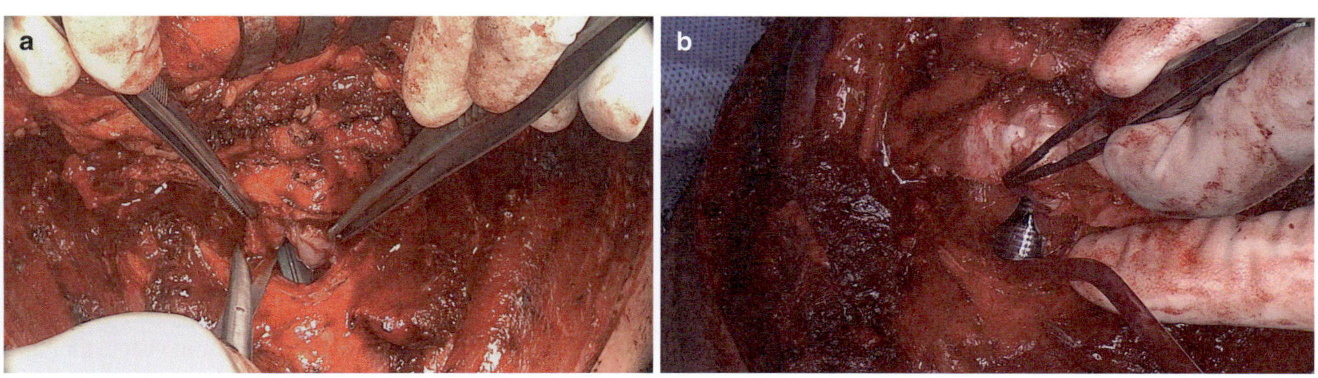

Fig. 5.9 (**a** and **b**) A detailed image showing the incisions through the ventricles up to the muscular process of the arytenoids

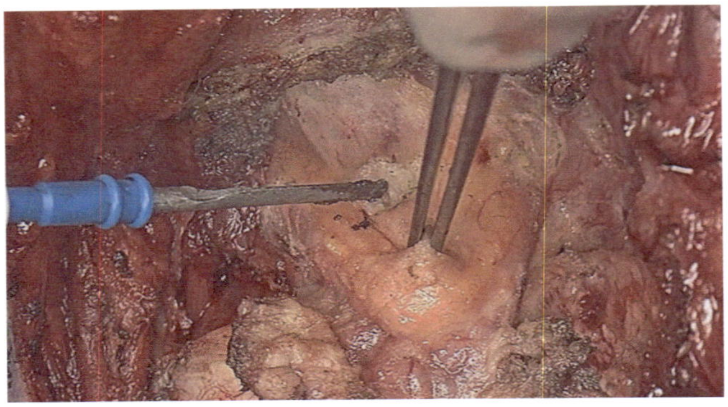

Fig. 5.10 Pre-epiglottic space removal

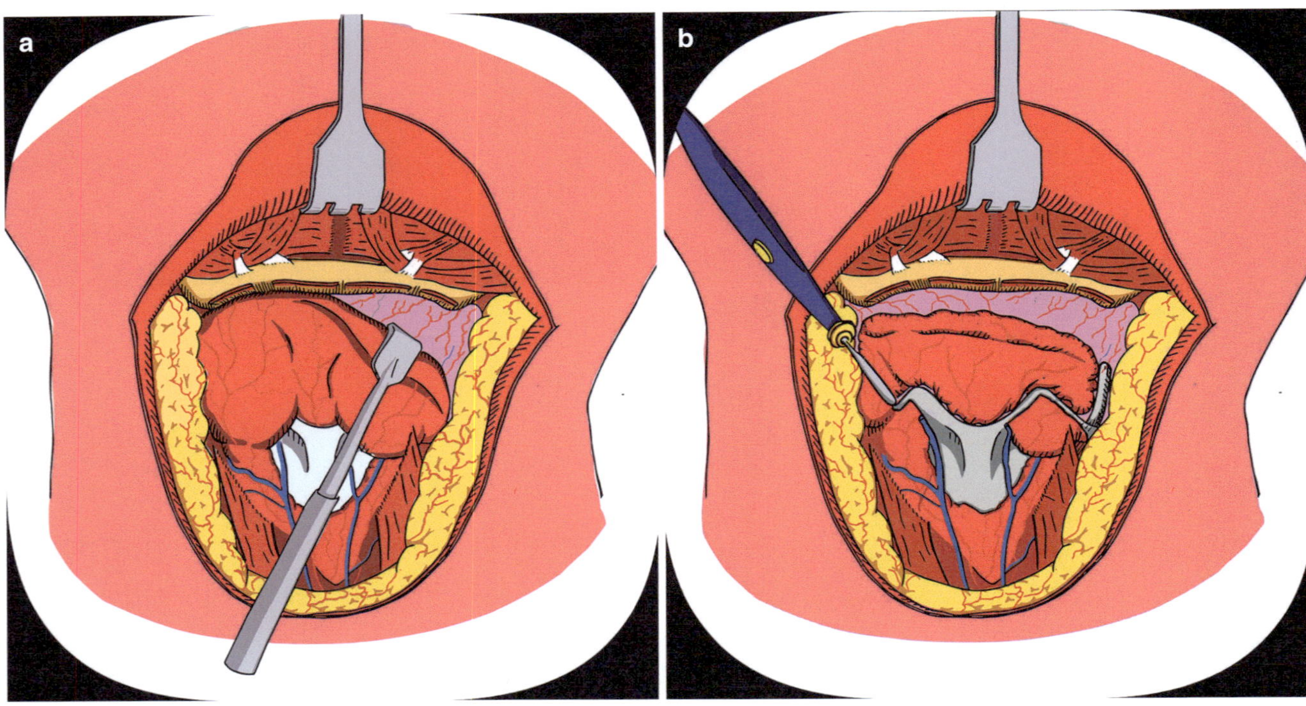

Fig. 5.11 Schematic drawings showing the pre-epiglottic space removal. (**a**) An incision with electrocautery is performed over the posterior edge of the hyoid bone to achieve a subperiosteal plane and detach the pre-epiglottic content from the deep plane. (**b**) The pre-epiglottic content is detached from the upper edges of the thyroid alae

margins. There are three commonly described routes of access: superiorly through the mucosa of the epiglottic valleculae, inferiorly through an incision just above the anterior commissure and laterally through the uninvolved pharyngeal mucosa near the great horn of the thyroid cartilage. To separate the supraglottis from the vocal cords, we first determine the height of the anterior commissure by making a small window in the anterior midline, at the level of the cartilaginous incision. A small opening is sufficient to identify the vocal cords and ventricle. One blade of the scissors is then placed in the ventricle and the other in the lateral surface of the thyroid cartilage. The incision runs from the anterior commissure to the vocal cord process of the arytenoid, along the floor of the ventricle. After the superior pharyngotomy has been performed, a third incision connects laterally the superior access to the ventricular incision. This incision passes transversely through the aryepiglottic fold, close to the anterior surface of the arytenoid cartilage, and joins the first incision at the level of the anterior aspect of the arytenoid. Now the supraglottis can be rotated medially allowing a complete view of the opposite side of the endolarynx with tumor in vision, facilitating resection. The opposite side of the supraglottis is separated from the larynx by cutting through the floor of the ventricle from the anterior commissure to the arytenoid. The incision is then passed upward along the anterior surface of the arytenoid, sectioning the aryepiglottic fold.

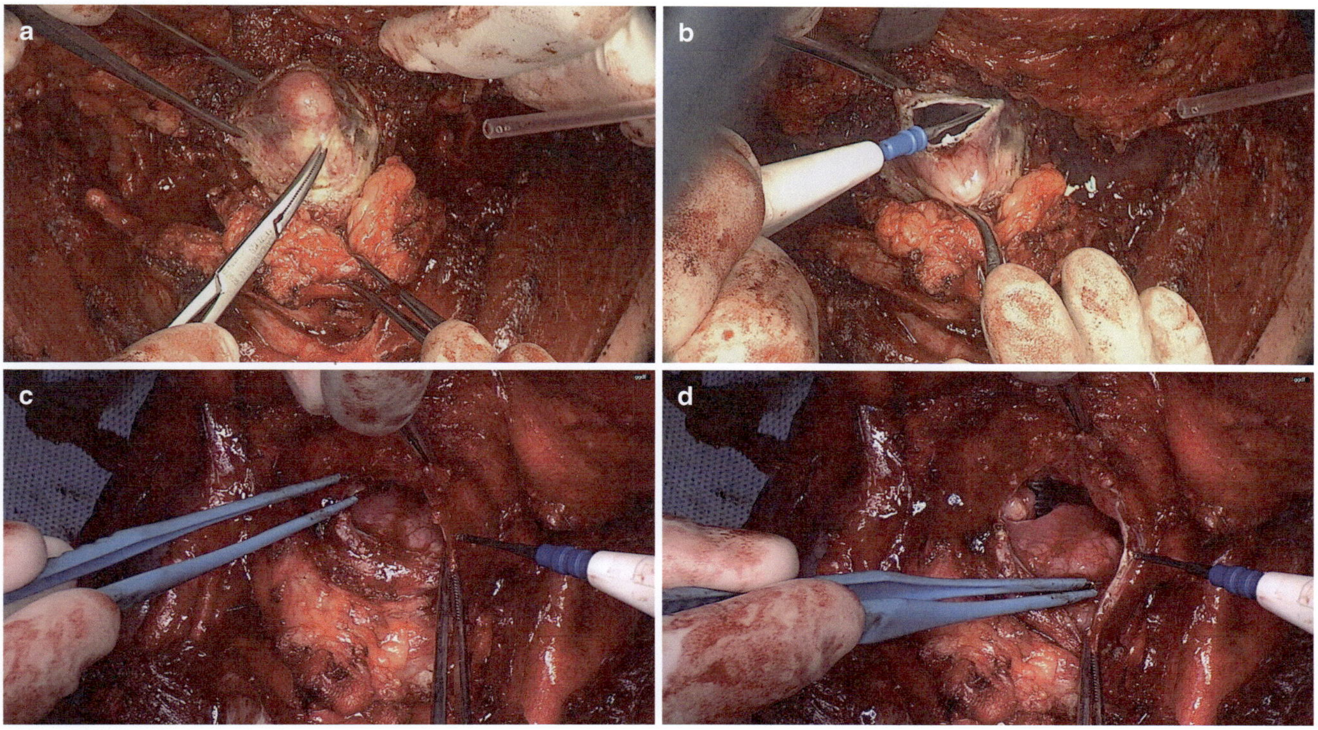

Fig. 5.12 (**a–d**) Supraepiglottic pharyngotomy to get the access to the endolarynx

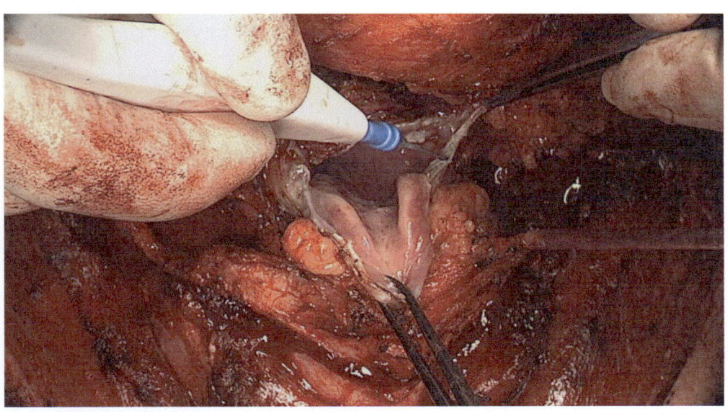

Fig. 5.13 The epiglottis is grasped with a clamp and rotated outward to provide direct visualization of the tumor extent inside the larynx

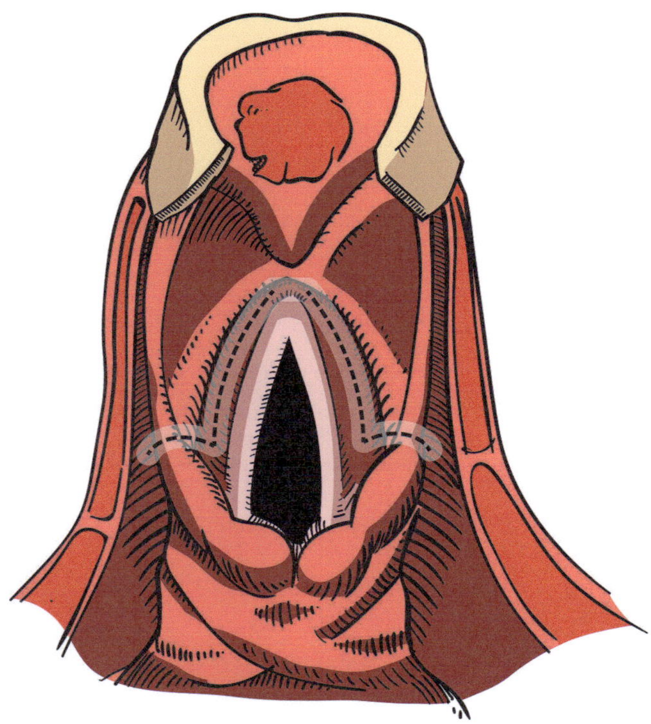

Fig. 5.14 Schematic drawing showing the view of the supraglottis of the first surgeon "from above." The dotted line shows the inferior limit of supraglottic resection

5.4.9 Reconstructive Phase: The Thyrohyoidopexy

Reconstruction or pexy can be done with different techniques. The goal is to correctly reapproximate the base of the tongue and the remaining glottic portion of the larynx to create a new functional swallowing unit. First, it is important to bend down patient's head and remove the roll under patient shoulders. If resection has been extended to an arytenoid cartilage and/or the medial aspect of pyriform

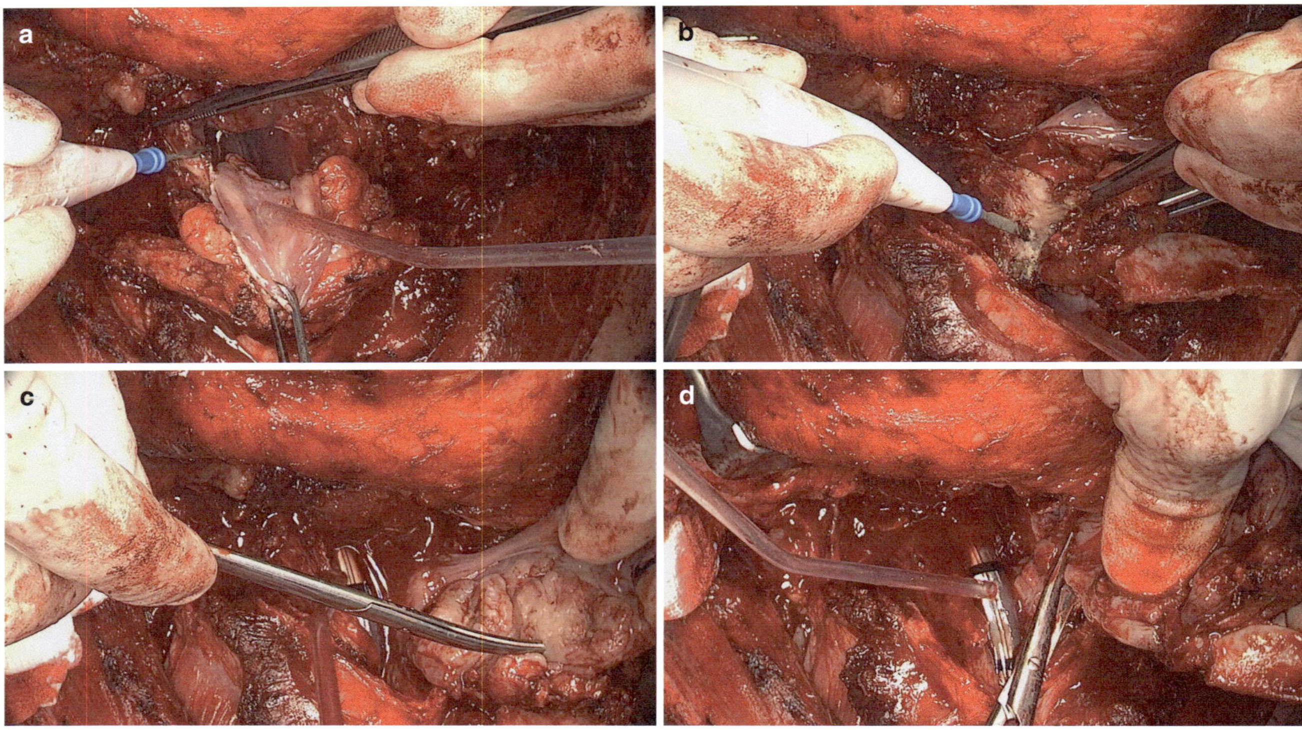

Fig. 5.15 (**a**–**d**) The supraglottic laryngectomy proceeds starting from the non-neoplastic side (right side) under direct vision along the aryepiglottic folds to the anterior aspect of vocal process of the arytenoids, which are preserved. The specimen is then pedicled on the affected side allowing a wide and direct view of tumor margins

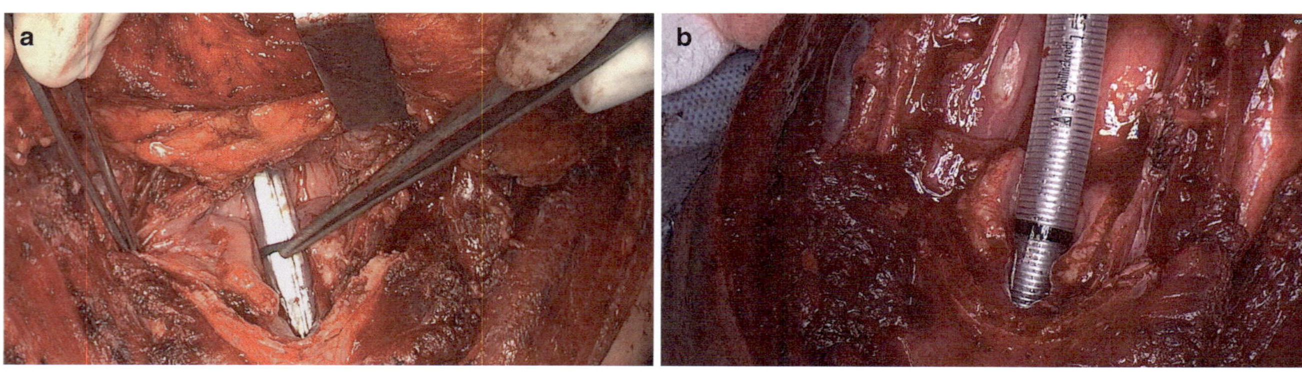

Fig. 5.16 (**a** and **b**) The surgical margins are checked intraoperatively

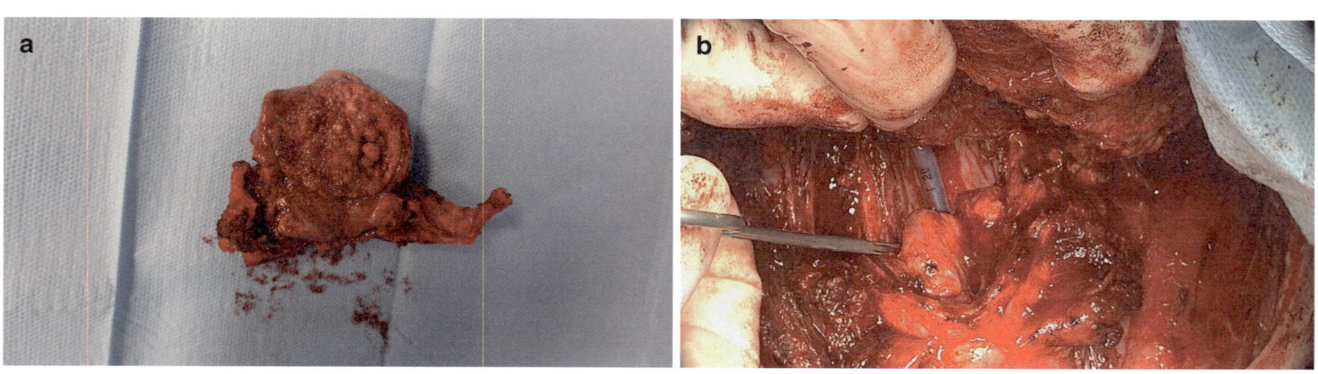

Fig. 5.17 (**a** and **b**) Supraglottic laryngectomy specimen (**a**). The two preserved cricoarytenoid units are visible on the surgical field (**b**)

sinus, it must be reconstructed before the pexy is performed. Otherwise, the pyriform sinus will not expand during swallowing leading patient to higher risks of inhalation. Thyrohyoidopexy is then performed. Three, 4 or 5 PDS or vicryl stiches can be positioned. Needle is first passed across the residual thyroid cartilage a few millimeters below the section line in a submucosal plane. It is important to include the submucosa of the residual larynx to achieve a proper pexy and reduce the possibility of postoperative fistula formation. Then, needle is passed deep in the base of tongue almost 2 cm above the hyoid bone in the central stitche(s). Care should be taken when placing the sutures around the lateral parts of hyoid body because of its close relationship to the lingual artery and hypoglossal nerve. In this setting, stitches should pass above the hyoid bone very close to it. We usually put 4 stiches for laryngopexy: 2 central and 2 lateral (Fig. 5.18). Each stitch is placed, but not tied. As soon as they are all placed, they are tied in sequence starting from the center (2 central stiches are tied together by two operators). Two or 3 simple knots are prepared before tied them (Fig. 5.19). At the end of thyrohyoidopexy, residual thyroid cartilage and hyoid bone are strictly tied together in a watertight fashion (Fig. 5.20) and strap muscles (if available) are sutured over it for protection.

5.4.10 Tracheostomy

When performing a tracheostomy, it is important to isolate the incision from the potential spaces on either side after neck dissection and from the pexy by suturing trachostoma in a 360 grades fashion. Failure to isolate the tracheostomy from the neck dissection may result in wound infection. For this reason, some surgeons prefer to create a separate incision between the sternal notch and the neck incision. We perform tracheostomy in the same neck incision, paying attention to separate it from the neck putting 10 stiches creating a temporary stoma (Fig. 5.21).

5.4.11 Skin Closure

A JP drain is placed where neck dissection has been performed and maintained to continuous suction to prevent postoperative hematoma. A layered closure of the skin is then performed.

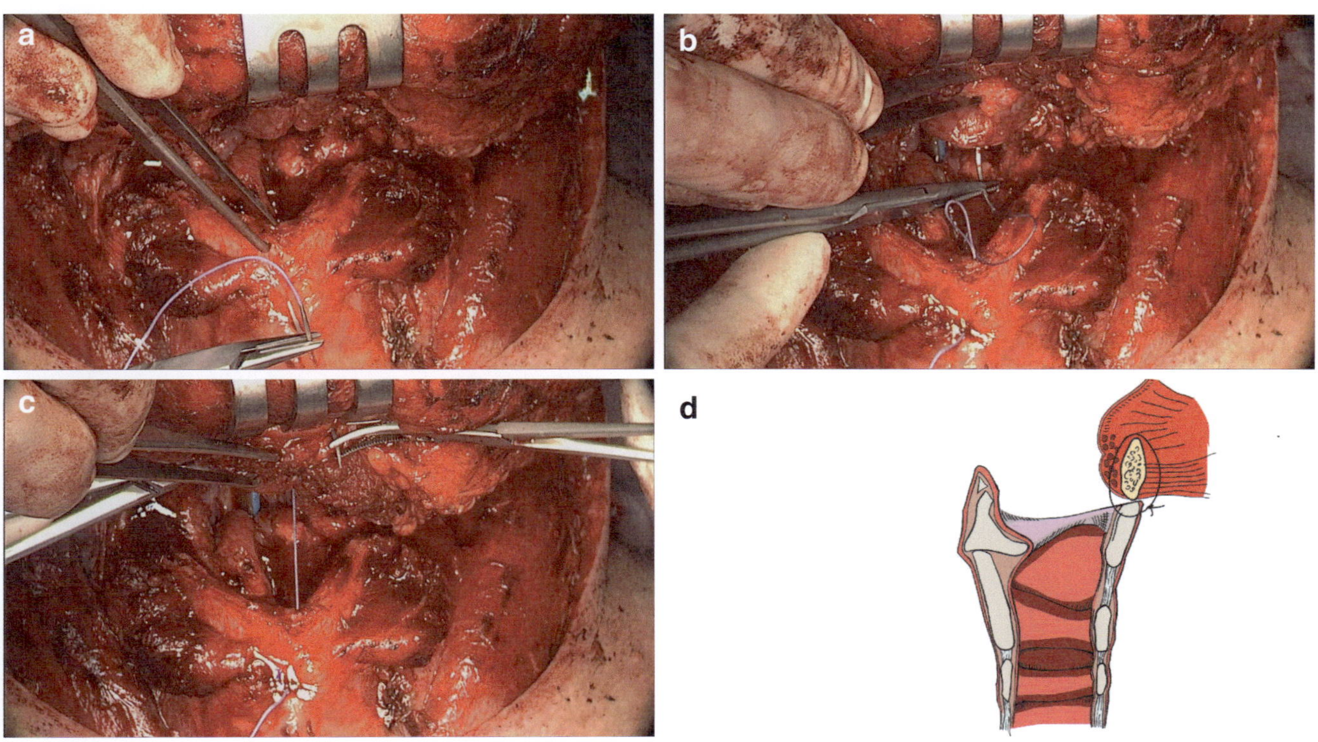

Fig. 5.18 (a–d) The thyrohyoidopexy. Needle is first passed across the residual thyroid cartilage (**a**) from the lower edge to the superior margin in a submucosal plane. Then, needle is passed deep in the base of tongue (**b**) and then across hyoid bone (**c**). A schematic drawing on the sagittal plane of the final pexy is shown (**d**)

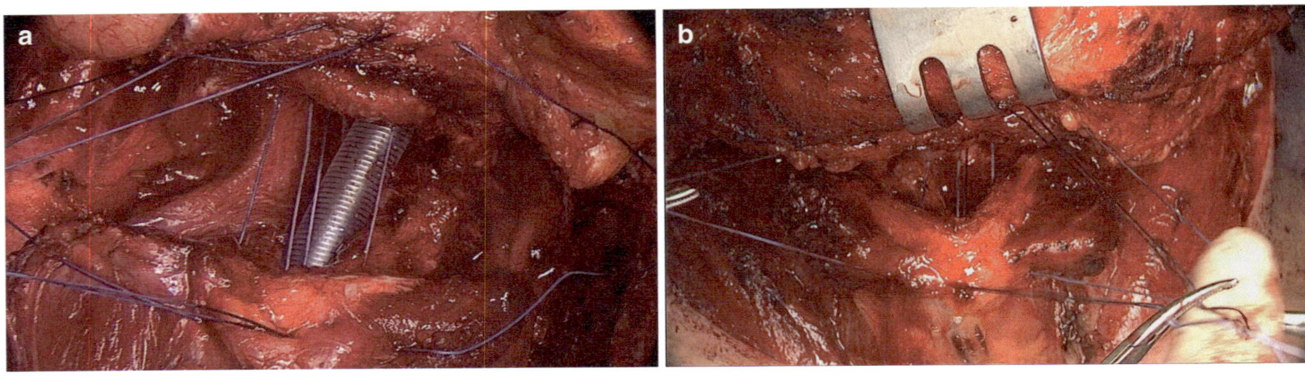

Fig. 5.19 (**a** and **b**) Thyro-hyoid stitches for the pexy are all prepared and ready to be tied starting from the central ones tied simultaneously

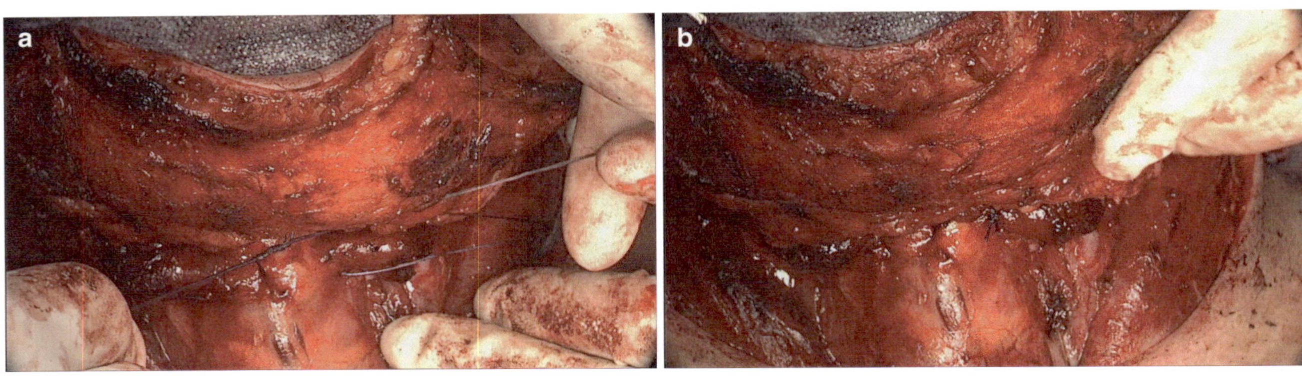

Fig. 5.20 (**a** and **b**) Thyrohyoidopexy. Final result

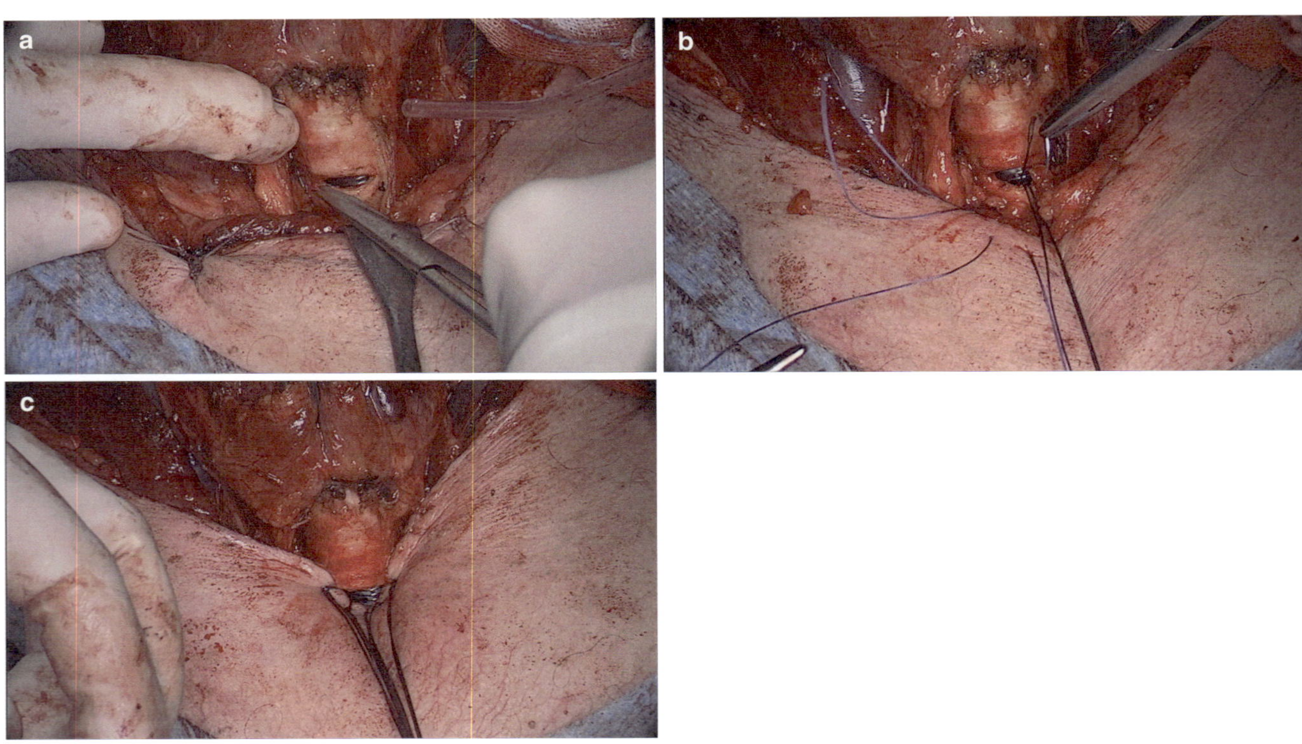

Fig. 5.21 (**a**–**c**) Temporary tracheostomy. It is performed below the usual level (**a**) (II–III tracheal ring). The trachea is anchored to the skin on the same incision line, taking care that the stoma is perfectly separated from the deep neck tissue to avoid infection (**b** and **c**)

5.5 Case Example

A 65-year-old man with a long history of tobacco smoking was admitted in the ENT department complaining of progressive hoarseness started 6 months before. The fiberoptic endoscopic laryngeal examination showed an ulcerated tissue along the laryngeal face of epiglottis and right ventricular fold. Glottic plane was not involved by the tumor and laryngeal mobility was not impaired as well (Fig. 5.22). Physical examination did not reveal any enlarged cervical lymph node. Contrast-enhanced CT scan showed an enhancing lesion involving the middle and inferior third of the epiglottis and extended to the right aryepiglottic and ventricular fold with 2.3 × 0.9 × 3 cm of dimension. One lymphadenopathy with suspected colliquate content was signaled at the right II level without radiological signs of extracapsular extension (Fig. 5.23). A diagnosis of undifferentiated (G3) squamous cell carcinoma (SCC) after a biopsy of the lesion. Clinical staging was T2 N1 M0.

Standard OPHL I with bilateral selective II-IV neck dissection was performed. The histopathological diagnosis confirmed the diagnosis of SCC G3 involving the epiglottis, the aryepiglottic fold, and ventricular fold mucosa without pre-epiglottic space involvement. Furthermore, squamous cell carcinoma cells were found inside one lymph node without extracapsular extension. Pathological staging was in accordance with clinical one, staging the cancer as pT2 pN1 cM0. The postoperative course was uneventful. Patient was discharged from the hospital after 17 days with complete oral alimentation. Due to the presence of lymph node metastasis, the patient was addressed to postoperative adjuvant therapy on local and regional sites of disease. At the last follow-up after 3 years, the patient maintained total oral feeding and was free-from disease clinically (Fig. 5.24) and radiologically.

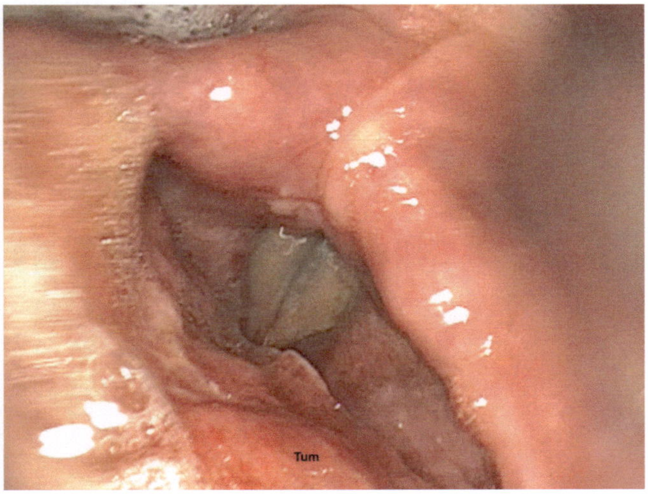

Fig. 5.22 Flexible endoscopic examination revealed an ulcerated tissue along the laryngeal face of epiglottis and right ventricular fold. *Tum* Tumor

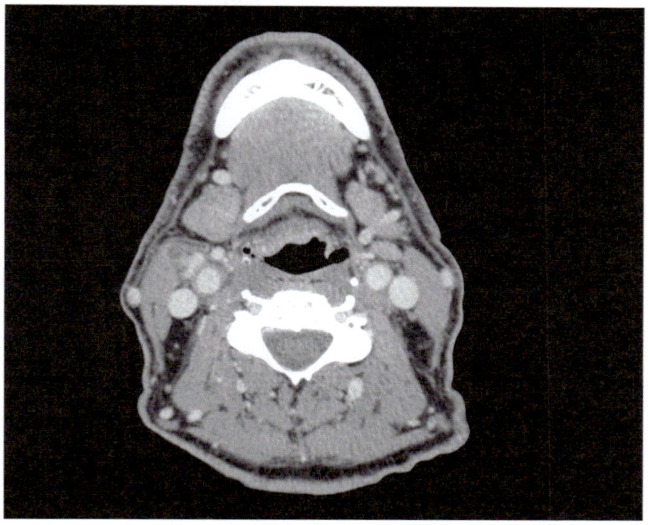

Fig. 5.23 Preoperative CT scan showing contrast-enhanced mass involving the laryngeal face of epiglottis and right aryepiglottic fold with a necrocolliquate node on the right side

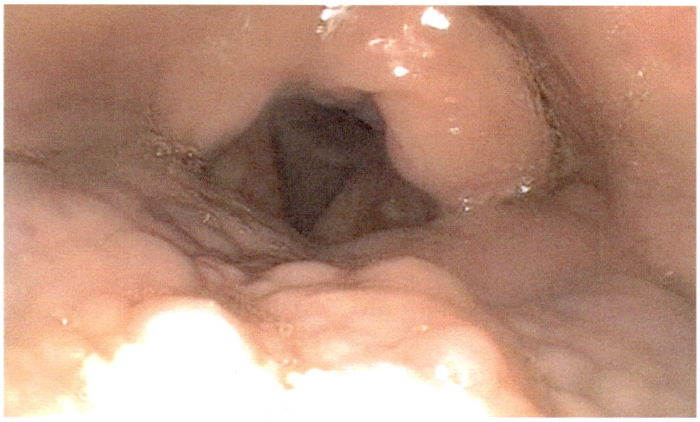

Fig. 5.24 Three years post-surgery flexible endoscopic examination shows well-functioning neolarynx with no signs of recurrence

5.6 Postoperative Care and Complications

Patients receive routine tracheostomy care. Drainage tubes are maintained until drainage is less than 30 ml/24 h. It is important to place a fenestrated tube without a cuff as soon as possible to avoid damage to the tracheal wall, early stimulate cough reflex when inhalation occurs, and allow early rehabilitation. During the fourth or fifth postoperative day patients usually begin swallowing training with speech-therapist with some exercises and usually start with semi-solid food in 6–7 postoperative days. Feeding tube is removed when the patient can eat without much difficulty. The tracheostomy tube is removed early to reduce cough and tracheal secretions when edema has decreased enough to allow normal breathing through the glottic opening also facilitating swallowing rehabilitation. This can be done in the first postoperative days, especially if a stoma is present. Swallowing rehabilitation is better with a close stoma because the tracheostomy is associated with a less effective cough, reduced larynx excursion movements, and decreased proprioception, which makes aspiration more likely. After overcoming the acute healing phase, patients with supraglottic laryngectomy have remarkably good voice and few dietary restrictions. Functional recovery is significantly, sometimes severely, compromised when postoperative radiation therapy is required. Radiation causes lymphedema and congestion, which can impair swallowing and lead to airway obstruction. For this reason, some surgeons prefer to mantain tracheostomy tube during radiation therapy. In case of OPHL type I extended to an arytenoid, a vocal fold or piriform sinus, swallowing rehabilitation can be more difficult. In some cases, arytenoid edema and immobility of the vocal cords cause airway obstruction and delays in decannulation (in the most severe cases, this results in the inability to decannulate).

Tips and Tricks

- Some authors suggest detaching the outer perichondrium of the superior aspect of the thyroid cartilage before cutting through it. Once the specimen has been removed, this outer perichondrium flap stays pedicled on the residual inferior half of the thyroid cartilage and is used to enforce the pexy at the end of the suture. Alternatively, we often reinforce the pexy with 3/0 Vicryl stitches passing through the outer perichondrium and around the hyoid bone.
- When dissecting through the pre-epiglottic space is very useful to pull the fatty tissue downward. In this way is much easier to identify the plane of valleculae submucosa without directly entering inside the pharyngeal lumen.
- When base of tongue resection is needed, it is very important to pull it behind the hyoid bone after pre-epiglottic space dissection. After the submucosa of valleculae has been identified, cautery is directed superiorly and posteriorly to the hyoid bone keeping a subperiosteal plane while pulling the base of tongue downward. Palpating the base of tongue during this maneuver is mandatory to identify a macroscopically free margin. When soft consistence of the base of tongue is finally identified, dissection is stopped, and base of tongue muscles and mucosa are transected with electrocautery from below to above entering the pharyngeal lumen in a more cranial site.
- The pexy can be additionally sealed by placing infrahyoid muscles (if preserved) onto it. Infrahyoid muscles should be sutured to the hyoid periosteum and the suprahyoid muscles.

References

1. Alonso JM. Conservative surgery of cancer of the larynx. Trans Am Acad Ophthalmol Otolaryngol. 1947;51:633–42.
2. Rizzotto G, Succo G, Lucioni M, Pazzaia T. Subtotal laryngectomy with tracheohyoidopexy: a possible alternative to total laryngectomy. Laryngoscope. 2006;116:1907–17.
3. Remacle M, Hantzakos A, Eckel H, Evrard AS, et al. Endoscopic supraglottic laryngectomy: a proposal for a classification by the working committee on nomenclature, European Laryngological Society. Eur Arch Otorrinolaringol. 2009;266:993–8.
4. Lee NK, Goepfert H, Wendt CD. Supraglottic laryngectomy for intermediate-stage cancer: U.T. MD Anderson Cancer Center experience with combined therapy. Laryngoscope. 1990;100:831.
5. Burstein FD, Calcaterra TC. Supraglottic laryngectomy: series report and analysis of results. Laryngoscope. 1985;95:833.
6. Piazza C, Peretti G, Cattaneo A, Garrubba F, de Zinis LO, Nicola P. Salvage surgery after radiotherapy for laryngeal cancer: from endoscopic resections to open-neck partial and total laryngectomies. Arch Otolaryngol Head Neck Surg. 2007;133:1037–43.
7. Pellini R, Pichi B, Ruscito P, Ceroni AR, Caliceti U, Rizzotto G, Pazzaia A, Laudadio P, Piazza C, Peretti G, Giannarelli D, Spriano G. Supracricoid partial laryngectomies after radiation failure: a multi-institutional series. Head Neck. 2008;30:372–9.
8. Hirano M, Kurita S, Matsuoka H, et al. Vocal fold fixation in laryngeal carcinomas. Acta Otolaryngol. 1991;111:449.
9. Succo G, Peretti G, Piazza C, et al. Open partial horizontal laryngectomies: a proposal for classification by the working committee on nomenclature of the European Laryngological Society. Eur Arch Otorrinolaringol. 2014;271(9):2489–96. https://doi.org/10.1007/s00405-014-3024-4.
10. Marandas P, Luboinski B, Leridant AM, et al. Functional surgery in cancer of the laryngeal vestibule. Apropos of 149 cases treated at the Institute Gustave-Roussy. Ann Otolaryngol Chir Cervicofac. 1987;104:259.
11. Brierley JD, Gospodarowicz MK, Wittekind C, editors. TNM classification of malignant tumours. 8th ed. Wiley-Blackwell; 2017. ISBN: 978-1-119-26357-9
12. Spriano G, Antognoni P, Piantanida R, Varinelli D, Luraghi R, Cerizza L, Tordiglione M. Conservative management of T1-T2N0 supraglottic cancer: a retrospective study. Am J Otolaryngol. 1997;18:299–305.
13. Lutz CK, Johnson JT, Wagner RL, et al. Supraglottic carcinoma: patterns of recurrence. Ann Otol Rhinol Laryngol. 1990;99:12.
14. Beckhardt RN, Murray JG, Ford CN, et al. Factors influencing functional outcome in supraglottic laryngectomy. Head Neck. 1994;16:232.
15. Bocca E. Supraglottic cancer. Laryngoscope. 1975;85:1318–26.

Open Partial Horizontal Laryngectomy Type II (OPHL 2)

6

Matteo Alicandri-Ciufelli, Alfredo Lo Manto, Matteo Fermi, Benedetta Mattei, Michael Ghirelli, and Francesco Mattioli

6.1 Introduction

Supracricoid partial laryngectomy (SCPL) was conceived in 1950 by Mayer and Rieder in Vienna and then updated by Labayle and Piquet in the early 1970s, thereby favoring its spread throughout France [1–3]. Professor Henri Laccourreye in the 1980s followed by Professors Rizzotto and Succo in 2006 standardized it distinguishing the reconstructive options in either cricohyoidopexy (CHP) or cricohyoidoepiglottopexy (CHEP), depending on whether the epiglottis was preserved or not [4, 5].

Nowadays, it is better to indicate SCPL as OPHL II following the last classification of the European Laryngological Society. This is based on the craniocaudal extent of laryngeal structures resected, instead of several different and heterogeneous variables. This classification identifies three variants:

- OPHL I (formerly defined horizontal supraglottic laryngectomy).
- OPHL II (previously called supracricoid laryngectomy).
- OPHL III (also named supratracheal laryngectomy).

M. Alicandri-Ciufelli (✉) · A. Lo Manto · F. Mattioli
Department of Otorhinolaryngology Head and Neck Surgery, University Hospital of Modena, Modena, Italy
e-mail: matteo.alicandri@unimore.it; francesco.mattioli@unimore.it

M. Fermi
Otorhinolaryngology Head and Neck Surgery, Azienda Ospedaliero Universitaria di Bologna IRCCS, Bologna, Italy

Alma Mater Studiorum, Università di Bologna, Bologna, Italy

M. Ghirelli
ENT Unit, AUSL Romagna, Ospedale Infermi di Rimini, Rimini, Italy

B. Mattei
Department of Medical and Surgical Sciences for Children and Adults, Cranio-Maxillo-Facial Surgery, University of Modena and Reggio Emilia, Modena, Italy

Use of suffixes “a” and “b” in Type II and III OPHLs reflects sparing or not of the suprahyoid epiglottis. Various extensions to one arytenoid, base of tongue, piriform sinus, and cricoarytenoid unit are indicated by abbreviations (Ary, BOT, PIr, and CAU, respectively) [6].

The strength of a partial approach to laryngeal surgery is that it is modular, allowing for a tailored treatment for each single patient, varying the extent of resection as the procedure goes while at the same time preserving disease-free structures. This is possible with removal of the neoplasm, in a step-by-step fashion, with progressive tissue exeresis checked with frozen sections, up to complete removal of the lesion [7].

As for the other approaches to partial laryngectomy, OPHL II is an organ-sparing procedure as it has the aim to preserve the three fundamental functions of the larynx, which are speech, swallowing, and breathing, still guaranteeing oncologically safe resection margins.

OPHL II involves the en bloc removal of the whole thyroid cartilage, both true and false cords, the ventricles, the paraglottic and pre-epiglottic spaces, sparing only the cricoid cartilage, hyoid bone, and at least one functional and mobile arytenoid. The basic principle of conservative laryngeal surgery is in fact the preservation of at least one functional cricoarytenoid unit. Finally, the epiglottis can be removed according to the chosen reconstruction type. The hyoid bone, the posterior lamina of the cricoid cartilage, and either one or both the arytenoid cartilages are always preserved instead.

6.2 Indications

Nowadays, OPHLs represent the first line surgical choice for conservative treatment of locally intermediate and selected advanced stage laryngeal cancers.

As mentioned above, the indication for this surgery is limited to laryngeal tumors in which the cricoid cartilage and at least one functional arytenoid unit can be preserved.

Contraindications are both tumor-related and patient-related. Patients who have, advanced N disease, tumors that

F. Mattioli et al. (eds.), *Atlas of Open Partial Horizontal Laryngectomy*, https://doi.org/10.1007/978-3-031-48023-2_6

extend to the subglottis, involve a fixed cricoarytenoid complex, have posterior commissure involvement, or have through-and-through cartilage involvement are not candidates for OPHL II. Patient-related contraindications are pulmonary compromise, extensive comorbidity, or are at high risk for aspiration [4, 8]. Previous CT-TR for laryngeal squamous cell carcinoma has been considered as absolute contraindications but it has been reported to be a valid option for surgical salvage in selected cases of laryngeal squamous cell carcinoma (LSCC) recurrence after RT.

Indications for OPHL II A:

- T1a–T1b glottic tumors in patients with inadequate laryngeal exposure.
- T2 glottic tumors with impaired vocal cord mobility, limited extension to supraglottis and/or subglottis (sempre sopra il limite superior della cartilagine cricoide).
- Selected T3 and T4a tumors anterior to a frontal plane passing through the vocal process of the arytenoid, perpendicular to the thyroid lamina (magic line) [9].
- Selected recurrences after Transoral Laryngeal Microsurgery (TLM) or after radiation therapy.

Indications for OPHL II B

- Selected T2 supraglottic tumors with invasion of the glottis.
- Selected T3 tumors with paraglottic space or pre-epiglottic space or inner cortex of thyroid cartilage involvement.

Indications for OPHL II + ary

- T3 tumors with involvement of the arytenoid cartilage without posterior paraglottic space or CAU involvement.

6.3 Surgical Steps

6.3.1 Patient Positioning and Surgical Setting

The patient lies on the bed with the head slightly extended. The orotracheal intubation is whenever possible performed, avoiding preoperative tracheostomy. Nasogastric tube is placed before starting surgery and secured to the nose tip.

6.3.2 Skin Incision

The procedure is started with a U-shaped apron incision beginning 2 cm cephalad from the sternum and extending laterally toward the hyoid bone following the sternocleidomastoid muscle. When a concurrent neck dissection is planned, the incision on that side is extended cranially up to the mastoid tip (Figs. 6.1 and 6.2).

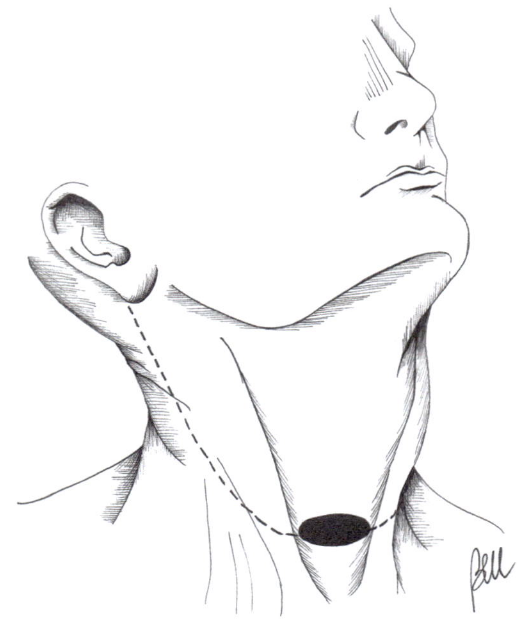

Fig. 6.1 Schematic drawing of the cervical incision encompassing the region for the tracheostomy

6.3.3 Subplatysmal Flap and Laryngotracheal Framework Skeletonization

A subplatysmal flap is raised up to the hyoid bone keeping the external jugular vein and the greater auricular nerve intact. The cranial insertion of the sternohyoid muscle is cut off the hyoid bone. When the tumor involves the anterior commissure and if there is a suspicion of transcartilaginous extension of the tumor (cT4a), it is mandatory to entirely remove the sternohyoid muscle (Fig. 6.3a, b). It represents in such case the anterior radicality margin.

Likewise, the thyrohyoid muscle is excised from the hyoid bone to expose the thyrohyoid membrane.

At the end of the above-mentioned maneuvers, the laryngotracheal framework is skeletonized (Fig. 6.3c, d).

During those steps, it is fundamental to avoid severing the suprahyoid muscle insertion off the hyoid bone, since these muscles are important to preserve the postoperative swallowing function.

6.3.4 Inferior Constrictor Muscle Section and Pyriform Sinus Isolation

The larynx is manually rotated toward the contralateral side to expose the posterior edge of the thyroid cartilage. The inferior pharyngeal constrictor muscle is dissected off the cartilage by means of a monopolar cautery taking utmost care not to injure the underlining pyriform sinus (Fig. 6.4). The inferior horn of the thyroid cartilage should be carefully exposed to prevent injury to the inferior laryngeal nerve.

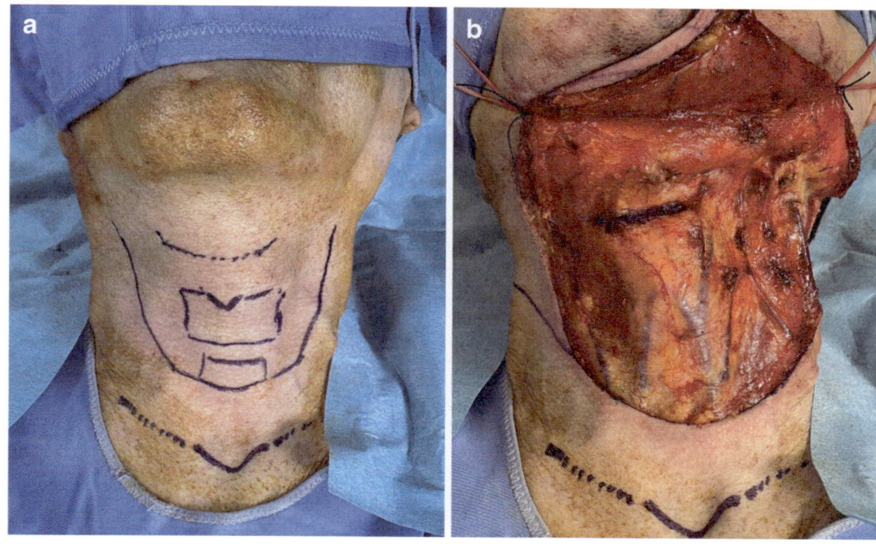

Fig. 6.2 (**a**) Skin incision landmarks. From the top to bottom: hyoid bone, thyroid cartilage, cricoid cartilage, sternal notch, and sterno-clavicular joints. (**b**) Subplatismatic flap with mastoid tip extension on the left

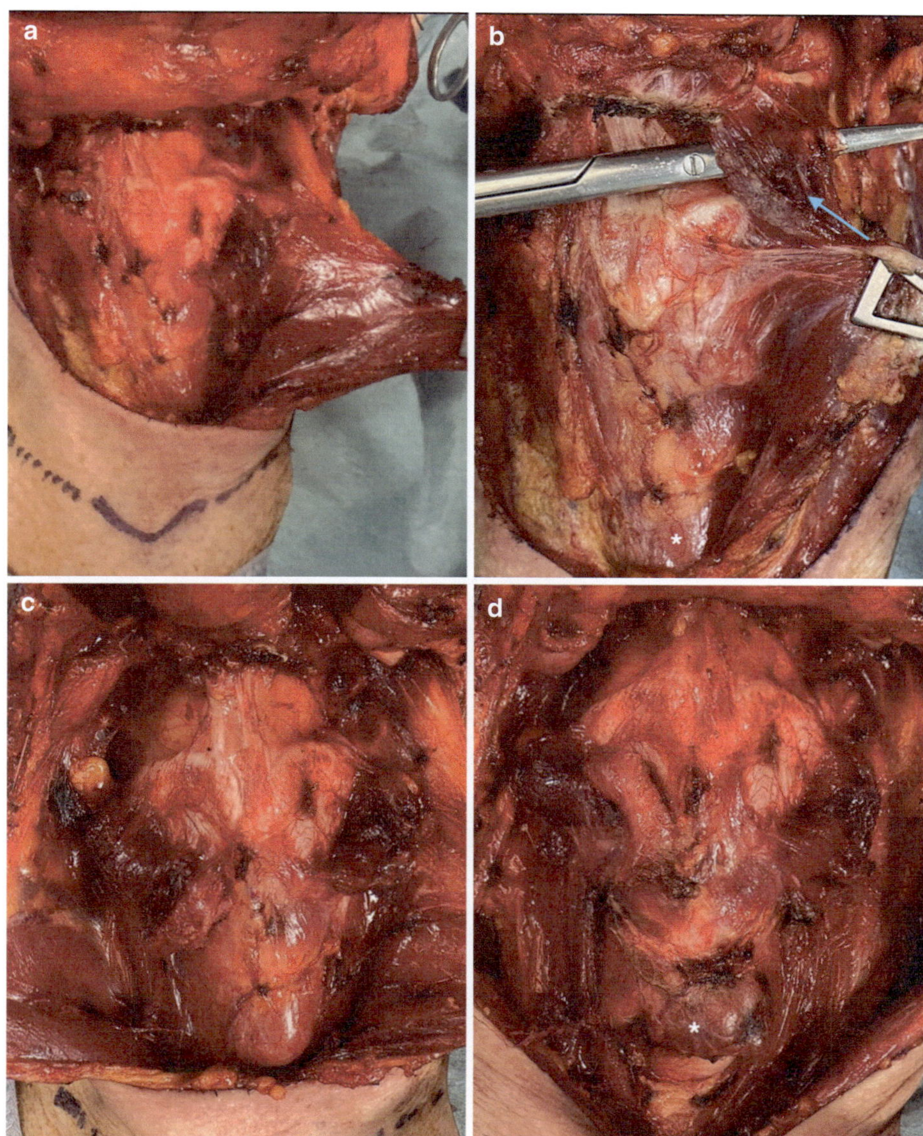

Fig. 6.3 Laryngotracheal framework skeletonization. (**a** and **b**) Detachment of the infrahyoid muscles from the hyoid bone (note how the scissors are positioned for the subsequent cut with a monopolar). (**c**, **d**) Exposure of the laryngotracheal framework. Blue arrows: Thyrohyoid muscle. White asterisk: thyroid gland

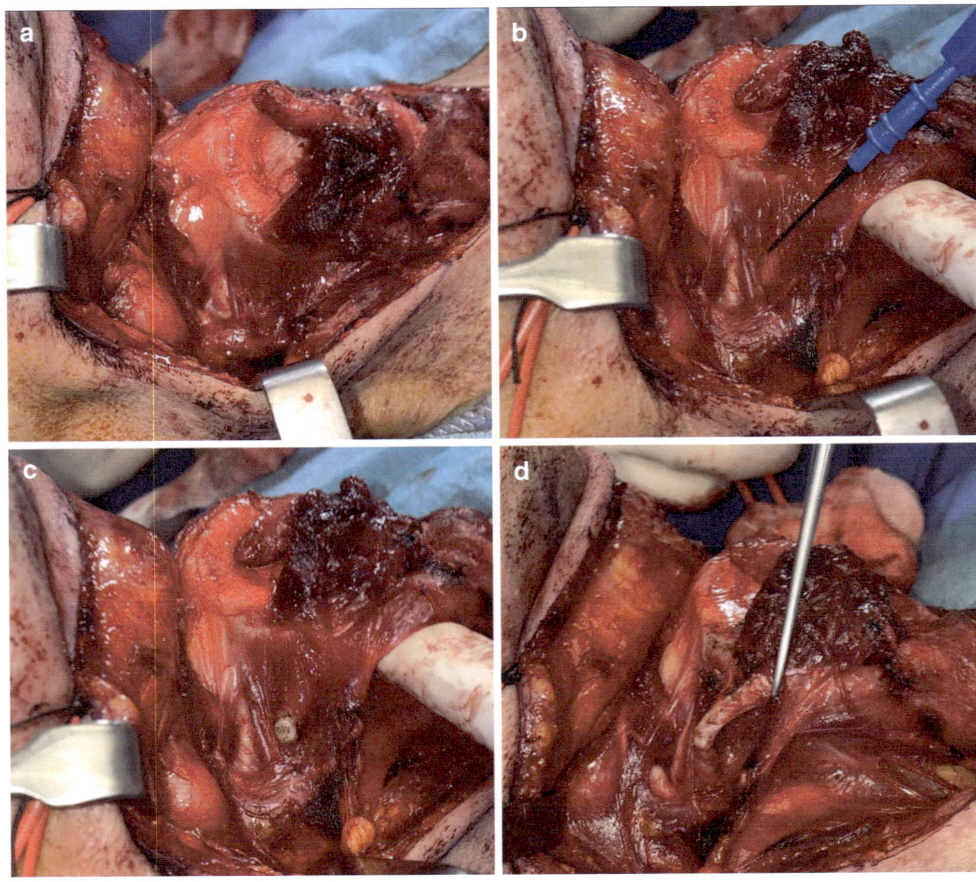

Fig. 6.4 (**a**) Lateral view of the thyroid cartilage. (**b**) Incision of the inferior pharyngeal muscle to better expose the lateral aspect of the thyroid cartilage. (**c**) Identification and incision of the thyro-hyoid ligament. (**d**) Elevation of the superior cornu by means of a hook

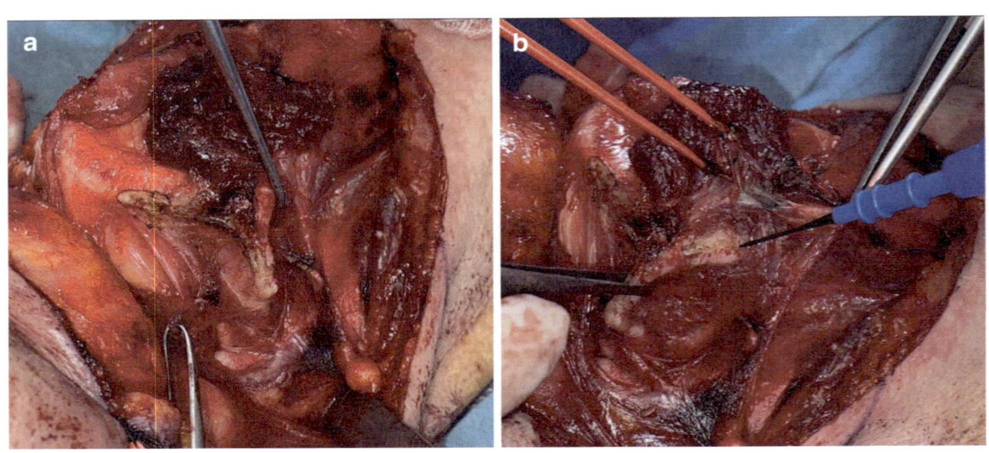

Fig. 6.5 (**a**) A hook is useful to medially tilt the larynx. (**b**) By means of monopolar, the lateral and superior aspect of the thyroid cartilage are dissected

The inner perichondrium of the thyroid cartilage is elevated to achieve a subperichondral detachment of the pyriform sinus from the inner aspect of the thyroid ala by means of a freer elevator or a cottonoid (Figs. 6.5 and 6.6). The same step is performed bilaterally.

6.3.5 Superior Laryngeal Pedicle Ligation and Nerve Identification

The superior laryngeal pedicle is found superolaterally with close relationship with the greater horn of the hyoid bone. Once it is identified, it should be craniocaudally dissected to

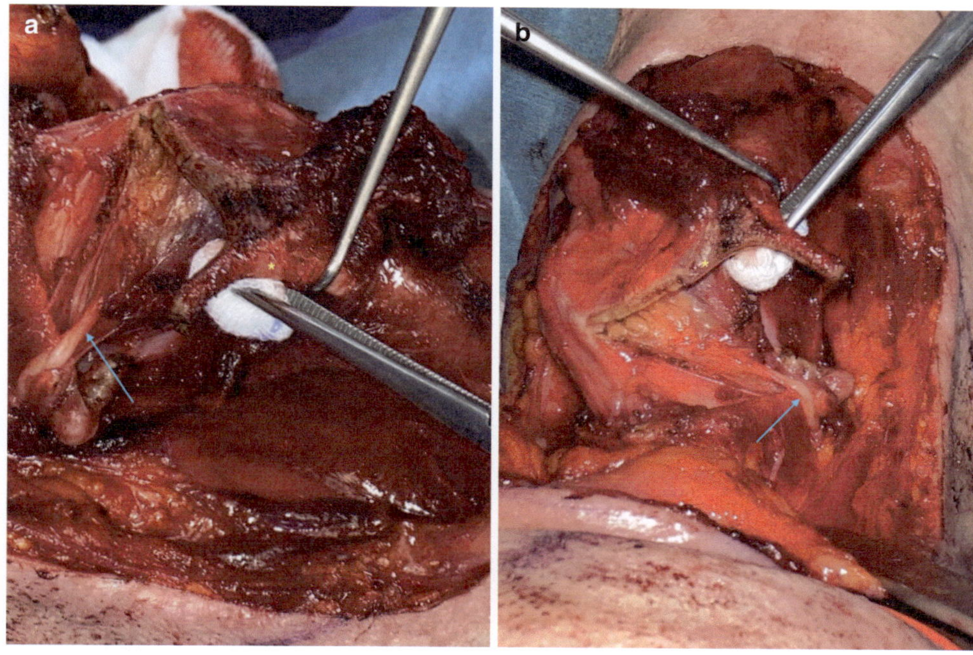

Fig. 6.6 (**a** and **b**) Subperichondrial detachment of the pyriform sinus from the inner aspect of the thyroid ala by means of a cottonoid. Blue arrows: superior laryngeal pedicle. Yellow asterisks: lateral aspect of thyroid cartilage

distinguish the superior laryngeal vascular pedicle (artery and vein) and the superior laryngeal nerve. The vascular pedicle is sectioned and ligated to limit bleeding during further laryngectomy steps. The superior laryngeal nerve is dissected until the lateral ramus of the internal branch which supplies the pyriform sinus is identified to preserve it during further surgical maneuvers (Figs. 6.7 and 6.8).

6.3.6 Inferior Laryngeal Nerve Protection

The inferior laryngeal nerve courses behind the inferior horn of the thyroid cartilage to reach the inferior margin of the cricoid cartilage, where its entry point lies.

Once the inferior horn of the thyroid cartilage is isolated, it can be sectioned by means of mayo scissors to keep it in the surgical field avoiding any damage to the inferior laryngeal nerve, when performing further laryngectomy steps (Figs. 6.9 and 6.10).

6.3.7 Pre-epiglottic Space Dissection (Optional)

The pre-epiglottic space is bounded by the thyrohyoid membrane anteriorly, by the thyroepiglottic ligament that connects with the epiglottis foot caudally, by the collagen fibers stretching from the tongue base to the hyoid bone. Posteriorly, at the level of the hyoid bone, the pre-epiglottic space continues from the lateral margins of the epiglottis toward the aryepiglottic folds and the superior paraglottic spaces, without borders.

The dissection of this space, which is mandatory during OPHL type 1, is optional during OPHL type 2 (Figs. 6.11 and 6.12).

The thyrohyoid membrane is incised in contact with the inner aspect of the hyoid bone to enter the pre-epiglottic space. The pre-epiglottic content is then detached from its upper and posterior attachments until it is dissected up to the epiglottis foot for further en bloc resection with whole specimen.

6.3.8 Pharyngotomy (Figs. 6.13 and 6.14)

6.3.8.1 Transepiglottic Pharyngotomy (OPHL 2A) (Fig. 6.14b)

The transepiglottic pharyngotomy is performed about 1 cm above the superior margin of the thyroid cartilage. This step is started at the midline. The incision should be performed parallel to the superior edge of the thyroid cartilage to preserve an adequate amount of suprahyoid epiglottis for further reconstructive steps. Once the access to the lumen is achieved, the pharyngotomy can be enlarged laterally in order improve the visualization on the endolarynx.

6.3.8.2 Supraepiglottic Pharyngotomy (OPHL 2B) (Fig. 6.14a)

The supraepiglottic pharyngotomy is performed about 1 cm below the inferior margin of the hyoid bone. The incision is started at the midline and should not involve the epiglottis which will be removed en bloc with the whole specimen. Once the access to the lumen is achieved, the pharyngotomy

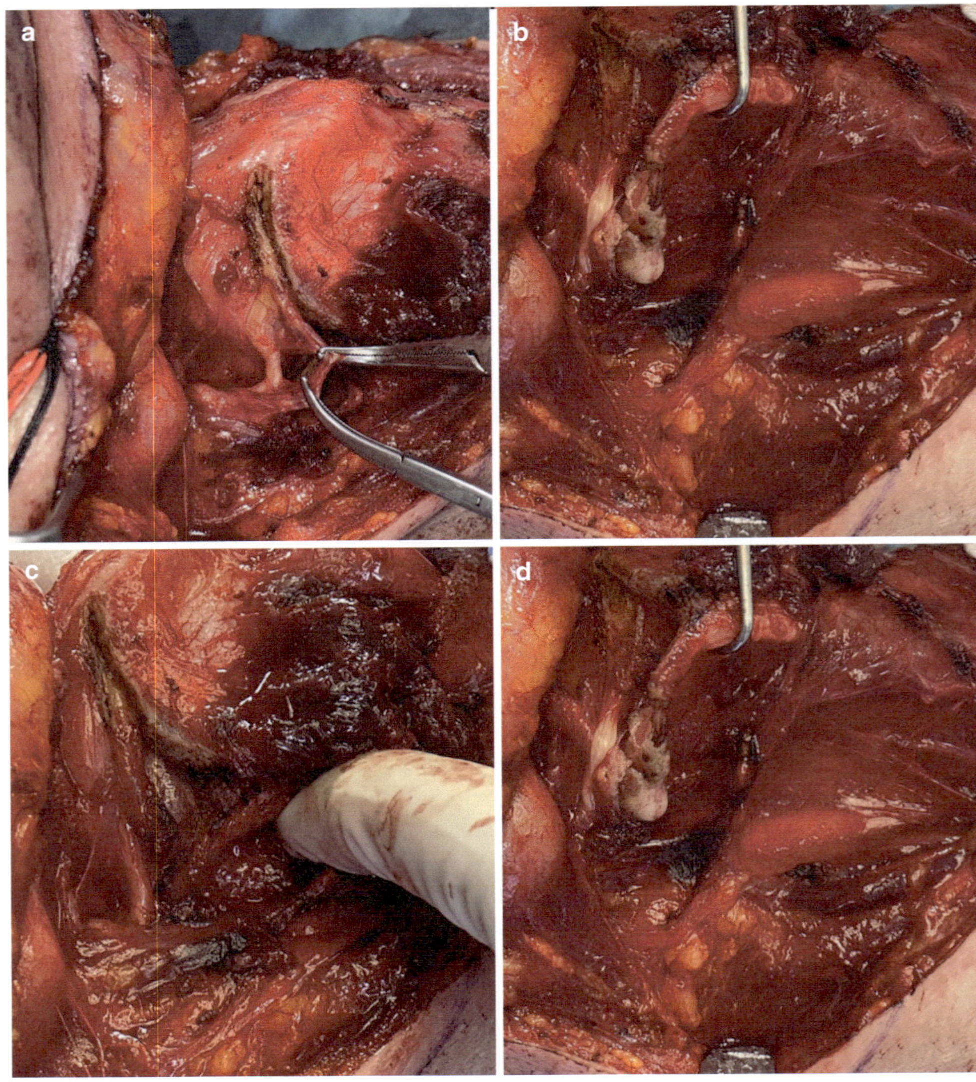

Fig. 6.7 (**a**) Identification of the superior laryngeal neurovascular pedicle. The artery and vein are dissected off the nerve and ligated. (**b**) When the larynx is medially tilted, the superior laryngeal nerve moves away from the superior horn of the thyroid cartilage

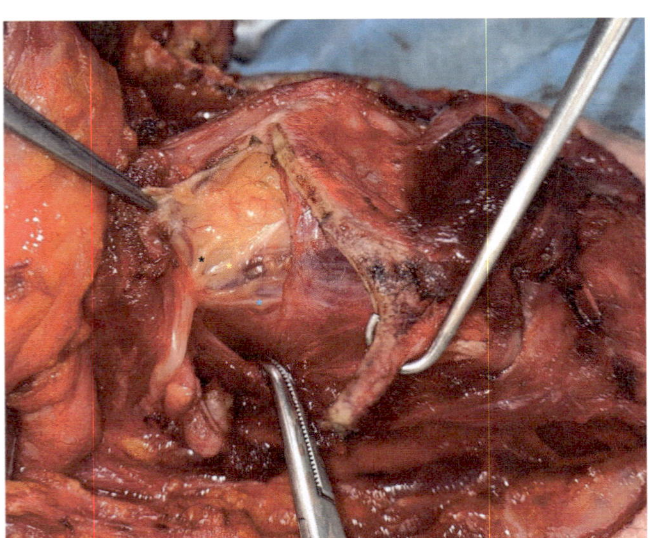

Fig. 6.8 (**a**) Focus on the superior laryngeal nerve at the entrance on the thyrohyoid membrane. *Black asterisk*: epiglottic branch. *Yellow asterisk*: arytenoid branch. *Blue arrow*: branch for the piriform sinus

can be enlarged laterally in order to improve the visualization on the endolarynx.

6.3.9 Cricothyroid Membrane Incision

The cricothyroid muscle can be detached off the anterior aspect of the cricoid ring, to remove it en bloc during the further surgical steps.

A horizontal cricothyroidotomy is performed along the superior border of the cricoid cartilage (Fig. 6.13a).

In case of subglottic extension, it is advisable to perform this step after the following step.

6.3.10 Laryngeal Dissection

The surgeon is now placed at the head of the bed. The incision is started on the unaffected side and extended through

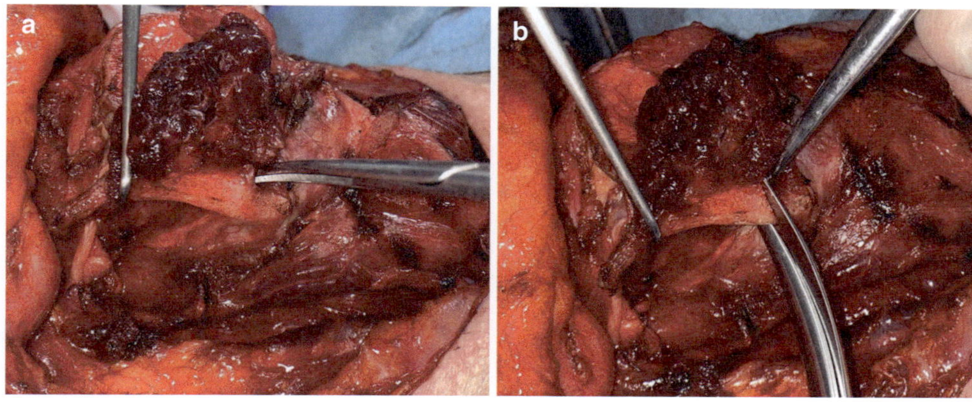

Fig. 6.9 (**a**) Scissors are placed at the angle between the lamina and the inferior horn of the thyroid cartilage. (**b**) The inferior horn is sectioned by means of mayo scissors

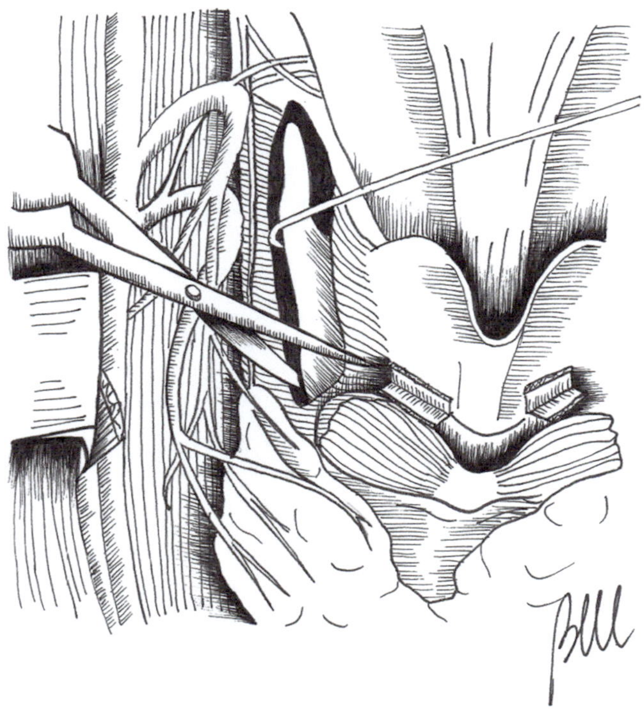

Fig. 6.10 Schematic representation of the inferior thyroid hornu section. Note the direction of the scissors that follow the inferior edge of the thyroid cartilage

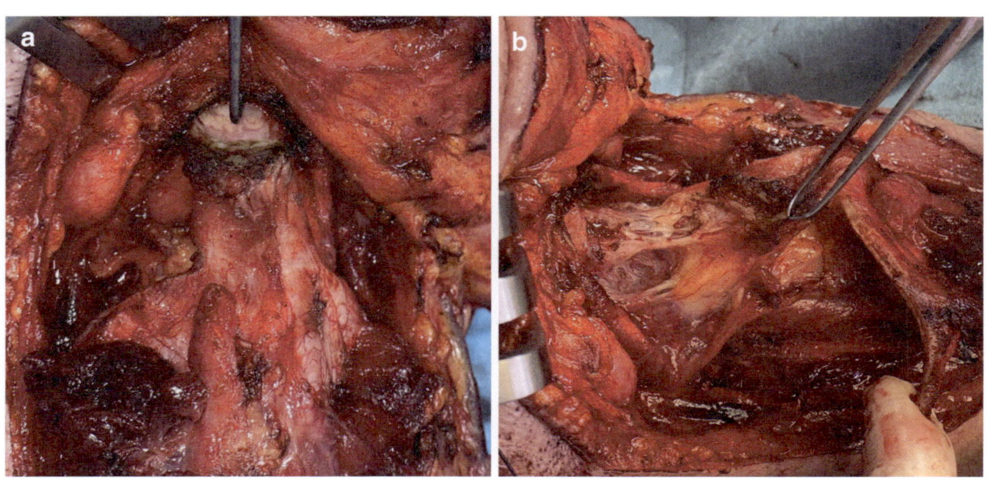

Fig. 6.11 (**a**) Frontal view of the larynx while elevating the hyoid bone by means of a hook to start the dissection of the pre-epiglottic space. (**b**) Lateral view of the larynx while dissecting the pre-epiglottic space. A good dissection plane between the pre-epiglottic space and the outer surface of the valleculae is found pushing down the pre-epiglottic fat by means of surgical forceps

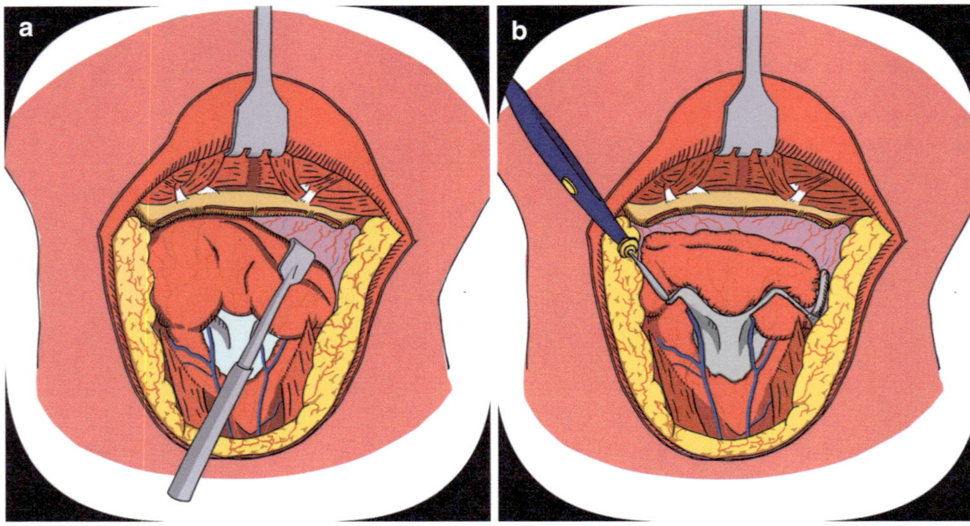

Fig. 6.12 Schematic representation of pre-epiglottic space dissection

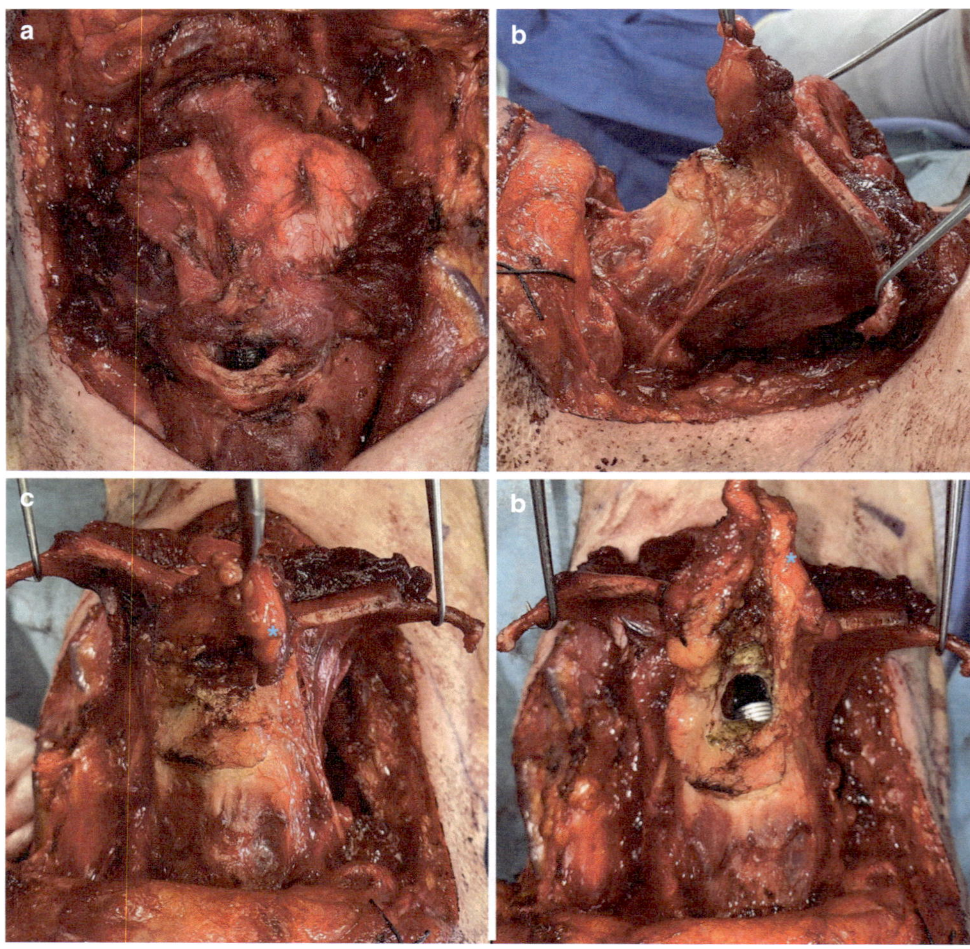

Fig. 6.13 (**a**) Horizontal incision is performed above the superior border of the cricoid cartilage. (**b**) The thyroid cartilage is fractured. (**c**) Cranio-superior view of the larynx. (**d**) Transepiglottic pharyngotomy. *Blue asterisk*: pre-epiglottic space

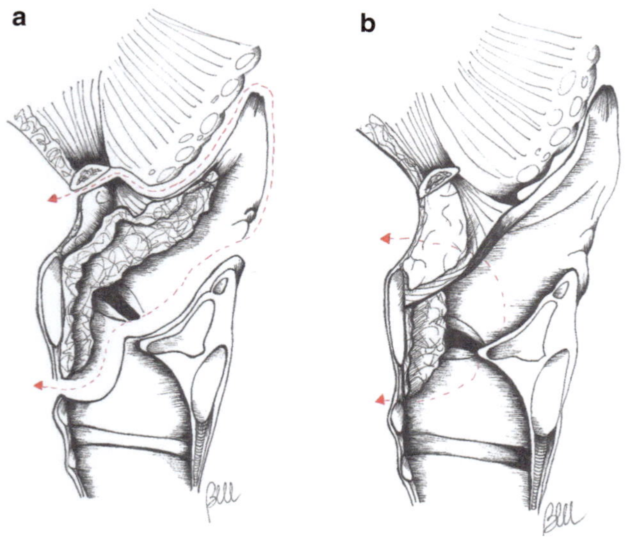

Fig. 6.14 Schematic representation of the superior pharyngotomy. (**a**) Supraepiglottic pharyngotomy. (**b**) Transepiglottic pharyngotomy

the aryepiglottic fold and the false vocal cord pointing the tip of the scissors toward the arytenoid. Then, the true vocal fold is cut off the vocal process of the arytenoid. The vertical incision is now connected to the horizontal cricothyroidotomy along the superior border of the cricoid cartilage.

The same steps are repeated on the affected side achieving a macroscopically safe margin if possible (Fig. 6.15).

6.3.10.1 Arytenoid Resection

When the tumor is in contact or involves the arytenoid, it is required to sacrifice the arytenoid cartilage.

If this is the case, it is important to preserve interarytenoid muscle and posterior arytenoid mucosa, for subsequent pyriform sinus reconstruction (Fig. 6.16).

6.3.11 Pyriform Sinus Reconstruction

A vicryl 3-0 stitch is placed through the anterior edge of the remaining arytenoid mucosa and then tied to the cricoid car-

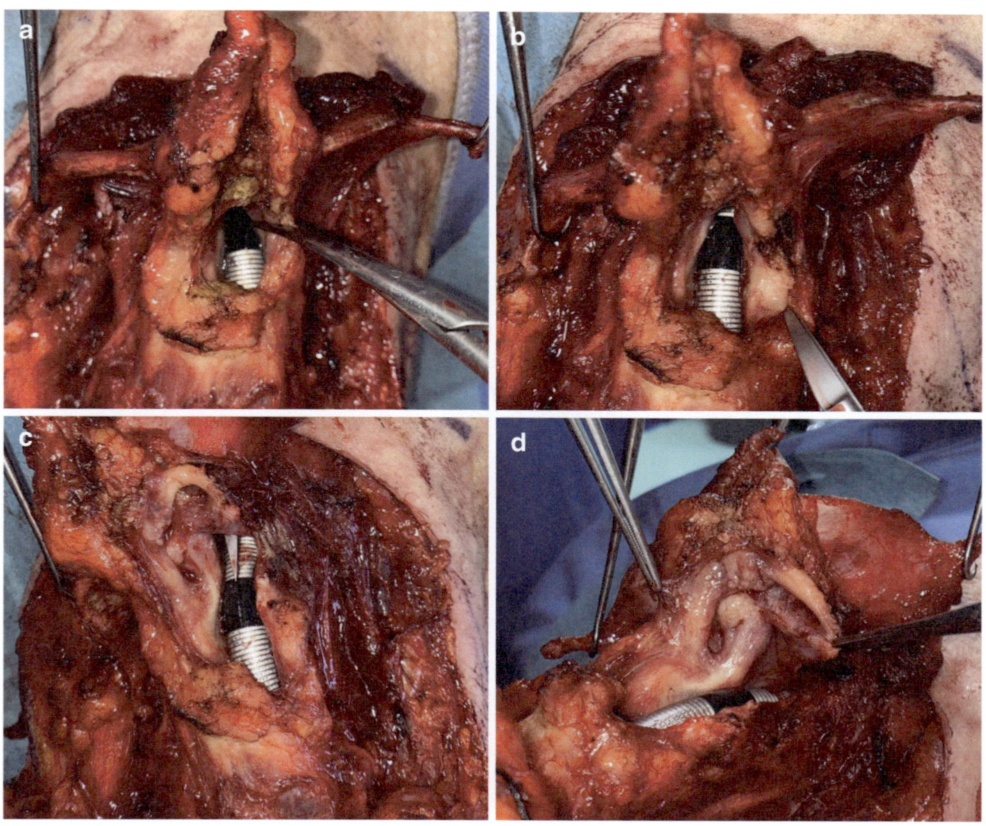

Fig. 6.15 (**a**) The incision is started on the unaffected side and extended through the aryepiglottic fold and the false vocal cord pointing the tip of the scissors toward and anteriorly the vocal process of the arytenoid. (**b**) Focus on the vocal process of the arytenoid on the unaffected side. (**c**) The lateral cut is continued to reach the inferior opening on the crico-thyroid membrane (scissors are introduced to guide the cut inferiorly). (**d**) When the larynx is opened on the unaffected side, a direct view of the tumor is achieved

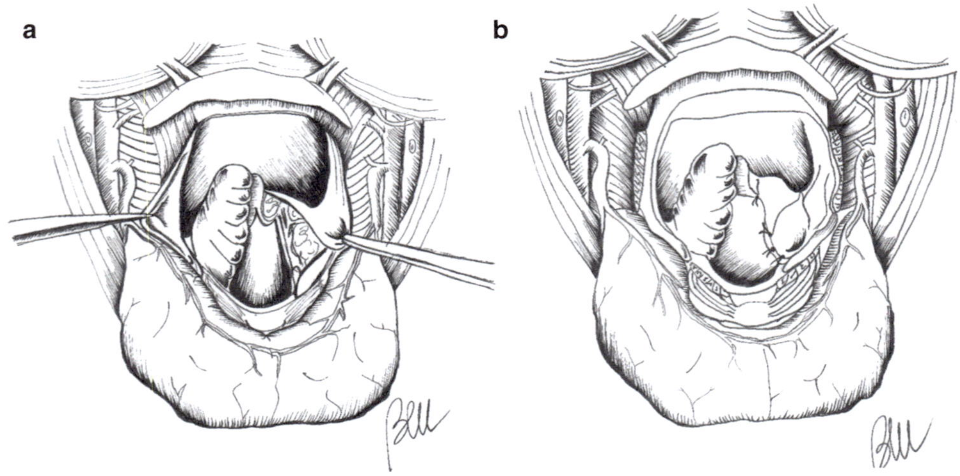

Fig. 6.16 Schematic drawing. (**a**) The left arytenoid has been resected leaving the mucosa of the anterior aspect of the pyriform sinus without any support. (**b**) Pyriform sinus reconstruction suturing the pyriform mucosal flap with the mucosa of the left subglottis

tilage with the aim to enlarge the pyriform sinus opening (Fig. 6.16).

6.3.12 Pexy

6.3.12.1 Crico—Hyoido—Epiglottopexy (OPHL 2A)

For the crico-hyoido-epiglottopexy, the remaining portion of the epiglottis as well as the hyoid bone is impacted to the cricoid cartilage by means of three (or more) PDS 1 stitches. The stiches are passed inferior to superior, submucosally around the cricoid ring and then to the epiglottis and around the hyoid bone.

The epiglottis is transfixed by the stitches about 5 mm above the inferior edge to avoid retroflexion of the cartilage that may determine further neoglottis stenosis.

The 1–2 central stitches are passed around the hyoid bone encompassing at least 1 cm of the base of the tongue to impact it to the hyoid bone and then to the pexy.

The lateral stitches are passed around and in close contact with the hyoid bone and, by doing this, preventing possible injuries to lingual arteries and hypoglossal nerves.

The two central stiches are tightened at the same time taking utmost care to ensure proper cricohyoid alignment. Lastly, the lateral stitches are closed.

6.3.12.2 Cricohyoidopexy (OPHL 2B)

For the cricohyoidopexy, the hyoid bone is impacted to the cricoid cartilage by means of three (or more) PDS 1 stitches. The stiches are passed inferior to superior, submucosally around the cricoid ring and then around the hyoid bone.

The 1–2 central stitches are passed around the hyoid bone encompassing at least 1 cm of the base of the tongue to impact it to the hyoid bone and then to the pexy.

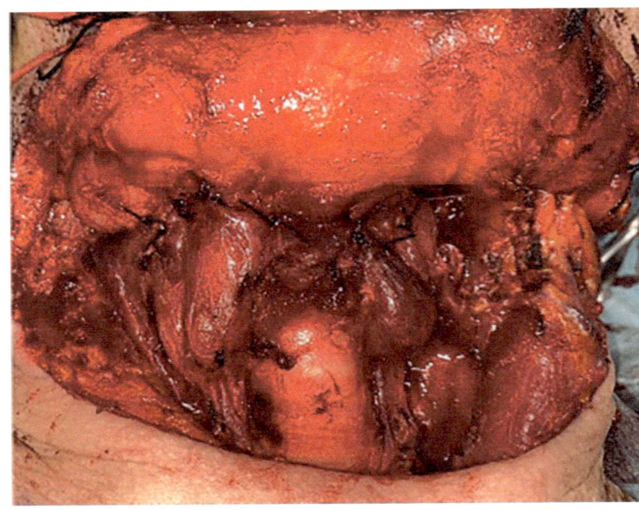

Fig. 6.17 The Crico-hyoido-epiglottopexy is complete. Thyroid gland is used to protect the line of the pexy

The lateral stitches are passed around and in close contact with the hyoid bone and, by doing this, preventing possible injuries to lingual arteries and hypoglossal nerves.

The two central stiches are tightened at the same time taking utmost care to ensure proper cricohyoid alignment. Lastly, the lateral stitches are closed.

6.3.13 Sternohyoid Muscle/Thyroid Gland Transposition

If available, the sternohyoid muscle can be sutured to the suprahyoid muscles in order to protect the pexy. Similarly inferior constrictor muscles can be sutured to the lateral edges of the sternohyoid muscle. This latter maneuver restores the physiologic position of the constrictor muscles, which is useful to restore the swallowing function (Fig. 6.17).

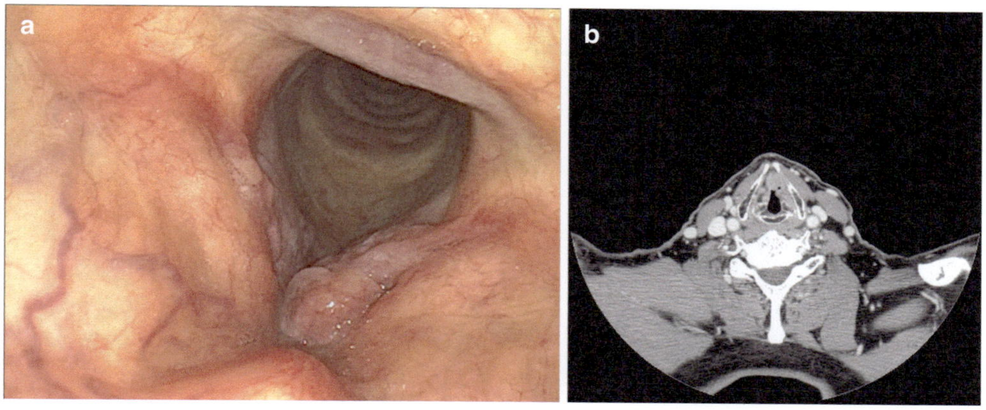

Fig. 6.18 Case example 1. (**a**) Fiberoptic endoscopic laryngeal. Red lesion with irregular surface of the two third of both vocal folds and the anterior commissure. The left vocal fold mobility was impaired while the arytenoid one was not. (**b**) CT scan with contrast showing a thickened left vocal fold with intense contrast enhancement involving the anterior commissure and the anterior two-thirds of the right vocal fold. The left paraglottic space seems to be interested

6.3.14 Tracheostomy

Prior to closure of skin flaps, the tracheostomy must be performed. The placement of skin incision for the tracheostomy tube is variable based on anatomy and surgeon's preference. Some surgeons prefer to place the tracheostomy through the midline of neck incision, and others prefer to create a separate midline incision in between the sternal notch and the neck incision. This latter option may reduce microbial contamination from the tracheostomy tube to the pexy site.

6.3.15 Skin Closure

A JP drainage is placed to prevent postoperative hematoma, especially in case of lateral neck dissection.

The platysma is reapproximated followed by careful closure of the skin.

6.4 Case Example 1 (Fig. 6.18)

A 67-year-old man with a long history of tobacco smoking was admitted in the ENT department complaining of progressive hoarseness, which started about 4 months earlier. The fiberoptic endoscopic laryngeal examination showed a red lesion with irregular surface of the two third of both vocal folds and the anterior commissure. The left vocal fold mobility was impaired while the arytenoid one was not. The right-side laryngeal mobility was not impaired as well. Physical examination did not reveal any enlarged cervical lymph node. Contrast-enhanced CT scan showed a thickened left vocal fold with intense contrast enhancement involving the anterior commissure and the anterior two-thirds of the right vocal fold. The left anterior paraglottic space seemed to be interested by the lesion and the radiologist suspected thyroid cartilage infiltration. No pathological lymph nodes were detected. A diagnosis of undifferentiated (G3) squamous cell carcinoma (SCC) was obtained with transoral microscopic biopsy. Clinical staging was T3 N0 M0.

An OPHL type II A was performed with bilateral elective neck dissection (II–IV). The histological diagnosis confirmed the diagnosis of SCC G3 involving the mucosa, the vocal muscle, the paraglottic space of the left vocal cord while the right vocal cord was interested up to the submucosal space. The inner cortex of the thyroid cartilage was infiltrated on this side and at the level of the anterior commissure. No pathological lymph nodes were found. Pathological staging was pT3 pN0 cM0. The patient was hospitalized for 16 days. After 7 days of nasogastric tube feeding and logopedic rehabilitation oral diet and speech were restored, the patient was discharged when autonomy in feeding was reached.

6.4.1 Case 2 (Fig. 6.19)

A 55-year-old man with a long-standing history of tobacco smoking and alcohol abuse presented to our clinic with a 2-month history of hoarseness and odynophagia starting one month before. Careful physical examination of the neck revealed a right level III palpable lymph node. A fiberoptic laryngeal evaluation was then performed revealing a pale lesion involving the entire right vocal cord from the arytenoid to the anterior commissure and the ipsilateral false fold. Both arytenoid and vocal fold's mobilities were impaired. The left side of the larynx was not affected. Contrast-enhanced CT scan showed a supraglottic mass extending

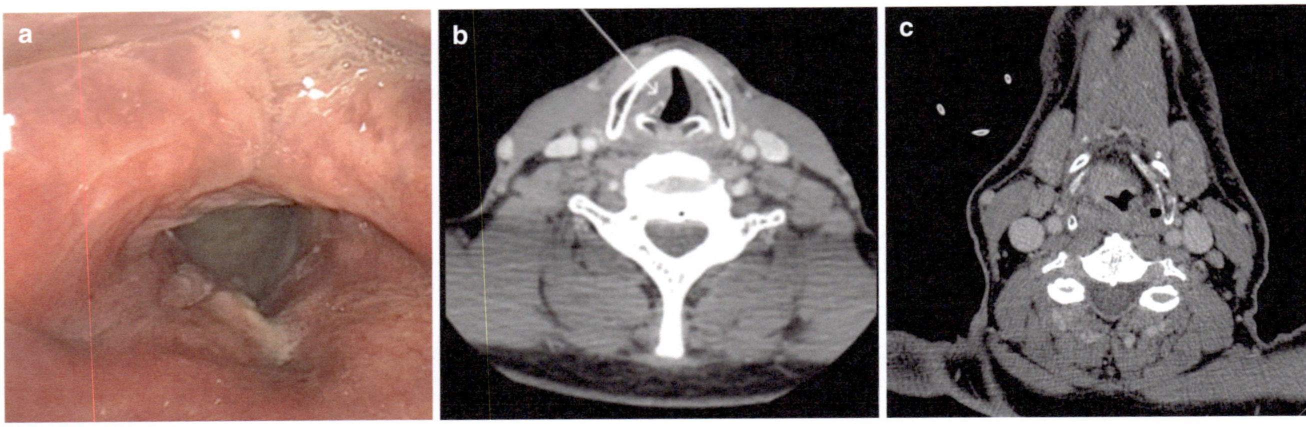

Fig. 6.19 Case example 2. (**a**) The fiberoptic laryngeal evaluation reveals a pale lesion involving the entire right vocal cord from the arytenoid to the anterior commissure and the ipsilateral false fold. Both arytenoid and vocal fold's mobility was impaired. (**b** and **c**) Supraglottic mass extending from the infrahyoid epiglottis and the right false vocal fold to the glottic plane, involving all the right vocal fold from the anterior commissure to the arytenoid and occupying the ipsilateral anterior and posterior paraglottic spaces

from the infrahyoid epiglottis and the right false vocal fold to the glottic plane, involving all the right vocal fold from the anterior commissure to the arytenoid and occupying the ipsilateral anterior and posterior paraglottic spaces. CT scan also confirmed the presence of a right cervical level III lymphadenopathy. Histological examination of the laryngeal lesion revealed a squamous cell carcinoma (SCC) of undifferentiated (G3) type. According to clinical and radiologic findings, the malignancy was staged as cT3 cN1 M0.

The patient underwent OPHL II B extended to the right arytenoid and bilateral neck dissection (II–IV). Histological examination of the surgical specimen confirmed the diagnosis of SCC G3 involving the mucosa of the right false and true vocal fold, the right laryngeal vestibule and the pre-epiglottic space. The right vocal muscle, paraglottic space, and arytenoid were involved as well. Only one pathological lymph node was found at right cervical level III. Pathological stage was T3 N1 cM0. The patient was hospitalized for a total of 14 days. After 8 days of nasogastric tube feeding and logopedic rehabilitation, oral diet and speech were restored. The patient was discharged when autonomy in feeding was reached.

6.5 Complications

Apart from the typical complications of any surgical procedure, such as wound infection, postoperative bleeding, and hematoma, there are specific complications for this type of surgery. The most important is certainly the pexy's rupture.

Dysphagia is the most frequently reported symptom and typically it is experienced between the seventh and the eighth postoperative day. When detachment of the pexy occurs, the residual portion of the larynx cannot move upwards and allow satisfactory swallowing for the patient, facilitating aspiration pneumonia.

When a rupture of the pexy is suspected, instrumental tests should be performed to confirm clinical suspicions.

FEES (functional endoscopic evaluation of swallowing) identifies the incorrect passage of the bolus in the digestive tract: if a rupture of the pexy is present, bolus penetrates the respiratory tract.

Laryngeal aspiration can be detected by a videofluorographic swallowing study (VFSS). This permits the visualization of bolus flow in real time in relation to structural movement throughout the upper aerodigestive tract and detection of the presence and timing of aspiration.

All these exams are useful options if a problem with the pexy is suspected but a CT scan is mandatory to have the final diagnosis. The CT scan (with 3D reconstructions) allows to confirm the suspicion if there is a gap of more than 3 cm between the lower border of the hyoid bone and the cricoid cartilage.

Sometimes the rupture of the pexy is not complete and a wait-and-see attitude can be undertaken if the patient has good neoglottic sensitivity and aspirations are not present.

Treatment is usually performed by revision surgery of the pexy line or by a laryngeal injection of Vox® Implants. In the revision surgery, the patient undergoes a second operation in which the region of the pexy is identified and a re-suturing of the pexy is performed. Sometimes, it is useful to administer a laryngeal injection of Vox® Implants when it is necessary to provide greater competence to the neoglottis. Only rarely is it necessary to perform a total laryngectomy [10].

Tips and Tricks

- Early identification of the superior laryngeal nerve is recommended to avoid its damage when sectioning the thyrohyoid ligament. In fact, it rarely crosses the big horn of the thyroid cartilage or the caudal part of the thyrohyoid ligament.

- Subperichondral dissection of pyriform sinus mucosa is recommended to prevent tearing it. Electrocautery can be used to detect the internal perichondrium at the posterior edge of the thyroid cartilage.
- The inferior horn of the thyroid cartilage should be sectioned to protect the recurrent laryngeal nerve close to its entry point. It is important to check the position of the scissors that should be parallel to the inferior limit of the thyroid laminae.
- The pexy can be additionally sealed by placing infrahyoid muscles (if preserved) onto it. Infrahyoid muscles should be sutured to the hyoid periosteum and the suprahyoid muscles.

References

1. Majer EH, Rieder W. Technic of laryngectomy permitting the conservation of respiratory permeability (cricohyoidopexy). Ann Otolaryngol. 1959;76:677–81.
2. Piquet JJ, Desaulty A, Decroix G. Crico-hyoido-epiglotto-pexy. Surgical technic and functional results. Ann Oto-Laryngol Chir Cervico Faciale Bull Soc Oto-Laryngol Hopitaux Paris. 1974;91(12):681–6.
3. Labayle J, Bismuth R. Total laryngectomy with reconstitution. Ann Oto-Laryngol Chir Cervico Faciale Bull Soc Oto-Laryngol Hopitaux Paris. 1971;88(4):219–28.
4. Laccourreye H, Laccourreye O, Weinstein G, Menard M, Brasnu D. Supracricoid laryngectomy with cricohyoidoepiglottopexy: a partial laryngeal procedure for glottic carcinoma. Ann Otol Rhinol Laryngol. 1990;99(6 Pt 1):421–6. https://doi.org/10.1177/000348949009900601.
5. Rizzotto G, Succo G, Lucioni M, Pazzaia T. Subtotal laryngectomy with tracheohyoidopexy: a possible alternative to total laryngectomy. Laryngoscope. 2006;116(10):1907–17. https://doi.org/10.1097/01.mlg.0000236085.85790.d5.
6. Succo G, Peretti G, Piazza C, et al. Open partial horizontal laryngectomies: a proposal for classification by the working committee on nomenclature of the European Laryngological Society. Eur Arch Otorrinolaringol. 2014;271(9):2489–96.
7. Bertolin A, Lionello M, Ghizzo M, et al. Modular approach in OPHL: are there preoperative predictors? Acta Otorhinolaryngol Ital. 2020;40(5):352–9.
8. Steuer CE, El-Deiry M, Parks JR, Higgins KA, Saba NF. An update on larynx cancer. CA Cancer J Clin. 2017;67(1):20.
9. Del Bon F, Piazza C, Lancini D, et al. Open partial horizontal laryngectomies for T3–T4 laryngeal cancer: prognostic impact of anterior vs. posterior laryngeal compartmentalization. Cancers. 2019;11(3):289. https://doi.org/10.3390/cancers11030289.
10. Ruberto M, Alicandri-Ciufelli M, Grammatica A, Marchioni D, Bergamini G, Presutti L. Partial laryngectomies: when the problem is the pexy. Acta Otorhinolaryngol Ital. 2014;34(4):247–52.

7 Open Partial Horizontal Laryngectomy Type III (OPHL 3)

Andy Bertolin, Benedetta Mattei, Alessandro Rosti, Erika Crosetti, and Marco Lionello

7.1 Introduction

In 1972, Serafini firstly described the supratracheal laryngectomy [1]. That procedure consisted of a subtotal laryngectomy with the preservation of the suprahyoid epiglottis and a pexy between the hyoid bone, the residual epiglottis, and the first tracheal ring (tracheo-hyoid-epiglottopexy, TIEP). Because of the removal of both arytenoids, the functional outcomes of this procedure were dismal, and the technique was early abandoned. Laccourreye et al. in 1996 described a modification of the conventional supracricoid partial laryngectomy, to remove the cricoid ring in case of anterior glottic-subglottic tumors [2]. Subsequently, in 2006, Rizzotto et al. refined and standardized this technique [3], pointing out that the functional success of the procedure was related to the preservation of at least one functional cricoarytenoid unit (CAU), represented by half of the cricoid plate with the corresponding arytenoid and cricoarytenoid joint, and the ipsilateral innervation provided by the inferior laryngeal nerve.

A. Bertolin
ENT Department Laryngeal Cancer Centre, Ospedale Civile di Vittorio Veneto, Vittorio Veneto, Italy

B. Mattei
Department of Medical and Surgical Sciences for Children and Adults, Cranio-Maxillo-Facial Surgery, University of Modena and Reggio Emilia, Modena, Italy

A. Rosti
Otorhinolaryngology Head and Neck Surgery, Azienda Ospedaliero Universitaria di Bologna IRCCS, Bologna, Italy

Alma Mater Studiorum—Università di Bologna, Bologna, Italy

E. Crosetti
ENT Department Head and Neck Cancer Unit, San Giovanni Bosco Hospital, Torino, Italy

M. Lionello (✉)
Otorhinolaryngology Unit, Ospedale Civile di Vittorio Veneto, Vittorio Veneto, Italy
e-mail: marco.lionello@aulss2.veneto.it

In 2014, Succo et al. proposed the current classification of the European Laryngological Society for open partial horizontal laryngectomies (OPHLs) based on the craniocaudal extent of laryngeal resection, defining three types: supraglottic laryngectomy (type I), supracricoid laryngectomy (type II), and supratracheal laryngectomy (type III) [4]. The classification foresees to specify the removed structure (i.e., OPHL III + right CAU = supratracheal laryngectomy with the sacrifice of the right cricoarytenoid unit).

One of the peculiarities of OPHLs is the possibility of intraoperatively modulating the procedure. According to the "modular" principle, the patients with glottic LSCC could be initially approached with supracricoid resection; the procedure could intraoperatively change to supratracheal laryngectomy, according to the macroscopic extension of the tumor and microscopic findings at frozen sections (positive or negative status of mucosal margins), with a progressive widening of the resection, sparing at least one cricoarytenoid unit [5].

The OPHL III may be considered a subtotal laryngectomy and could be considered for the treatment of selected intermediate-to-advanced laryngeal cancers with subglottic extension and/or for tumors with posterior extension through the thyro-cricoarytenoid space (TCAS) [6].

7.2 Indications

1. Anterior/lateral glottic-subglottic cT2 tumors spreading closed to the cricoid ring
2. Glottic-subglottic cT3 tumors spreading within the paraglottic space between the conus elasticus and, laterally, the perichondrium of the thyroid cartilage. Typical clinical features are fixed vocal cord, fixed arytenoid, and subglottic swelling
3. Transglottic cT3 tumors spreading superiorly in the superior paraglottic space and inferiorly toward the subglottic area. In these cases, the vocal cord and arytenoid are both fixed.
4. Selected anterior cT4a tumors with limited extra laryngeal extension.

F. Mattioli et al. (eds.), *Atlas of Open Partial Horizontal Laryngectomy*, https://doi.org/10.1007/978-3-031-48023-2_7

7.3 Contraindications

1. Supraglottic T4a tumors reaching the base of the tongue or invading the hyoid bone
2. Glottic-subglottic T3 tumors with posterior commissure involvement, involvement of both the arytenoids, massive invasion of the paraglottic space reaching the posterior cricoarytenoid muscle, and the piriform sinus submucosa
3. Glottic-subglottic T4a tumors with massive cricoid invasion or involvement of the retrocricoid area or reaching the first tracheal ring
4. N3 lymph node metastases

General patient-related contraindications include alcohol and drug abuse or major comorbidities such as heart failure, lung diseases, diabetes mellitus, or severe neurocognitive decline (low-performance status).

7.4 Surgical Technique

The patient is supine, with the neck placed in slight extension using a shoulder roll. The Andrè's incision of the skin is chosen when a neck dissection was scheduled, in order to obtain a U-shaped apron flap (Figs. 7.1 and 7.2a).

The flap is arisen at least 2–3 cm above the hyoid bone (Fig. 7.2b). The infrahyoid muscles are routinely removed, together with the central compartment lymphatics from the hyoid bone to the thyroid isthmus, including the Delphian lymph nodes. For patients with subglottic extension, an ipsilateral paratracheal neck dissection (PTND) should be performed, given the high rate of occult metastasis in level VI. The thyroid gland is isolated, and the anterior wall of the trachea is dissected, to facilitate the subsequent tracheohyoidopexy. The larynx is rotated exposing the constrictor muscles and the superior laryngeal pedicle that is left above the superior cornu of the thyroid cartilage. The inferior pharyngeal constrictors are then incised along the lateral edge of the thyroid cartilage (Fig. 7.3).

The thyrohyoid ligament is sectioned with a scissor closed to the superior thyroid horn, while rotating the larynx, to avoid any injury of the superior laryngeal pedicle (Fig. 7.4). The superior laryngeal pedicle can be also identified before sectioning the thyrohyoid ligament. The vascular pedicle can be ligated, and the superior laryngeal nerve must be preserved (Fig. 7.5).

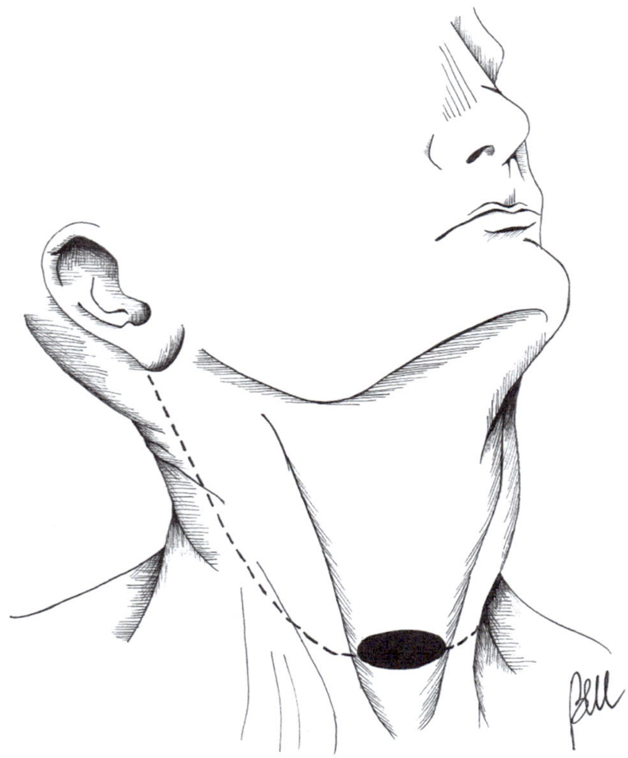

Fig. 7.1 Bimastoid cervical incision with temporary tracheotomy included (Paul-Andrè incision)

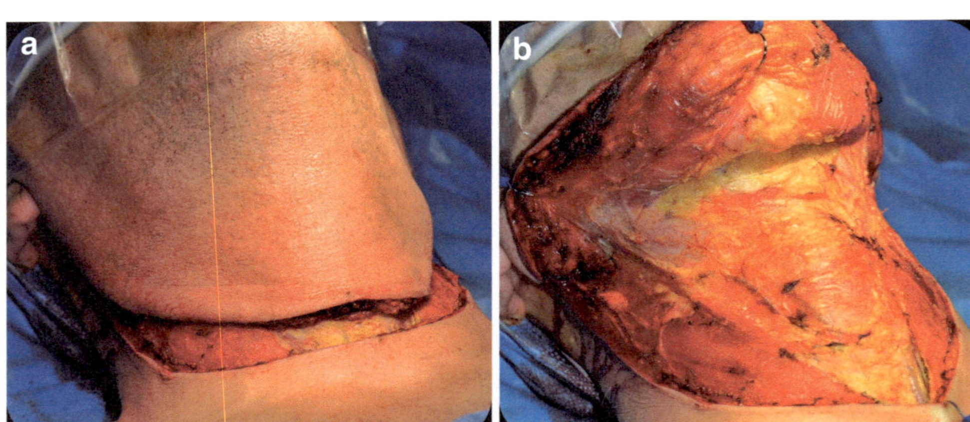

Fig. 7.2 (**a**) Paul-Andre's cutaneous incision. (**b**) Subplatismatic flap elevation until 2–3 cm above the hyoid bone

A blunt subperichondrial bilateral release of the pyriform sinus and paraglottic spaces from the thyroid cartilage is carried out (Fig. 7.6).

On the side of the cricoarytenoid unit to be spared, the inferior cornu of the thyroid cartilage is sectioned to spare the underlying recurrent laryngeal nerve (Fig. 7.7).

The inferior access to the airway is between the cricoid and the first tracheal ring, allowing to check the distance from the tumor (Fig. 7.8).

Superiorly, a horizontal incision is carried out below the hyoid bone, tangential to the superior border of the thyroid cartilage (Fig. 7.9).

In the case of glottic-subglottic tumors, the pre-epiglottic space is partially removed and a transepiglottic laryngotomy is performed, preserving the suprahyoid portion of the epiglottis (OPHL type IIIa) (Fig. 7.10a). In the case of anterior transglottic tumors with higher cranial extension, the epiglottis can be completely removed, with en bloc removal of the pre-epiglottic space (OPHL type IIIb) (Fig. 7.10b).

The dissection proceeds on the side not involved or less involved by the tumor, through the aryepiglottic fold, the false vocal cord (just anterior to the body of the arytenoid cartilage), the thyroarytenoid muscle (anterior to the vocal process of the arytenoid), and the conus elasticus, including the lateral cricoarytenoid muscle (Fig. 7.11).

On this side, the CAU is spared, taking care to preserve the superior laryngeal nerves by following the lateral edges of the

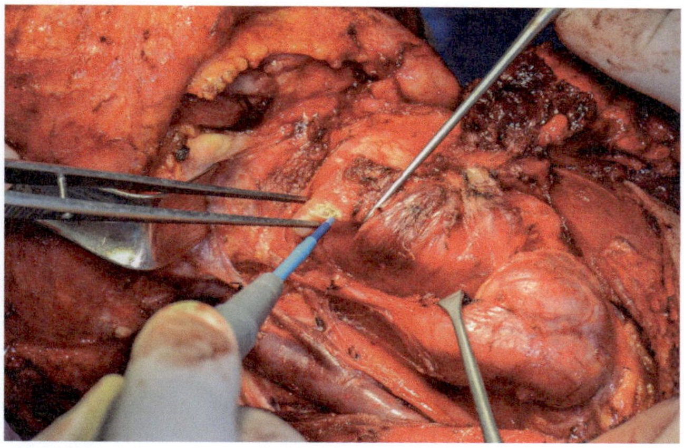

Fig. 7.3 Right side. Inferior pharyngeal constrictor detachment from lateral edge of thyroid cartilage, starting from superior horn. Please note the rotation and anteriorization of laryngotracheal framework to displace the superior laryngeal pedicle over the cartilaginous structure

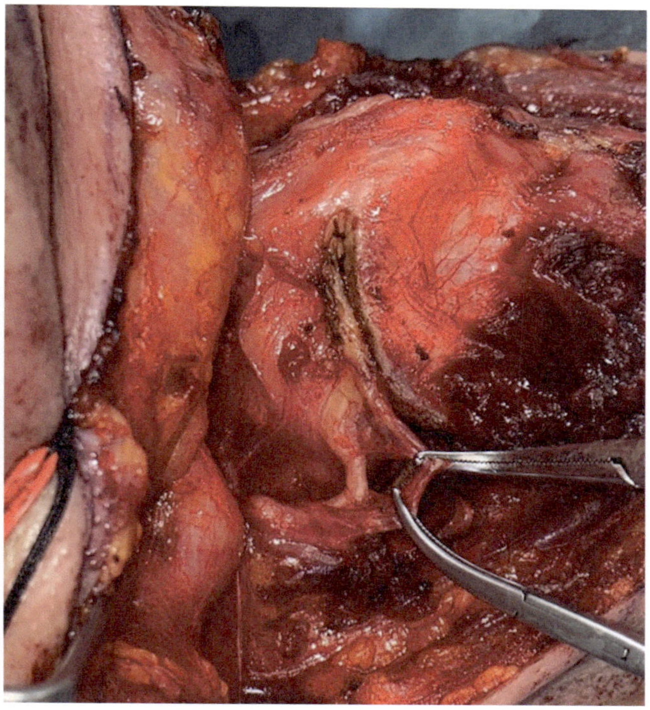

Fig. 7.5 Right side. Superior laryngeal vascular pedicle ligation and section. Notice the relationship between the vascular pedicle and the superior laryngeal nerve lying medially

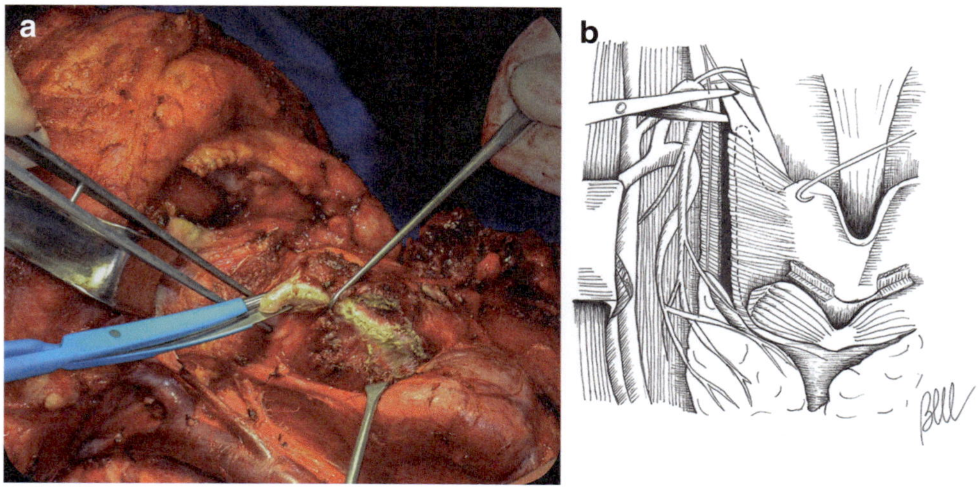

Fig. 7.4 Right side. (**a**) Thyro-hyoid ligament section. Keep in mind the cutting line parallel to the superior horn of the thyroid cartilage to prevent any damage to the superior laryngeal pedicle. (**b**) Schematic drawing showing the transection of the thyro-hyoid ligament

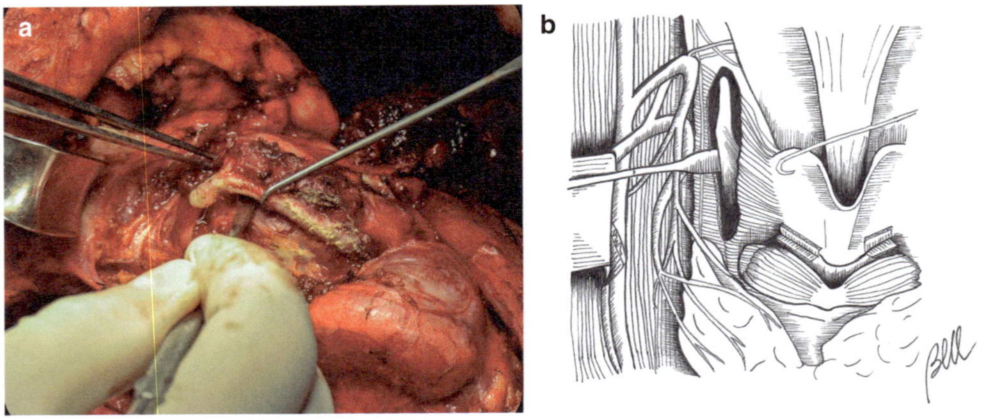

Fig. 7.6 Right side. (**a**) Blunt subperichondrial dissection of pyriform sinus and paraglottic space from internal lamina of the thyroid cartilage. (**b**) Schematic drawing of the blunt subperichondrial dissection

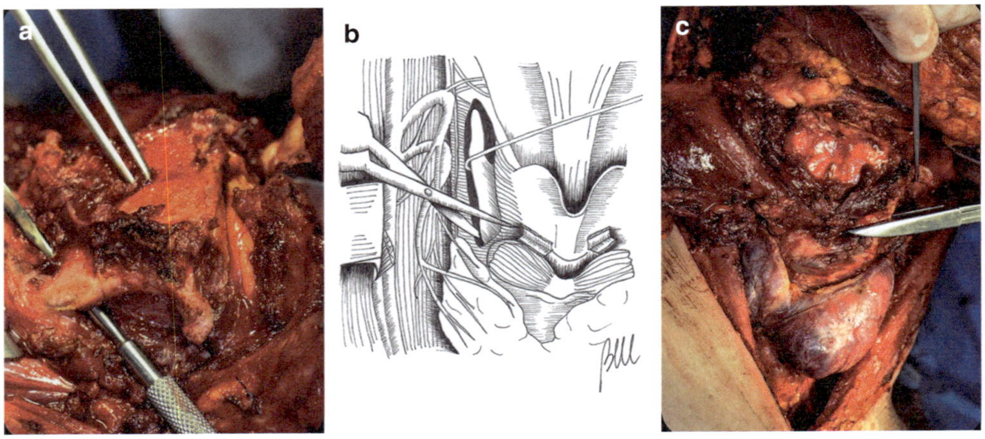

Fig. 7.7 (**a**) Left side. Inferior thyroid cornu skeletonization. (**b**) Right side. Section of the inferior cornu. Notice the direction of the scissors parallel to the inferior edge of thyroid lamina, to protect the recurrent laryngeal nerve and its entry point. (**c**) Left side. Section of the inferior cornu

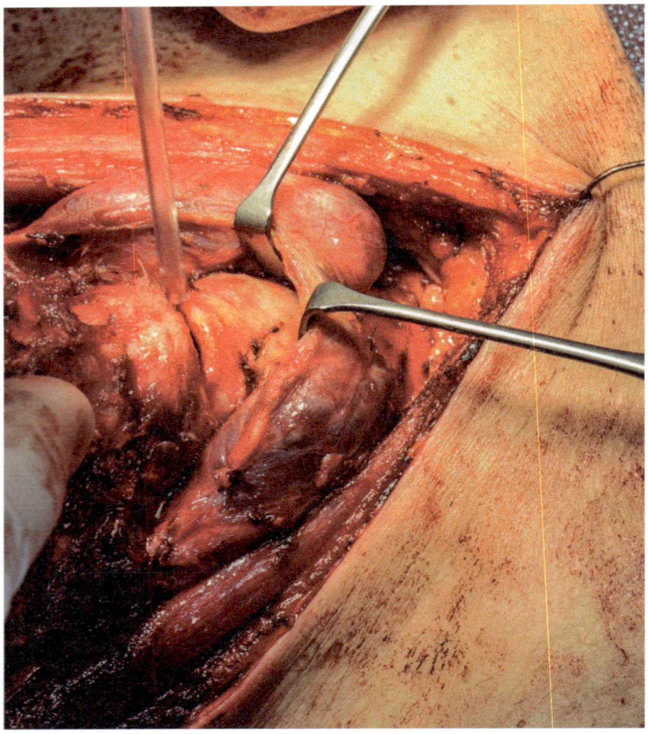

Fig. 7.8 Caudal access to the airway between the cricoid ring and first tracheal ring. Notice the preliminary detachment of thyroid isthmus to enhance the access to this anatomic area

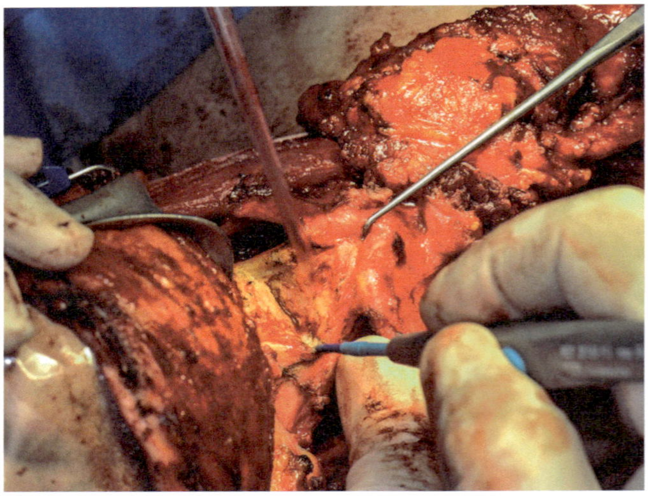

Fig. 7.9 Transepiglottic pharyngotomy to achieve cranial access to the larynx

epiglottis. Therefore, the vertical incision reaches the horizontal cricotracheotomy encompassing the whole subglottic mucosa, cutting the cricoid in front of the junction between the ring and plate, preserving the recurrent laryngeal nerve, which runs more posteriorly (Fig. 7.11b). To improve visualization of the larynx, the thyroid cartilage can be fractured along the midline.

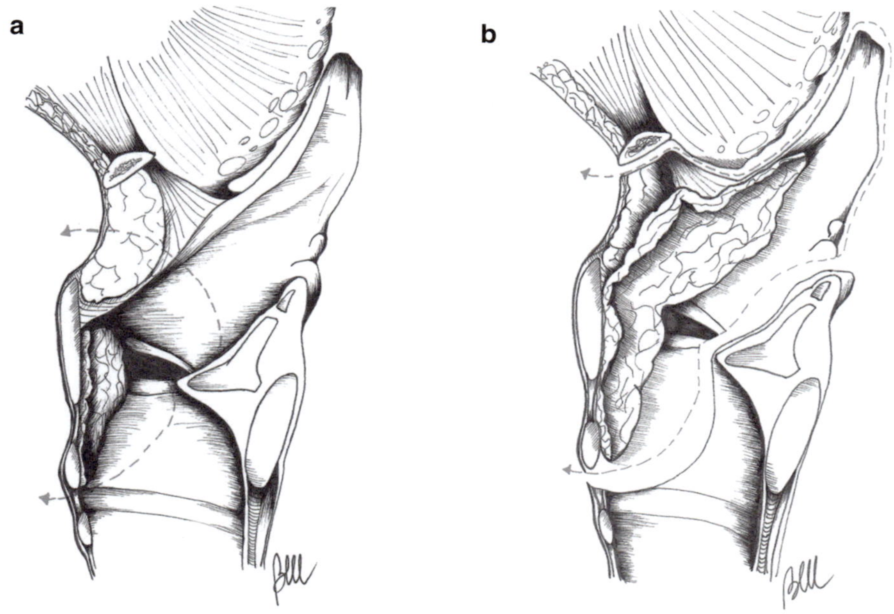

Fig 7.10 (**a**) Schematic drawing showing the transepiglottic resection line preserving the suprahyoid part of the epiglottis (OPHL IIIA). (**b**) Schematic drawing showing the supraepiglottic resection line to achieve en bloc removal of epiglottis and pre-epiglottic space (OPHL IIIB)

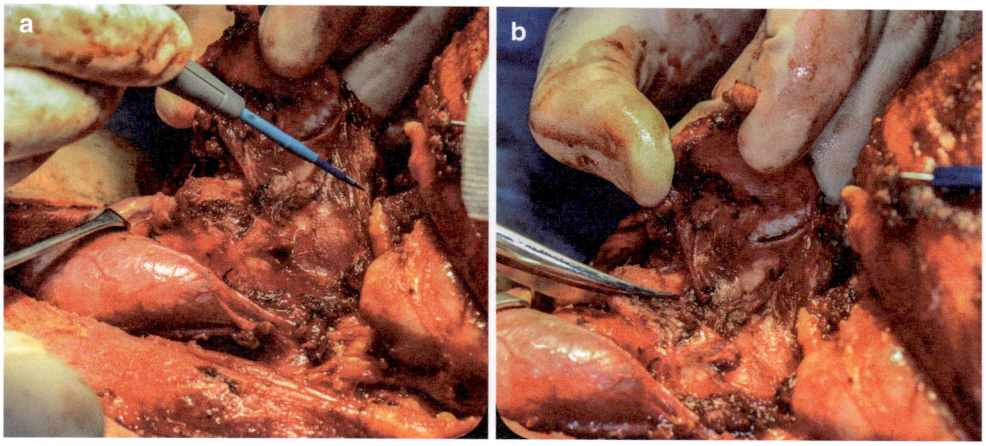

Fig. 7.11 (**a**) Left Side. Aryepiglottic fold section starting from the side not involved and proceeding through the false cord and thyroarytenoid muscle just anteriorly to the vocal process. To achieve a better exposure, thyroid cartilage can be fractured along the midline. (**b**) Left side. Section of cricoid ring at the junction between ring and plate to protect the inferior laryngeal nerve

According to the "modular" principle, it is possible to start with a supracricoid resection; the procedure could intraoperatively change to supratracheal laryngectomy, according to the macroscopic extension of the tumor and microscopic findings at frozen sections.

The resection is completed by sectioning the cricoid plate on the midline and dissecting the pyriform sinus and postcricoid mucosa. To avoid any injury to the hypopharyngeal mucosa, the surgeon puts a finger into the pyriform sinus (inside-out technique) (Fig. 7.12).

On the side of the tumor, to achieve an oncologic margin, the resection should encompass the en bloc removal of the cricoid ring, half cricoid plate, and cricopharyngeal muscle insertion.

The resection margins are always checked with frozen sections (Fig. 7.13). A temporary tracheostomy is now performed between the fifth and sixth tracheal ring and the endotracheal tube is moved through the tracheostomy.

When both the CAUs can be spared, the airway is directly reconstructed with a symmetrical tracheohyoidopexy (Fig. 7.14).

In other cases, the pyriform sinus on the side of the sacrificed CAU is first reconstructed by suturing the hypopharyngeal mucosa to the tracheal mucosa with 4/0 Vicryl (Fig. 7.15).

The pexy is now performed with 2/0 Vicryl by suturing the remaining portion of the epiglottis and the hyoid bone to the trachea. At least 3 stitches must be placed. The first double stitch at the midline superiorly enters longitudinally the suprahyoid epiglottis and encompasses 10–15 mm of the base of tongue muscles (Fig. 7.16, 7.17, and 7.18).

The two paramedian sutures are superiorly passed close to the hyoid bone, to avoid any injury to the lingual arteries and the hypoglossal nerve (Fig. 7.19).

On the side of the sacrificed cricoarytenoid unit, further stitches can be tied to strengthen the reconstruction by

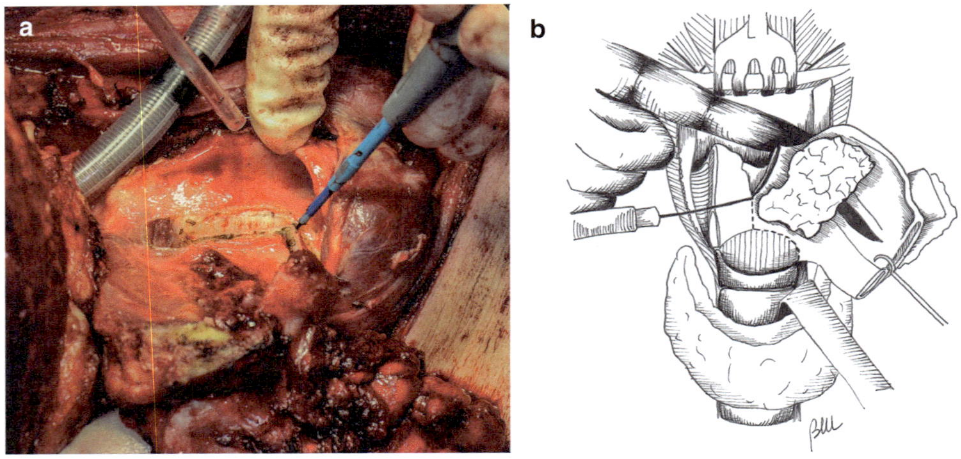

Fig. 7.12 (**a**) Right side. Section of the cricoid plate on the midline and dissection of the pyriform sinus mucosa. Notice the temporary removal of the oro-tracheal tube to perform the en bloc resection. (**b**) Schematic drawing showing the same surgical step on the left side. Notice the position of index finger into the pyriform sinus to protect it from accidental hypopharyngeal injuries (inside-out technique)

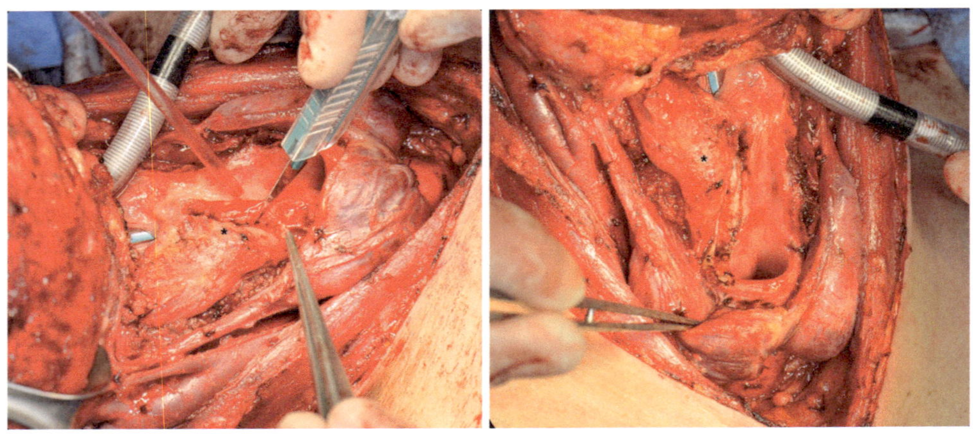

Fig. 7.13 Sampling of the margins on the posterior commissure for frozen section pathological assessment. *Right pyriform sinus mucosa

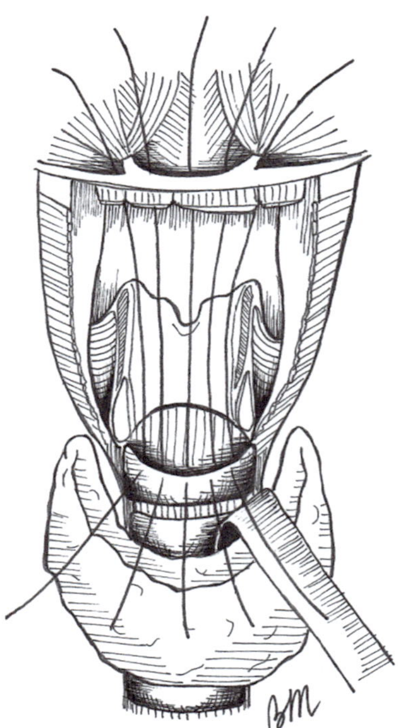

Fig. 7.14 Symmetrical reconstruction of the trachea-hyoidopexy in case of bilateral CAU sparing (OPHL IIIB)

anchoring the hypopharyngeal mucosa. At fixation, the sutures are tightened symmetrically after removing the shoulder roll and flexing the head, to avoid excessive traction on the tracheal stump. The tracheohyoidoepiglottopexy is further stabilized by thyroid gland suspension to the supra-hyoid muscles using 0 Vicryl stitches (Fig. 7.20).

One suction drain is inserted on each side, providing negative pressure. Finally, the superior edge of the tracheostomy is tied, and the incision is closed in layers. A nasogastric feeding tube (NFT) is positioned in all cases.

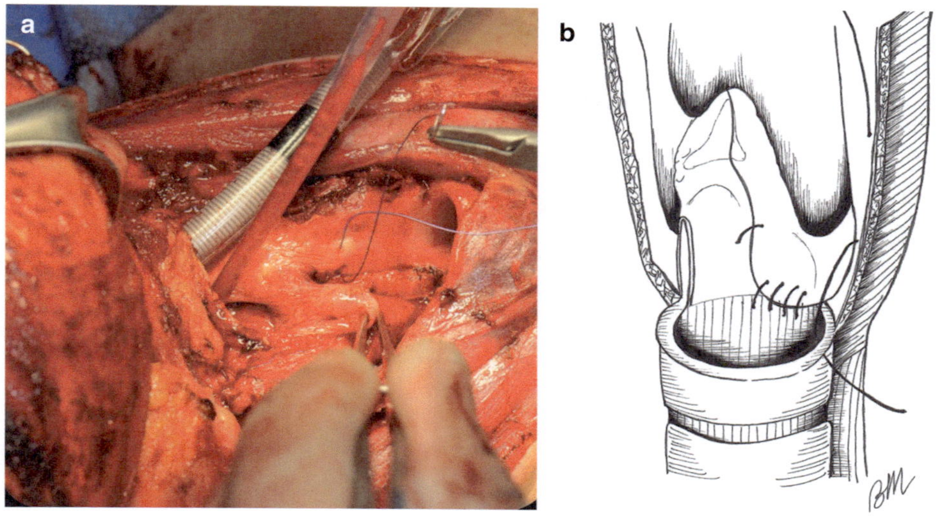

Fig. 7.15 (**a**) Right side: Reconstruction of the pyriform sinus through single-stitches direct suture of hypopharyngeal and tracheal mucosa, after right cricoarytenoid unit resection. (**b**) Schematic drawing showing final result after left pyriform sinus reconstruction

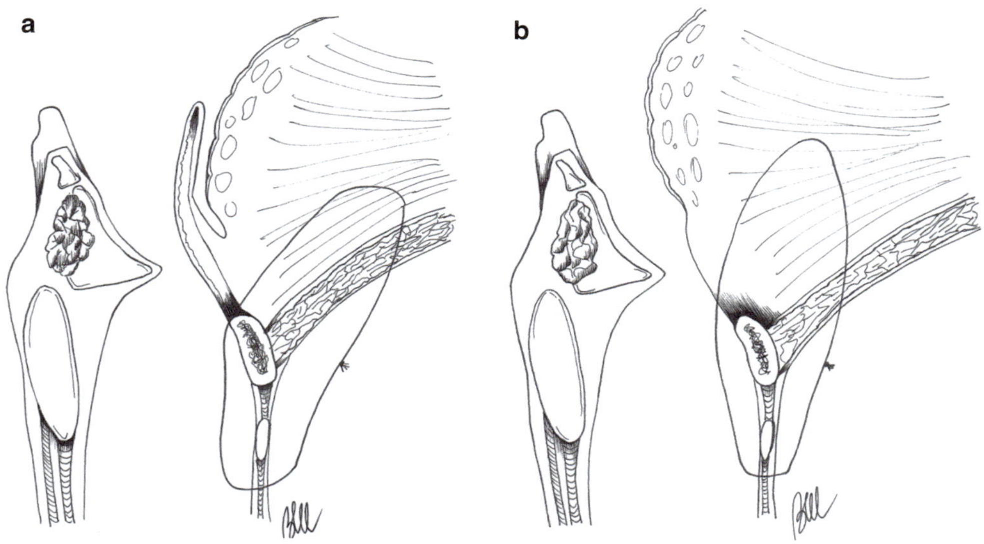

Fig. 7.16 Examples of median stitches of the pexy in OPHL IIIA (**a**) and OPHL IIIB (**b**) in case of suprahyoid epiglottis spared (**a**), the median stitch encompasses both the epiglottis with the hyoid bone and 10–15 mm of base of tongue

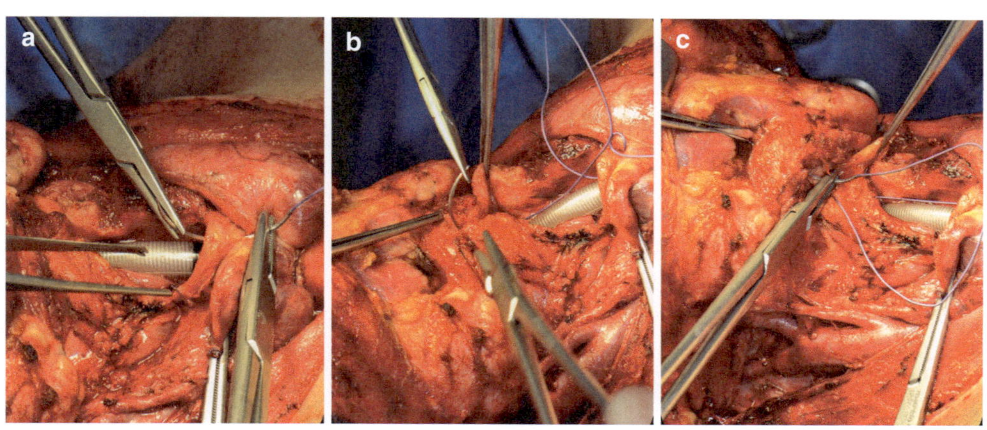

Fig. 7.17 (**a**) Inferiorly, the stitch should pass in a submucosal layer around the tracheal ring. (**b**) Then, the stitch should pass through the suprahyoid epiglottis (OPHL IIIA). (**c**) Lastly, the stitch should encompass the base of the tongue for at least 10–15 mm

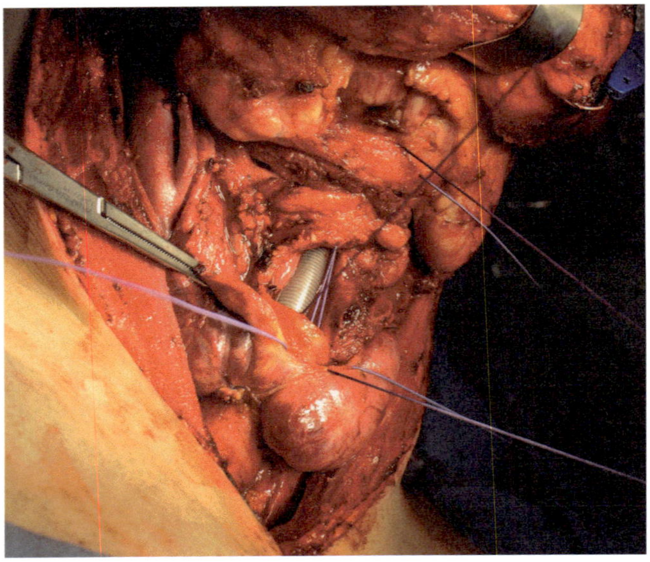

Fig. 7.18 Consider the possibility to pass a double stitch over the median part of the pexy in order to achieve more stability

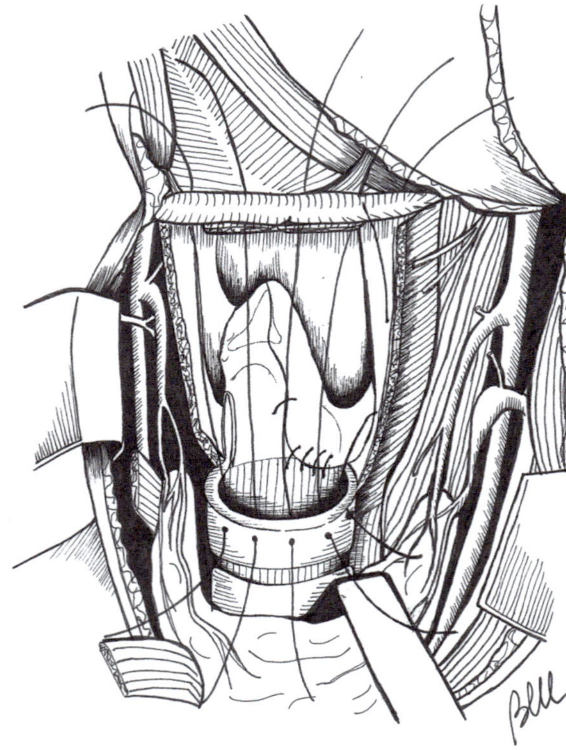

Fig. 7.19 Schematic drawing showing the stitches over the pexy (OPHL IIIB+ left CAU). Notice that the lateral stitches should enclose only the hyoid bone to prevent damage to the lingual artery or hypoglossal nervous branches

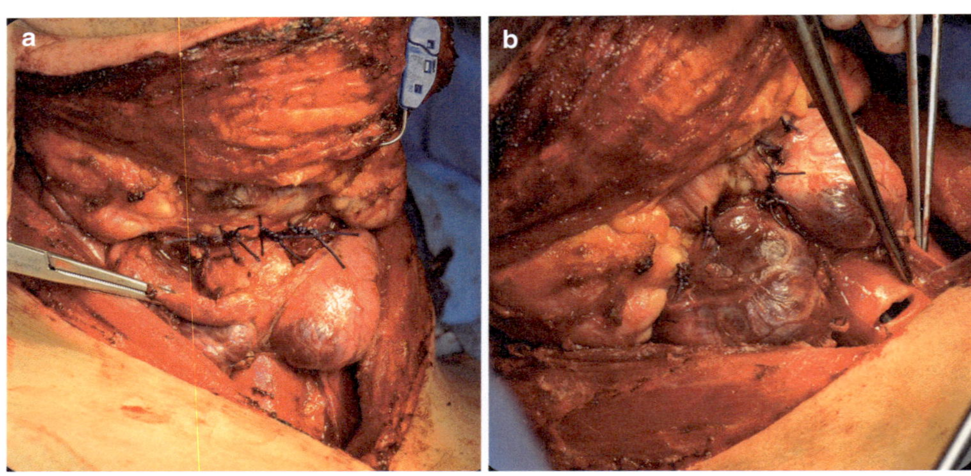

Fig. 7.20 (**a**) Final aspect after tightening of the pexy surgical knots. (**b**) Thyroid gland suspension to protect and seal the tracheo-hyoido(epiglotto)pexy. Temporary tracheostomy

7.5 Oncologic Outcomes

A proper patient selection leads to satisfactory oncologic outcomes for OPHL type III. In a multicentric series, Succo et al. [7] reported 5 years overall survival (OS) of 78%, disease-specific survival (DSS) of 90%, locoregional control (LRC) of 73%, and local control (LC) of 80% in a cohort of 148 patients treated with OPHL type III for locally intermediate-to-advanced laryngeal carcinoma. Furthermore, the study demonstrated that the glottic/transglottic pT3 category with subglottic extension represents the actual core group for type III OPHL, showing a 5-year OS and DSS of 85.3% and 91.1%, respectively. In selected pT4a cases, OPHL type III showed a 5-year OS and DSS of 73.2% OS and 88.1%, respectively, outcomes comparable with those achievable by total laryngectomy, and howsoever higher in comparison with that achievable with radiotherapy and/or chemoradiotherapy (28–38%) [8, 9].

7.6 Functional Outcomes

The functional success of OPHL is mainly related to the recovery of swallowing and breathing function and is defined by the decannulation rate that ranges from 60% to 90%, after OPHL type III [10].

The reported preliminary functional outcomes after OPHL type III showed that, although swallowing was acceptably restored, the voice quality resulted to be significantly worsened. Nonetheless, the oral communication and the quality of life were satisfactory [11].

Although infrequent, persistent dysphagia represents the most common long-term complication after OPHLs. In most of the cases, however, it is well tolerated by patients [12–14]. Slight dysphagia can be conservatively managed with swallowing rehabilitation by a trained speech therapist. In selected cases, the injection laryngoplasty aims at improving the sphincteric action of the larynx [13, 15]. Aspiration pneumonia was observed as both acute complication (3.5%) and late sequela (8.5%) after OPHL type III [7].

On the other hand, laryngeal postoperative laryngeal obstruction (POLO) is the most common late sequela (18%) occurring after OPHL type III, due to laryngeal soft tissues stenosis. In most cases, it can be safely managed with transoral laser microsurgery [16].

7.7 Complications

From our previous multi-institutional study [7], acute postoperative complications occurred in 7% of cases during hospital stay (Table 7.1) and there were no perioperative deaths. The mean hospitalization time for patients with acute complications (37 ± 6 days) was significantly longer than that for patients who did not experience acute complications (25 ± 5 days). Late sequelae following discharge were observed in 28% of cases (Table 7.1). In most of cases, these were successfully treated with transoral CO_2 laser surgery for managing postoperative laryngeal obstruction (89%), injective laryngoplasty using Vox-implants for dysphagia correction (8%), or total laryngectomy for persistent dysphagia (2%).

Table 7.1 Acute postoperative complications and late sequelae

Acute complications	
Cervical bleeding	1/142 (0.7%)
Wound infection	2/142 (1.4%)
Aspiration pneumonia	5/142 (3.5%)
Other	2/142 (1.4%)
Late sequelae	
Laryngeal soft tissue stenosis	25/142 (17.6%)
Dyspnea	3/142 (2.1%)
Aspiration pneumonia	12/142 (8.5%)

Tips and Tricks

- Removal of all strap muscles is preferable to clear any microscopic disease. We have found that sacrifice of these structures does not adversely affect functional recovery in terms of swallowing.
- In cases of tumors with subglottic extension, an ipsilateral paratracheal neck dissection should be performed, given the high rate of occult metastasis in level VI.
- In order not to damage the hypopharyngeal mucosa during tumor resection, it is useful to digitally relax the ipsilateral pyriform sinus allowing a safe dissection along the submucosa (inside-out technique).
- Temporary tracheostomy is performed after resection, while waiting for frozen section results.
- Before proceeding to the pexy, the pyriform sinus on the side of the sacrificed cricoarytenoid unit is reconstructed, suturing the hypopharyngeal mucosa to the tracheal mucosa with 4/0 Vicryl.
- During tracheohyoidoepiglottopexy, the first double stitch at the midline superiorly enters longitudinally and not crosswise the suprahyoid epiglottis, in order to avoid an erroneous postoperative swinging of the epiglottis that could determine a postoperative obstruction of the neoglottis.
- The tracheohyoidoepiglottopexy is finally stabilized by thyroid gland suspension to the suprahyoid muscles using 0 Vicryl stitches.

7.8 Clinical Case 1 (Fig. 7.21)

A 60-year-old man was submitted to supratracheal laryngectomy with sacrifice of the right cricoarytenoid unit (OPHL IIIa + right CAU) and right selective neck dissection for a cT3N2a right glottic squamous cell carcinoma. The image shows a detail of the preoperative flexible laryngoscopy (a): a right cordo-ventricular exophytic lesion involves the anterior commissure and extension to the hypoglottic region. The right arytenoid and vocal cord were fixed. The preoperative contrastenhanced CT scans showed a clear invasion of the inferior paraglottic space with erosion of the thyroid cartilage (b), and invasion of the right thyro cricoarytenoid space (c).

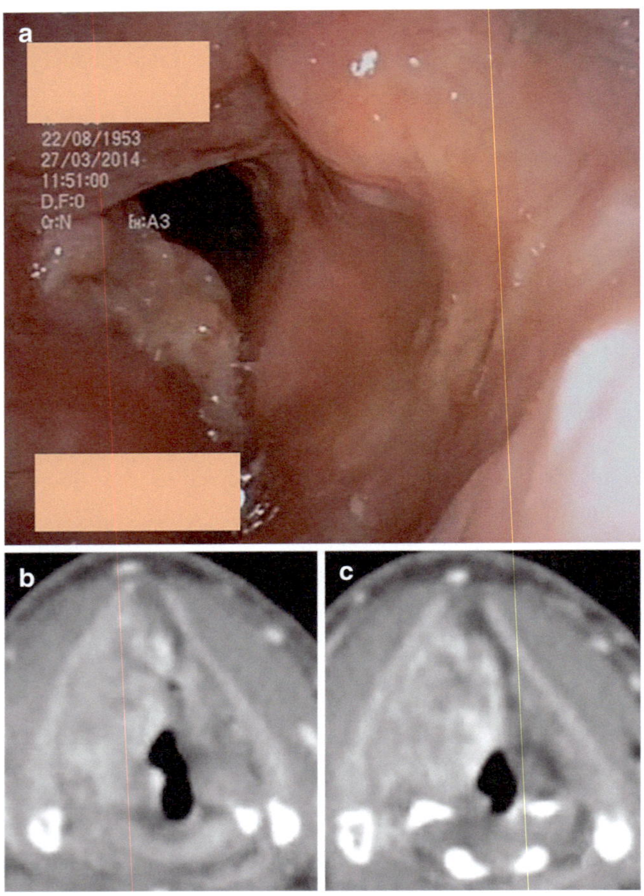

Fig. 7.21 (**a**) Endoscopic view of a right cordo-ventricular exophytic lesion involving the anterior commissure and extending toward the vocal process with right arytenoid and vocal cord fixation. (**b**) Invasion of the inferior paraglottic space at the contrast-enhanced CT scan with erosion of the thyroid cartilage. (**c**) Invasion of the thyro-cricoarytenoid space (TCAS)

7.9 Clinical Case 2 (Fig. 7.22)

A 66-year-old man was submitted to supratracheal laryngectomy with sacrifice of the right cricoarytenoid unit (OPHL IIIa + right CAU) and right selective neck dissection for a cT3N1 right glottic squamous cell carcinoma. The image shows a detail of the preoperative flexible laryngoscopy (a): a right glottic-subglottic ulcerated lesion determined an impaired mobility of the right arytenoid and vocal cord. The preoperative contrast-enhanced CT scans showed the invasion of the right posterior conus elasticus with sclerosis of the right portion of the cricoid plate (b), and invasion of the right inferior paraglottic space and thyro-cricoarytenoid space, with clear sclerosis of the right arytenoid cartilage (c)

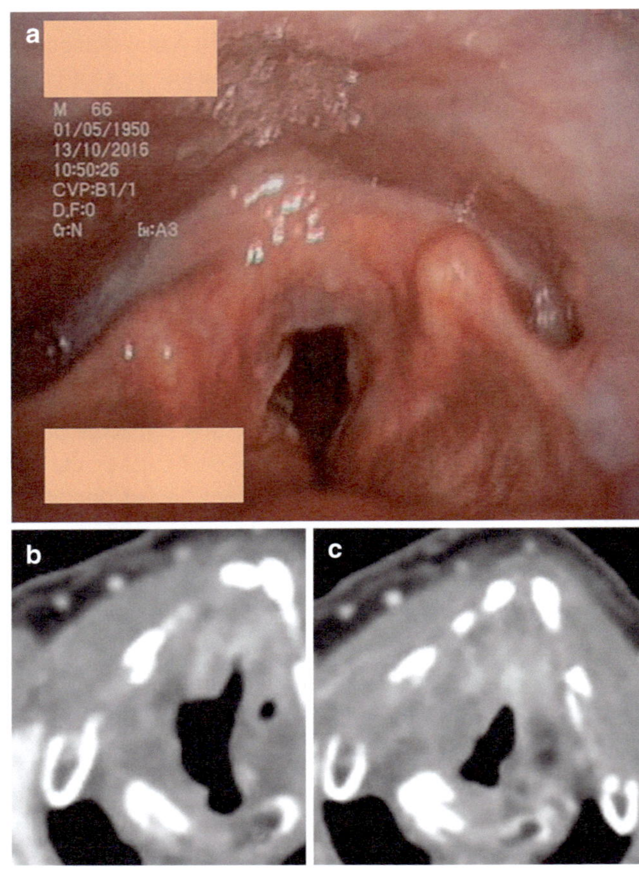

Fig. 7.22 (**a**) Endoscopic view of a right glottic-subglottic ulcerated lesion with impaired mobility of the right arytenoid and vocal cord. (**b**) Invasion of the right posterior conus elasticus with sclerosis of the right portion of the cricoid plate. (**c**) Invasion of the right inferior paraglottic space and thyro-cricoarytenoid space, with sclerosis of the right arytenoid cartilage

References

1. Serafini I. Reconstructive laryngectomy. Rev Laryngol Otol Rhinol. 1972;93:23–32.
2. Laccourreye O, Brasnu D, Jouffre V, et al. Supra-cricoid partial laryngectomy extended to the anterior arch of the cricoid with tracheo-crico-hyoido-epiglottopexy. Oncologic and functional results. Ann Otolaryngol Chir Cervicofac. 1996;113:15–9.
3. Rizzotto G, Succo G, Lucioni M, Pazzaia T. Subtotal laryngectomy with tracheohyoidopexy: a possible alternative to total laryngectomy. Laryngoscope. 2006;116:1907–17.
4. Succo G, Peretti G, Piazza C, et al. Open partial horizontal laryngectomies: a proposal for classification by the working committee on nomenclature of the European Laryngological Society. Eur Arch Otorhinolaryngol. 2014;271:2489–96.
5. Bertolin A, Lionello M, Ghizzo M, et al. Modular approach in OPHL: are there preoperative predictors? Acta Otorhinolaryngol Ital. 2020;40(5):352–9. https://doi.org/10.14639/0392-100X-N0782.
6. Lucioni M, Lionello M, Guida F, Sovran F, Canal F, Rizzotto G, Bertolin A. The thyro-cricoarytenoid space (TCAS): clinical and prognostic implications in laryngeal cancer. Acta Otorhinolaryngol Ital. 2020;40(2):106–12.
7. Succo G, Bussi M, Presutti L, et al. Supratracheal laryngectomy: current indications and contraindications. Acta Otorhinolaryngol Ital. 2015;35:146–56. Review
8. Forastiere AA, Zhang Q, Weber RS, et al. Long-term results of RTOG 91-11: a comparison of three nonsurgical treatment strategies to preserve the larynx in patients with locally advanced larynx cancer. J Clin Oncol. 2013;31:845–52.
9. Wolf G. Reexamining the treatment of advanced laryngeal cancer: the VA laryngeal cancer study revisited. Head Neck. 2010;32:7–14.
10. Rizzotto G, Crosetti E, Lucioni M, Succo G. Subtotal laryngectomy: outcomes of 469 patients and proposal of a comprehensive and simplified classification of surgical procedures. Eur Arch Otorhinolaryngol. 2012;269(6):1635–46.
11. Schindler A, Fantini M, Pizzorni N, et al. Swallowing, voice, and quality of life after supratracheal laryngectomy: preliminary long-term results. Head Neck. 2015;37:557–66.
12. Benito J, Holsinger FC, Perez-Martin A, et al. Aspiration after supracricoid partial laryngectomy: incidence, risk factors, management, and outcomes. Head Neck. 2011;33:679–85.
13. Ricci Maccarini A, Stacchini M, Salsi D, et al. Surgical rehabilitation of dysphagia after partial laryngectomy. Acta Otorhinolaryngol Ital. 2007;27:294–8.
14. de Virgilio A, Greco A, de Vincentiis M. The role of cricohyoido-epiglottopexy in the era of transoral laser surgery and radio/chemotherapy. Acta Otorhinolaryngol Ital. 2014;34:209.
15. Bergamini G, Alicandri-Ciufelli M, Molteni G, De Siati DR, Luppi MP, Marchioni D, Presutti L. Rehabilitation of swallowing with polydimethylsiloxane injections in patients who underwent partial laryngectomy. Head Neck. 2009;31(8):1022–30.
16. Lucioni M, Bertolin A, Lionello M, Giacomelli L, Ghirardo G, Rizzotto G, Marioni G. Transoral laser microsurgery for managing laryngeal stenosis after reconstructive partial laryngectomies. Laryngoscope. 2017;127(2):359–65.

Management and Treatment of Neck Lymph Nodes in Laryngeal Carcinoma

8

Gabriele Molteni, Gennaro Confuorto, Davide Dal Molin, and Andrea Sacchetto

8.1 Lymphatic Drainage Pattern of the Larynx

The expected lymphatic drainage of the different sites of the upper aerodigestive tract dates to the historical works of Lindberg and Byers and correlates with the anatomic dissections of Rouviere. These works suggested that there are predictable and specific pathways of lymphatic drainage within the sites of the upper aerodigestive tract (Fig. 8.1).

However, there is some variability within each site.

Laryngeal subsites (supraglottis, glottis, and subglottis) differ markedly in terms of risk of lymph node metastasis, spread pattern to regional lymph nodes, and overall prognosis. Malignant tumors of supraglottic origin have a greater tendency to loco-regional extension, while the percentage of lymph node metastasis in exclusively glottic or subglottic carcinomas is less marked. The site, or even better the subsite, of origin of the tumor is one of the factors determining the behavior of laryngeal cancer. There are certainly other factors, both known and unknown, that influence the behavior and local and distant extension of the tumor. Among the main risk factors reported in the literature are the degree of tumor differentiation, T size, the presence of lymph node inflammatory reaction, and vascular and perineural invasion.

The supraglottis is the most common origin of laryngeal cancers and, according to the literature, between 30% and 60% of supraglottic cancers develop cervical metastases [1, 2]. Indeed, the anatomic triangular area between the false vocal fold, aryepiglottic fold, and the epiglottis has the highest density of lymphatic vessels. Moreover, this subsite has a high propensity for bilateral lymph node involvement due to its midline location [3, 4]. The endolaryngeal lymphatic drainage is separated into two components, a superficial and deep system. The superficial submucosal system consists of many vessels and anastomoses also crossing the midline, so tumors involving the supraglottic larynx are at risk for

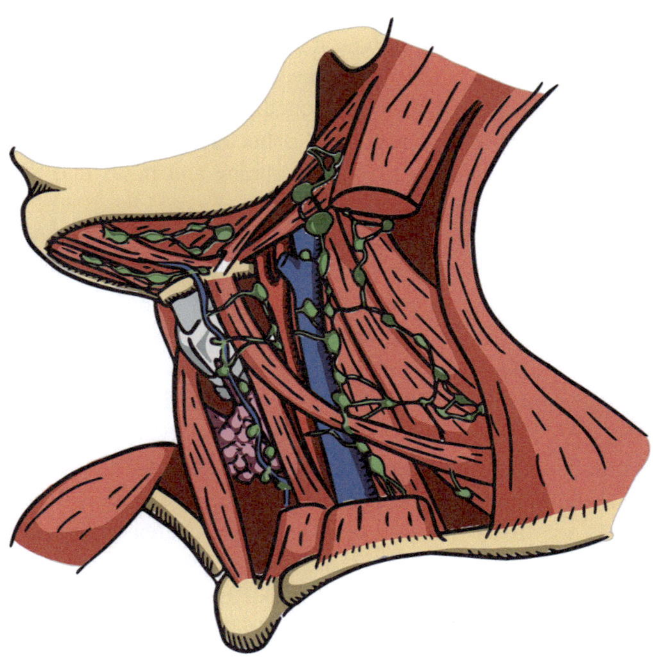

Fig. 8.1 Schematic drawing of cervical lymphatic system. Cervical lymph nodes of the lateral, central, and submandibular compartment are represented

G. Molteni (✉)
Department of Otorhinolaryngology—Head and Neck Surgery, Azienda Ospedaliero Universitaria di Bologna IRCCS, Bologna, Italy

Alma Mater Studiorum—Università di Bologna, Bologna, Italy
e-mail: g.molteni@unibo.it

G. Confuorto · A. Sacchetto
Division of Otorhinolaryngology—Head and Neck Surgery, University Hospital of Verona Borgo Trento, Verona, Italy

Department of Surgery, Dentistry, Paediatrics and Gynaecology, University of Verona, Verona, Italy

D. Dal Molin
Department of Otorhinolaryngology—Head and Neck Surgery, Azienda Ospedaliero Universitaria di Bologna IRCCS, Bologna, Italy
e-mail: davide.dalmolin@studio.unibo.it

F. Mattioli et al. (eds.), *Atlas of Open Partial Horizontal Laryngectomy*, https://doi.org/10.1007/978-3-031-48023-2_8

crossed lymphatic drainage. The deep lymphatic flow is from above to below (the unidirectional flow is favored by the presence of numerous valves within the lymphatic vessels) and has an ipsilateral direction, from medial to lateral. The deep system forms a drainage pedicle at the level of the anterior portion of the aryepiglottic fold; this pedicle converges with the lymphatic drainage originating from the hypopharynx. The lymphatic drainage vessels then exit through the thyrohyoid membrane [5, 6]. Subsequently, a component of lymphatic drainage moves superiorly toward the subdigastric triangle to drain into Kuttner's (or Chaissaignac's or subdigastric) lymph node. Another component extends transversely by taking the pathway of the thyro-linguo-facial trunk and drains into lymph nodes located at the junction of level II and III. Occasionally, there is a third component that drains directly to lymph nodes of level III [7].

On the ipsilateral side, levels II (67%) and III (48%) are most likely at risk for developing nodal metastases. Level at highest risk for metastases on the contralateral side is group II (21%) [8].

There is a paucity of lymphatics draining the glottic region. The poor development of the glottic lymphatic network constitutes a natural barrier between supraglottic and subglottic lymphatics; therefore, the main factors for the development of lymph node metastases from this subsite are the extension to neighboring areas and the invasion of paraglottic space and the cricoid region by the neoplasm. The superficial mucosal lymphatic vessels form a continuous layer along the true vocal cords and drain through the cricothyroid membrane to the level II and to the Delphian lymph node. In cases of squamous carcinoma limited to the glottic larynx, bilateral or contralateral metastases are rare because the true vocal folds are nearly devoid of lymphatics [9, 10].

Subglottic lymphatics come together to form 3 collectors: an anterior and two posterolateral collectors. The anterior collector crosses the cricothyroid membrane and flows into the Delphian lymph node, from where it is directed partly to the pretracheal lymph nodes and partly laterally to the lymph nodes of the internal jugular vein (level IV). The posterolateral collectors cross the cricotracheal ligament and, passing below the thyroid, head to the VI and VII levels lymph nodes [9] (Fig. 8.2).

The distribution of metastatic nodes by level confirms that the process of metastasis follows a predictable pattern (Fig. 8.3). The presence of skip metastasis in the lymph nodes is rare, especially when compared to other sites in the head and neck region such as the tongue and oral mucosa. Levels II, III, and IV are firstly involved by metastases, whereas metastatic lymph nodes at levels I and V are usually found together with the former levels and are reported in <10% of cases.

Level I may be rarely involved (1–2%), and usually in cases of extensive involvement along the jugular chain, often only in patients with cN2 or cN3 disease.

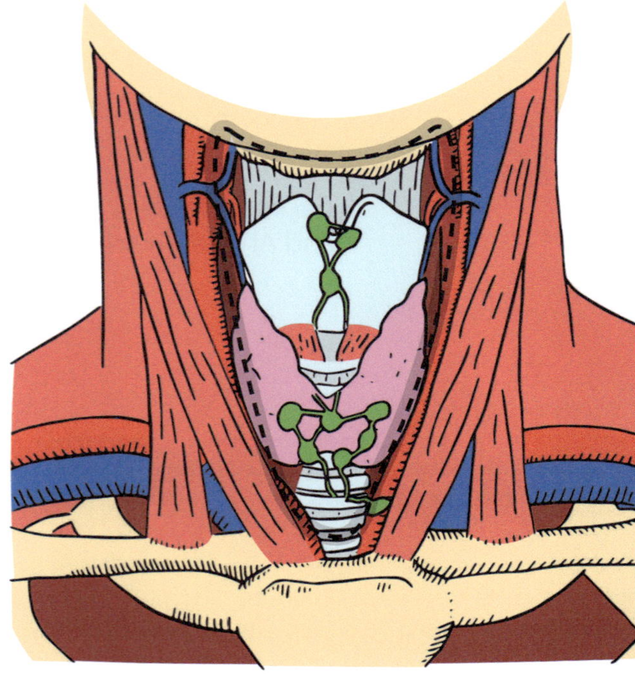

Fig. 8.2 Schematic drawing of lymph nodes distribution in the central compartment of the neck. Prelaryngeal, perithyroidal, and paratracheal lymph nodes are represented

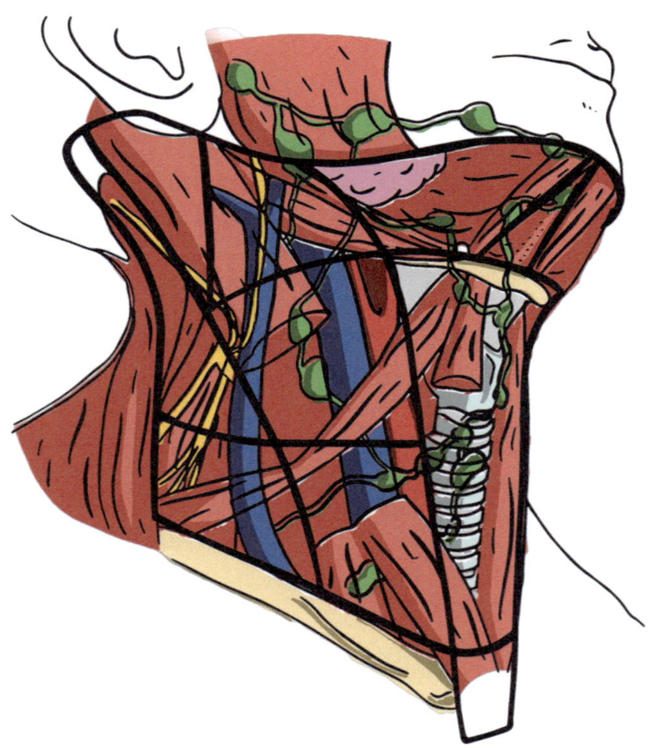

Fig. 8.3 Schematic drawing of the subdivision of cervical lymph node levels according to Robbins' classification

The dissection of the anterior aspect of level I is not routinely indicated, since nodal involvement of the submandibular and, even more, of the submental triangle is rare.

Lymphatic metastases are found in level V in 1% or less of the cases. The extremely rare involvement of the posterior triangle means that prophylactic dissection of this level is not necessary [11, 12].

The connection between the lymphatic networks of the hemilarynx at both supraglottic and subglottic levels has been demonstrated to be an anatomical prerequisite for the possibility of metastasis to contralateral cervical lymph nodes.

However, strictly lateral tumors that drained into ipsilateral lymphatic vessels were seen with contralateral metastases in 5% of the patients only. A higher prevalence was observed only when central and lateral neoplasms were grouped together. The rare involvement of the contralateral side of the neck in strictly lateral lesions suggests that bilateral elective treatment of the neck may be reserved for central tumors [13].

8.2 Central Compartment (Level VI)

Controversies still exist about the management of the central compartment lymph nodes (level VI). The anatomical boundaries of this lymph node level, also called the anterior compartment of the neck or paratracheal lymph nodes, are represented by the medial edge of the common carotid artery (lateral border), the tracheal wall (medial border), the inferior cricoid edge (cranial border), and the suprasternal notch (caudal border) [14, 15] (Figs. 8.4 and 8.5).

Although paratracheal lymph nodes are not included in radical, modified radical, or selective dissection of the lateral neck, the reported prevalence of paratracheal lymph node metastasis in laryngeal cancer ranges between 9% and 27%. Tumor extension to the subglottic region correlates most strongly with metastasis to lymph node level VI, and paratracheal lymph nodes' metastases may develop independently from lymph node metastases in other levels [16, 17].

The higher rate of paratracheal metastasis is found in cases of tumors with anterolateral subglottic extension, because of the numerous efferent lymphatics draining from the anterolateral subglottis into paratracheal lymph nodes. On the contrary, the patients with posterolateral subglottic extension showed higher rates of lateral cervical lymph node involvement, which may suggest a prominent lymphatic drainage from such posterior subglottic areas to the homolateral lateral cervical lymph nodes [9]. Almost invariably, the subglottis is reached by tumors arising in the glottis or supraglottis through a caudal transglottic growth or paraglottic space invasion. Involvement of the subglottis seems to be associated with a relatively high frequency of lymphatic spread to the paratracheal lymph nodes and stomal recurrences which significantly affect patients' survival [17, 18].

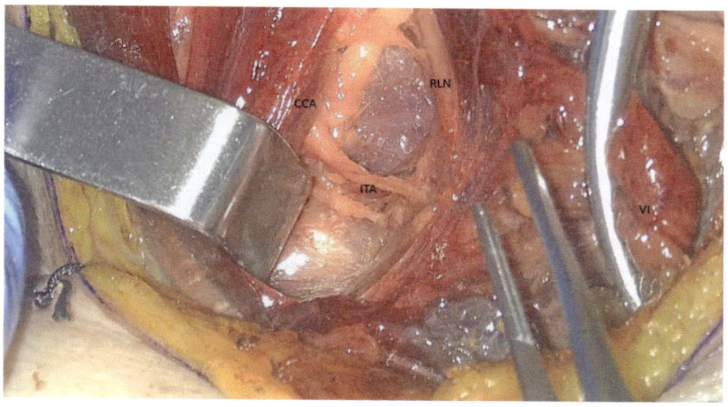

Fig. 8.4 Cadaveric dissection: main landmarks of the VI level of cervical lymph nodes. *CCA* common carotid artery, *ITA* inferior thyroidal artery, *RLN* recurrent laryngeal nerve

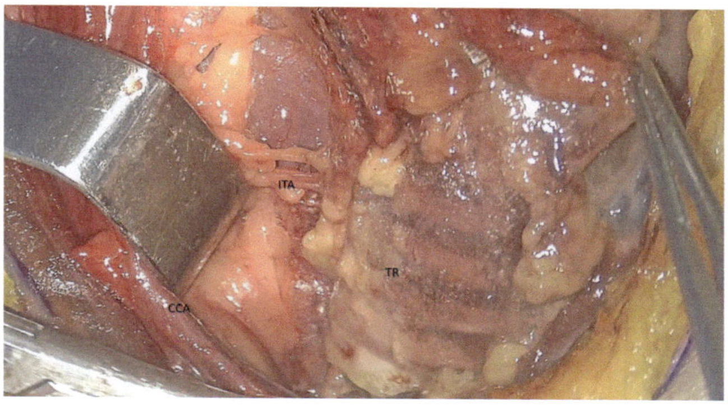

Fig. 8.5 Cadaveric dissection: central compartment of the neck after removal of the VI level of cervical lymph nodes. *CCA* common carotid artery, *ITA* inferior thyroidal artery, *TR* trachea

Such findings may confirm the prophylactic and therapeutic role of paratracheal lymph node neck dissection in advanced (T3–T4) laryngeal carcinomas with anterior subglottic extension. In cases of tumors confined to one side of the larynx, the surgical treatment should include the ipsilateral paratracheal nodes, whereas in tumors involving both sides of the larynx, a bilateral paratracheal lymph node neck dissection should be performed. The dissection of the VI level is also indicated in case of subglottis involvement with clinically apparent node metastases in the lateral compartment of the neck, especially in case of an anteroinferior subglottic involvement [19].

The most frequently and universally used oncological staging system is the TNM system of the Union Internationale Contre le Cancer (UICC) and the American Joint Committee on Cancer (AJCC). The TNM system describes the extent of the primary tumor (T), the presence and extent of metastasis to regional lymph nodes (N), and the possible presence of distant metastases (M). When staging is performed prior to treatment of the disease, it is referred to as cTNM (clinical

TNM); when staging is performed after histopathological examination of a surgical specimen it is referred to as pTNM (pathologic TNM). Combinations of T, N, and M with similar prognosis are then grouped into stages numbered I to IV; increasing stage is associated with a worse prognosis.

The most significant change in N classification occurred in the latest edition, published in 2017, with the introduction of the Extra Nodal Extension (ENE) criterion, a factor that determines the transition to N3b stage. ENE represents one of the most significant negative prognostic factors for laryngeal squamous cell carcinomas, significantly reduces overall survival and local disease control, and increases the risk of distant metastasis.

8.3 Management of the Clinically Negative Neck

Since metastatic nodal disease is the most important prognostic factor for laryngeal cancer [20], the aim of neck treatment should be to remove any potential metastatic lymph nodes. However, there are still debates on many aspects of neck management, such as when and how to treat the neck in patients with laryngeal carcinoma without clinical evidence of metastatic involvement (elective treatment of the neck). In addition, there is no general consensus on which type of neck dissection is more adequate whenever the surgeon is faced with an evident metastatic lymph node involvement (therapeutic treatment of the neck).

The detection of cervical lymph node dissemination is difficult to evaluate in the absence of clinically or radiologically evident metastases, and it is a major challenge to the head and neck oncology because of its prognostic and therapeutic implications. Even the most sensitive and technologically advanced diagnostic procedures (CT, MRI, ultrasound, ultrasound-guided FNAC, SPECT, PET-CT, lymphangiography, radioimmunoscintigraphy, and radionuclide scanning) may be unable to reveal occult micrometastases preoperatively. According to the literature, 25% of clinically N0 necks have occult metastases [21, 22]. The metastasis rate of cN0 cervical lymph nodes appears to be closely related to T staging and tends to increase with the progress of T staging and with lower differentiated carcinoma [23].

Therapeutic decisions regarding the neck must also be undertaken according to the size, site, phenotype, and treatment plan for the primary cancer. As stated by several studies, elective neck dissection is strongly suggested if the risk of cervical LNMs is >15–20%. The therapeutic role of cervical dissection is manifested in the reduction of the rate of recurrence and distant metastases [24]. The role of elective treatment of the neck in laryngeal cancer continues to be controversial, and variations in type and extent of surgical dissection have evolved. The current surgical strategies used for the treatment of cN0 laryngeal carcinoma are summarized in Table 8.1.

Table 8.1 Surgical strategies for elective neck dissection in cN0 laryngeal carcinoma

	Ipsilateral neck	Contralateral neck
Supraglottic T2/T4	II–IV	II-IV
Glottic T3/T4	II–IV, VI	
Transglottic (FVC and glottis)	II–IV, VI	
Subglottic T3/T4	II–IV, VI	VI
Intraoperative N+ staging	RND/MND	RND/MND

RND radical neck dissection, *MND* modified neck dissection

Prophylactic neck dissection has been recommended for the N0 neck in patients with T2–T4 supraglottic cancers [24–26], T3–T4 glottic cancers [24, 27–31], T3–T4 subglottic cancers [24, 31–33], and in patients with recurrent supraglottic and advanced glottic cancers treated by radiotherapy and salvaged by laryngectomy [34].

The location of cervical lymph node metastases is closely linked with the site of the primary lesion. As previously described, the supraglottic area is richly supplied with lymphatics, and tumors of the supraglottic region metastasize in 25–75% of cases when all stages are considered. Moreover, bilateral metastases are more common than other subsites, as the supraglottis is a midline structure [2, 35]. Several studies reported a high incidence of recurrence on the contralateral side of the neck in patients affected by supraglottic cancer treated by unilateral neck dissection, and an improvement in overall survival and local-regional control is achieved when patients are treated with bilateral neck dissection. Consequently, elective bilateral neck dissection including nodes level II–III–IV is strongly suggested in the management of the cervical lymphatics in patients with supraglottic cancer, with an observed decrease in loco-regional recurrence, confirming the oncologic reliability of the use of neck dissection in N0 patients [36] (Figs. 8.6, 8.7, and 8.8).

The nodes at high risk for T3 and T4 glottic cancers include level II–III–IV and VI, and metastases in the ipsilateral paratracheal nodes are found in <10%. Contralateral metastases are very rare in advanced glottic cancers as well [28, 37]. Glottic, transglottic, and subglottic cancers may also metastasize to precricoid or prelaryngeal lymph node or Delphian and sub-Delphian nodes in the anterior tracheal compartment of level VI [32].

The carcinoma of the subglottis has a 65% incidence of occult paratracheal nodal metastasis and may involve the thyroid gland by direct extension and/or by lymphatic spread. An inadequate treatment of the paratracheal lymphatics and of the thyroid gland is probably the principal cause of peristomal recurrence in patients with subglottic cancer [38–40]. There is a general advice for a policy of ipsilateral selective neck dissection including levels II–III–IV and ipsilateral VI level for the management of T3 and T4 glottic cancer. In cases of

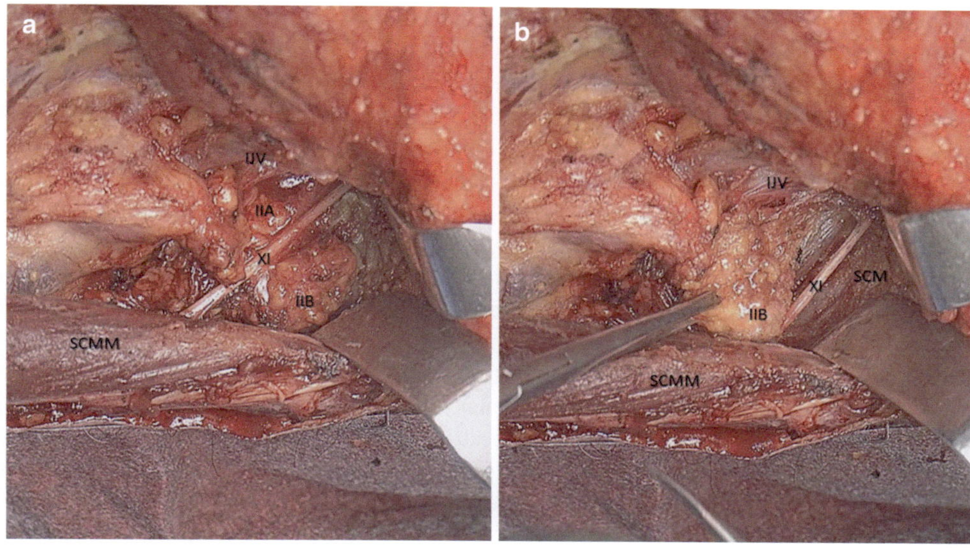

Fig. 8.6 Panel A: intraoperative image of II level of cervical lymph nodes dissection. *IJV* internal jugular vein, *SCMM* sternocleidomastoid muscle, *XI* XI cranial nerve, *IIA* cervical level IIA, *IIB* cervical level IIB. Panel B: intraoperative image after complete dissection of cervical lymph nodes level IIB. *IJV* internal jugular vein, *SCMM* sternocleidomastoid muscle, *XI* XI cranial nerve, *IIB* cervical level IIB, *SCM* splenius capitis muscle

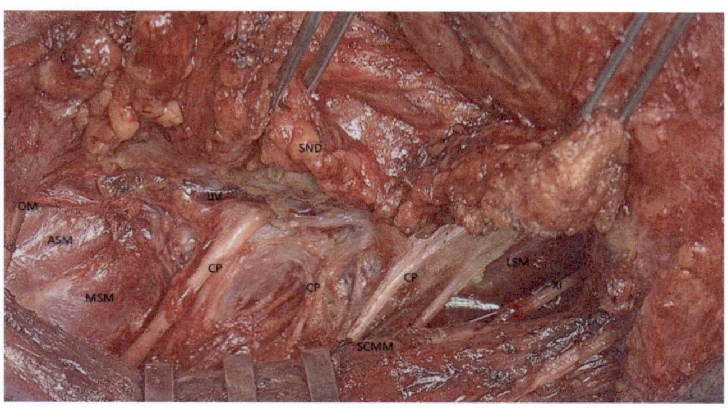

Fig. 8.7 Intraoperative image of selective neck dissection levels II, III, and IV. *SND* selective neck dissection, *IJV* internal jugular vein, *SCMM* sternocleidomastoid muscle, *XI* XI cranial nerve, *CP* cervicalis plexus, *OM* omohyoid muscle, *LSM* levator scapulae muscle, *ASM* anterior scalene muscle, *MSM* medial scalene muscle

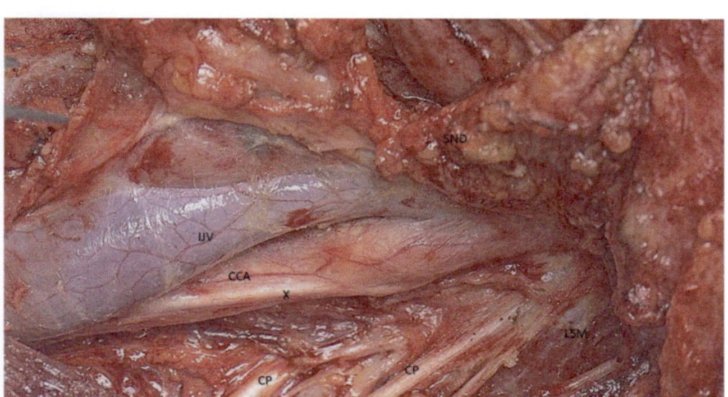

Fig. 8.8 Intraoperative image of selective neck dissection levels II, III, and IV after skeletonization of cervical neurovascular bundle. *SND* selective neck dissection, *IJV* internal jugular vein, *CCA* common carotid artery, *X* X cranial nerve, *CP* cervicalis plexus, *LSM* levator scapulae muscle

subglottic lesions, an ipsilateral hemithyroidectomy with contralateral VI level dissection is performed in addition [41].

Nowadays, a conventional or modified radical neck dissection is not indicated for elective surgical treatment of the neck in patients with supraglottic and transglottic squamous cell carcinoma. According to several studies, the 5-year overall survival rate and neck recurrence are not influenced by the type of neck dissection, and selective neck dissection is associated with lower morbidity and less postoperative injuries than radical dissection in experienced hands [42]. Recently, complete functional neck dissection has been considered an unnecessarily extensive procedure for treatment of the clinically negative neck as levels I and V are rarely involved, particularly in the absence of clinically or radiologically apparent neck metastases [43]. Thus, selective lateral neck dissection can be considered a valid treatment in laryngeal cancer since it includes dissection of levels II–IV, removing only those lymph node groups that are at highest risk of metastases [44].

8.4 Management of the Clinically Positive Neck

In clinically N-positive neck patients affected by laryngeal carcinoma, the presence of histologically confirmed metastasis is associated with a high risk of recurrence, varying from 3% for single metastasis to 33.3% for multiple, and a decrease in the survival rate of up to 50% [45]. The type of treatment of clinically positive necks must be based on the extent and location of metastases.

As the goal of neck dissection is to remove all clinically evident metastatic nodal disease and all the nodal groups at greatest risk, conservative modifications of the traditional radical neck dissection may be indicated according to the stage and location of metastatic lymph nodes, as well as the characteristics of the primary tumor.

While complete conventional or modified radical neck dissections (with inclusion of level VI as indicated) constitute appropriate treatment for many patients, selective neck dissection of levels II–III and IV (including resection of accessory nerve, sternocleidomastoid muscle, or internal jugular vein as necessary) may offer a more efficient and effective treatment tailored to the requirements of any particular situation [46]. This type of neck dissection has generally not been advocated for the management of more advanced nodal status, although data in the literature support the concept that selective neck dissection and modified radical neck dissection give the same results of radical neck dissection in N1–N2 patients [47].

The use of intraoperative diagnosis during neck dissection is still debated.

Intraoperative diagnosis of occult metastasis in the clinically N0 neck has a sensitivity of 44% and a specificity of 63% when reliance is placed on the surgeon's ability to evaluate lymph nodes by inspection and palpation only. Frozen section diagnosis of malignancy has a sensitivity and specificity of 100% per suspicious node. In some institutions, the sampling of suspicious nodes during elective neck dissection for intraoperative frozen section exams is a routine procedure. If a metastasis is diagnosed by frozen section, then the elective neck dissection is converted to a therapeutic neck dissection, usually modified radical neck dissection type I [48].

When surgery is selected as the treatment of choice for carcinoma of the larynx, it is extremely important to know and recognize which tumor and patient-related variables may lead to surgical treatment failure. In recent years, particular attention has been paid to the concept of lymph node ratio (LNR) or lymph node density (LND). This term refers to the ratio of lymph nodes positive for metastases to the number of total lymph nodes removed during surgery. It is therefore an index that can only be calculated after lymph node emptying surgery and therefore influences post-treatment staging. Numerous studies have recently recognized its importance as a prognostic factor for numerous malignancies of the body such as bladder [49], stomach, colorectal, and oral cavity [50, 51]. On the basis of these results, some authors have therefore sought to understand the prognostic value of NDI in predicting cancer-related mortality in patients with laryngeal cancer and positive laterocervical lymph nodes (pN+). The studies conducted by Ryu et al. [52], Kunzel et al. [53], and Imre et al. [54] highlighted LND as an important independent prognostic predictor of overall survival and disease-free survival in patients with pN+ squamous cell carcinoma of the larynx. Other authors have focused their research on the relationship between the number of lymph node metastases and survival of patients with these tumors. The exact number of lymph nodes involved by metastases in the TNM classification of cervical-facial cancers is not considered. Recent studies have investigated this variable both in cancers of the oral cavity [55] and in carcinomas of the larynx and hypopharynx [56]. The latter, a retrospective study of more than 8000 patients, showed that the number of metastatic lymph nodes is an independent factor associated with mortality. Comparison with current TNM staging also showed that lymph node size and contralaterality have no independent prognostic value when compared with the number of metastases. The authors therefore proposed a different lymph node staging that, in their opinion, allows a better stratification of patients with laryngeal carcinoma. Finally, the prognostic role of LNR and the number of metastatic lymph nodes (NPLN) in laryngeal carcinoma were recently investigated by Molteni et al. [57]. In a large, multicenter retrospective study, the potential predictive role of these two factors was demonstrated, suggesting their integration into pTNM staging to allow better risk stratification of recurrence and cancer-related death in this group of patients.

References

1. Esposito ED, Motta S, Cassiano B, Motta G. Occult lymph node metastases in supraglottic cancers of the larynx. Otolaryngol Head Neck Surg. 2001;124:253–7.
2. Sinard RJ, Netterville JL, Garrett CG, Ossoff RH. Cancer of the larynx. In: Myers EN, Suen JY, editors. Cancer of the head and neck. 3rd ed. Philadelphia: Saunders; 1996. p. 381–421.
3. Redaelli de Zinis LO, Nicolai P, Tomenzoli D, et al. The distribution of lymph node metastases in supraglottic squamous cell carcinoma: therapeutic implications. Head Neck. 2002;24(10):913–20.
4. Welsh LW. The normal human laryngeal lymphatics. Ann Otol Rhinol Laryngol. 1964;73:569–82.
5. Werner LA, Schunke M, Lippert BM, Koeleman H, Gottschlich S, Tillmann B. Das Laryngeal Lymphgrfabsytem des Menschen. HNO. 1995;43:523–31.
6. Beck C, Mann W. The inner laryngeal lymphatics. Acta Otorhinolaryngol Stockh. 1980;89:265–70.
7. Robbins KT, Medina JE, Wolfe GT, et al. Standardizing neck dissection terminology. Arch Otolaryngol Head Neck Surg. 1991;117:601–5.
8. Redaelli de Zinis LO, Nicolai P, Tomenzoli D, Ghizzardi D, Trimarchi M, Cappiello J, Peretti G, Antonino R, Antonelli AR. The distribution of lymph node metastases in supraglottic squamous cell carcinoma: therapeutic implications. Head Neck. 2002;24(10):913–20.
9. Rouviere H. Anatomy of the human lymphatic system. J Anat. 1939;73(Pt 4):675.
10. Byers RM, Wolf PF, Ballantyne AJ. Rationale for elective modified neck dissection. Head Neck Surg. 1988;10:160–7.
11. Candela FC, Kothari K, Shah JP. Patterns of cervical node metastases from squamous carcinoma of the larynx. Arch Otolaryngol Head Neck Surg. 1990;116:432–5.
12. Buckley JG, MacLennan K. Cervical node metastases in laryngeal and hypopharyngeal cancer: a prospective analysis of prevalence and distribution. Head Neck. 2000;22:380–5.

13. Guney E, Yigitbasi OG. Management of N0 neck in T1–T2 unilateral supraglottic cancer. Ann Otol Rhinol Laryngol. 1999;108:998–1003.
14. Robbins KT, Shaha AR, Medina JE, et al. Consensus statement on the classification and terminology of neck dissection. Arch Otolaryngol Head Neck Surg. 2008;134(5):536–8.
15. Robbins KT, Clayman G, Levine PA, et al. Neck dissection classification update: revisions proposed by the American Head and Neck Society and the American Academy of Otolaryngology-Head and Neck Surgery. Arch Otolaryngol Head Neck Surg. 2002;128:751–8.
16. de Bree R, Leemans CR, Silver CE, et al. Paratracheal lymph node dissection in cancer of the larynx, hypopharynx, and cervical esophagus: the need for guidelines. Head Neck. 2011;33(6):912–6.
17. Chiesa F, Tradati N, Calabrese L, et al. Surgical treatment of laryngeal carcinoma with subglottis involvement. Oncol Rep. 2001;8(1):137–40.
18. Medina JE, Ferlito A, Robbins KT, et al. Central compartment dissection in laryngeal cancer. Head Neck. 2011;33(5):746–52.
19. Plaat RE, de Bree R, Kuik DJ, et al. Prognostic importance of paratracheal lymph node metastases. Laryngoscope. 2005;115(5):894–8.
20. Grandi C, Mingardo M, Guzzo M, Licitra L, Podrecca S, Molinari R. Prognostic significance of lymphatic spread in head and neck carcinoma: therapeutic implications. Head Neck Surg. 1985;8:67–73.
21. Van den Brekel MWM, van der Waal I, Meijer CJLM, Freeman JL, Castelijns JA, Snow GB. The incidence of micrometastases in neck dissection specimens obtained from elective neck dissections. Laryngoscope. 1996;106:987–91.
22. Ferlito A, Rinaldo A. False negative conventional histology of lymph nodes in patients with head and neck cancer. ORL J Otorhinolaryngol Relat Spec. 2000;62:112–4.
23. Ma H, Lian M, Feng L, Li P, Hou L, Chen X, Huang Z, Fang J. Factors contributing to lymph node occult metastasis in supraglottic laryngeal carcinoma cT2–T4 N0M0 and metastasis predictive equation. Chin J Cancer Res. 2014;26(6):685–91.
24. Pillsbury HC 3rd, Clark M. A rationale for therapy of the N0 neck. Laryngoscope. 1997;107:1294–315.
25. Gavilan C, Gavilan J. Five-year results of functional neck dissection for cancer of the larynx. Arch Otolaryngol Head Neck Surg. 1989;114:1193–6.
26. Herranz-Gonzalez J, Gavilan J, Martinez-Vidal J, Gavilan C. Supraglottic laryngectomy: functional and oncologic results. Ann Otol Rhinol Laryngol. 1996;105:18–22.
27. Yuen A, Medina JE, Goepfert H, Fletcher G. Management of stage T3 and T4 glottic carcinomas. Am J Surg. 1984;148:467–72.
28. Johnson JT. Carcinoma of the larynx: selective approach to the management of cervical lymphatics. Ear Nose Throat J. 1994;73:303–5.
29. Hao SP, Myers EN, Johnson JT. T3 glottic carcinoma revisited—transglottis vs. pure glottic carcinoma. Arch Otolaryngol Head Neck Surg. 1995;121:166–70.
30. Yang CY, Andersen PE, Everts EC, Cohen JI. Nodal disease in purely glottic carcinoma: is elective neck treatment worthwhile? Laryngoscope. 1998;108:1006–8.
31. Myers EN, Fagan JJ. Management of the neck cancer of the larynx. Ann Otol Rhinol Laryngol. 1999;108:828–32.
32. Dahm JD, Sessions DG, Paniello RC, Harvey J. Primary subglottic cancer. Laryngoscope. 1998;108:741–6.
33. Ferlito A, Rinaldo A. The pathology and management of subglottic cancer. Eur Arch Otorrinolaringol. 2000;257:168–73.
34. Wax MK, Touma BJ. Management of the N0 neck during salvage laryngectomy. Laryngoscope. 1999;109:4–7.
35. Marks JE, Devineni VR, Harvey J, Sessions DG. The risk of contralateral lymphatic metastases for cancers of the larynx and pharynx. Am J Otolaryngol. 1992;13:34–9.
36. Lutz CK, Johnson JT, Wagner RL, Myers EN. Supraglottic carcinoma: patterns of recurrence. Ann Otol Rhinol Laryngol. 1990;99:12–7.
37. Shenoy A, Nanjundappa A, Kumar P, Kumar RV, Reddy BKM, Kannan V, Anantha N. Interjugular neck dissection and postoperative irradiation for neck control in advanced glottic cancers—are we justified? J Laryngol Otol. 1994;108:26–9.
38. Harrison DFN. The pathology and management of subglottic cancer. Ann Otol Rhinol Laryngol. 1971;80:6–12.
39. Jones AS, Stell PM. Is laterality important in neck node métastases in head and neck cancer? Clin Otolaryngol. 1991;16:261–5.
40. Fagan JJ, Loock JW. Tracheostomy and peristomal recurrence. Clin Otolaryngol. 1996;21:328–30.
41. Fagan JJ, Kaye PV. Management of the thyroid gland with laryngectomy for cT3 glottic carcinoma. Clin Otolaryngol. 1997;22:7–12.
42. Brazilian Head and Neck Cancer Study Group. End results of a prospective trial on elective lateral neck dissection vs. type III modified radical neck dissection in the management of supraglottic and transglottic carcinomas. Head Neck. 1999;21:694–702.
43. Ferlito A, Rinaldo A. Level I dissection for laryngeal and hypopharyngeal cancer: is it indicated? J Laryngol Otol. 1998;112:438–40.
44. Jesse RH, Ballantyne AJ, Larson D. Radical or modified neck dissection: a therapeutic dilemma. Am J Surg. 1978;136:516–9.
45. Moe K, Wolf GT, Fisher SG, et al. Regional metastasis in patients with advanced laryngeal cancer. Arch Otolaryngol Head Neck Surg. 1996;122:644–8.
46. Bhattacharyya N. The effects of more conservative neck dissections and radiotherapy on nodal yields from the neck. Arch Otolaryngol Head Neck Surg. 1998;124:412–6.
47. Shah JP, Medina JE, Shaha AR, Schantz SP, Marti JR. Cervical lymph node metastasis. Curr Probl Surg. 1993;30:284–1335.
48. Rassekh CH, Johnson JT, Myers EN. Accuracy of intraoperative staging of the NO neck in squamous cell carcinoma. Laryngoscope. 1995;105:1334–6.
49. Kassouf W, Agarwal PK, Herr HW, et al. Lymph node density is superior to TNM nodal status in predicting disease-specific survival after radical cystectomy for bladder cancer: analysis of pooled data from MDACC and MSKCC. J Clin Oncol. 2008;26:121–6.
50. Shrime MG, Bachar G, Lea J, et al. Nodal ratio as an independent predictor of survival in squamous cell carcinoma of the oral cavity. Head Neck. 2009;31:1482–8.
51. Kim SY, Nam SY, Choi SH, Cho KJ, Roh JL. Prognostic value of lymph node density in node-positive patients with oral squamous cell carcinoma. Ann Surg Oncol. 2011;18:2310–7.
52. Ryu IS, Roh JL, Cho KJ, et al. Lymph node density as an independent predictor of cancer-specific mortality in patients with lymph node-positive laryngeal squamous cell carcinoma after laryngectomy. Head Neck. 2015;37(9):1319–25.
53. Künzel J, Mantsopoulos K, Psychogios G, et al. Lymph node ratio is of limited value for the decision-making process in the treatment of patients with laryngeal cancer. Eur Arch Otorrinolaringol. 2015;272(2):453–61.
54. Imre A, Pinar E, Dincer E, et al. Lymph node density in node-positive laryngeal carcinoma: analysis of prognostic value for survival. Otolaryngol Head Neck Surg. 2016;155(5):797–804.
55. Ho AS, Kim S, Tighiouart M, et al. Metastatic lymph node burden and survival in oral cavity cancer. J Clin Oncol. 2017;35(31):3601–9.
56. Ho AS, Kim S, Tighiouart M, et al. Association of quantitative metastatic lymph node burden with survival in hypopharyngeal and laryngeal cancer. JAMA Oncol. 2018;4(7):985–9.
57. Molteni G, Nocini R, Mattioli F, et al. Impact of lymph node ratio and number of lymph node metastases on survival and recurrence in laryngeal squamous cell carcinoma. Head Neck. 2023:1–20. https://doi.org/10.1002/hed.27471.

9 Postoperative Management and Rehabilitation After OPHL

Marco Bonali, Matteo Miglio, Maria Pia Luppi, Davide Dal Molin, and Claudio Melchiorri

9.1 Postoperative Management

Although postsurgical management may vary among different institutions, there are some common topics that characterize patients undergoing Open Partial Horizontal Laryngectomies (OPHLs). Herein, we discuss the management of these postoperative issues.

9.1.1 Tracheotomy vs Tracheostomy

At the end of the OPHL procedure, a tracheotomy is performed. The choice between suturing the trachea to the skin or performing a tracheotomy depends essentially on the possibility to have a 24/24 doctor in the department and on nursing staff experience; in case of accidental decannulation or in case of complications (such as bleeding), the first goal is to secure the airway. Besides, the final goal for these patients is tracheal decannulation.

Different skin incisions for tracheo(s)tomy are codified. Some surgeons prefer to create a separate midline incision in between the sternal notch and the neck incision while others prefer to place the tracheostomy through the midline of the neck incision. The first option may reduce microbial contamination from the tracheostomy tube to the pexy site [1].

M. Bonali · M. Miglio (✉) · M. P. Luppi · C. Melchiorri
Department of Otolaryngology—Head and Neck Surgery, University Hospital of Modena, Azienda Ospedaliero-Universitaria di Modena, Largo del Pozzo, Modena, Italy

D. Dal Molin
Department of Otorhinolaryngology—Head and Neck Surgery, Azienda Ospedaliero Universitaria di Bologna IRCCS, Bologna, Italy

9.1.2 Tracheostomy Tube Management

After surgery, a cuffed tracheostomy tube, which allows breathing only from tracheostomy, is placed. If there are no major contraindications (copiousness of salivary secretions, bleeding, the need for positive-pressure ventilation), the cuff is deflated during the first postoperative day. Around the second or third postoperative day, the tracheostomy tube is replaced with a fenestrated one. In the case of a patient with a tracheotomy, it is important to do this maneuver with an aspirator, the Killian forceps on the one hand, and the cannula with the obturator ready on the other. Once the fenestrated tracheostomy tube is in place, it is essential that the patient learns immediately how to phonate and begin the breathing exercises; this aspect helps to reduce the neoglottic postoperative edema. During the following days, usually around the 4th–fifth-day post-op, the patient starts to use occlusion cap. The latter is adopted at the beginning during the day, then also at the night, and eventually 24/24.

If there isn't the histological diagnosis yet, the patients are discharged with the tracheostomy, as they may undergo adjuvant therapy, depending on tumor staging. Maintaining the tracheostomy is a safety decision to ensure an airway flow, due to the possibility to have mucosal toxicity and adverse reactions caused by chemo- and radiotherapy.

The timing of decannulation is another debated issue regarding swallowing rehabilitation; in some institutions, patients do not begin swallowing exercises until the tracheostomy tube is removed and the stoma is closed.

9.1.3 Nasogastric Tube

Nasogastric tube (NGT) is a medical device that is placed during surgery to enterally feed the patient during postoperative days. The timing of its removal is usually established by the therapist and the ENT surgeon. It's preferable to take it out as soon as possible, because the continuous lying on the crico-arytenoid joint may lead to anchylosis of the joint

F. Mattioli et al. (eds.), *Atlas of Open Partial Horizontal Laryngectomy*, https://doi.org/10.1007/978-3-031-48023-2_9

itself, with a consequent functional impact on the residual larynx. Moreover, it is considered a foreign body that reduces the caliber of the aero-digestive tract.

In case of accidental removal of the feeding tube (e.g., during the first postoperative days), it should be replaced under flexible laryngoscopy guide, to prevent risky maneuver on the pexy region. Other feeding possibilities during the postoperative period are PICC (Peripherally Inserted Central Catheter) or PEG (Percutaneous Endoscopic Gastrostomy).

9.1.4 Generic Postsurgical Management

During hospital stay, the patient is medicated daily basis to prevent complications such as wound infections, peristomitis, pressure lesions, etc.

In addition to this common protocol, a compressive bandage around the neck is applied just for 4–5 days, to reduce the risk of neck swelling.

Desuture is usually done after 10–12 days.

During the first couple of days after decannulation, the tracheotomy is simply closed with compressive medication to heal it by secondary intention. In case of a tracheostomy, it's necessary to perform a plasty of the stoma. It's advisable to use a horizontal mattress suture to evert the skin edges. Throughout the healing period of the stoma, it's essential to avoid an airflow leak from the wound. Therefore, patients are advised to compress the sutured stoma whenever they talk or cough.

In patients undergoing adjuvant radiotherapy or in long-standing tracheostomies, it would be difficult to close the stoma in the outpatient clinic. In these selected cases, the closure of the tracheo-cutaneous fistula is generally performed in the operating room, using local or pedunculated flaps.

9.2 Rehabilitation

Even if OPHLs are conservative surgical techniques, the voice and swallowing functions are modified after the procedure [2]. To have a minimum impact on Quality of Life (QoL), patients need rehabilitation training which begins in the following days after surgery (Fig. 9.1).

Rehabilitation goals include the restoration of airflow through neo-glottis, resulting in faster reduction of postsurgical edema, and the activation of swallowing mechanisms to improve deglutition and reduction of NGT permanence. The removal of this device allows a better arytenoid mobilization, resulting in a restoration of sphincteric function and leading to airway protection and good voice quality [3].

In absence of surgical or medical contraindications, around the fifth postoperative day, patients begin respiration exercises, closing the tracheostomy tube few hours a day, and muscular training. Between the sixth and eighth postoperative days, they start working on swallowing and arytenoid mobilization.

9.2.1 Muscular Training

Muscular training consists of some exercises concerning the main muscular groups involved in speech and swallowing processes, such as head and neck, shoulder, lips, and tongue. Relevance should also be given to the stimulation of pharynx contraction, provoking pharyngeal (or gag) reflex, using a tongue depressor or mouth mirror, and to laryngeal elevation. In fact, after surgery, the relationship between laryngeal elevation and the opening of the upper esophageal sphincter is no longer physiological; therefore, it is important to focus on the stimulus of the elevation of laryngeal residue [4]. Nevertheless, these maneuvers may be limited by the presence of tracheostomy tube.

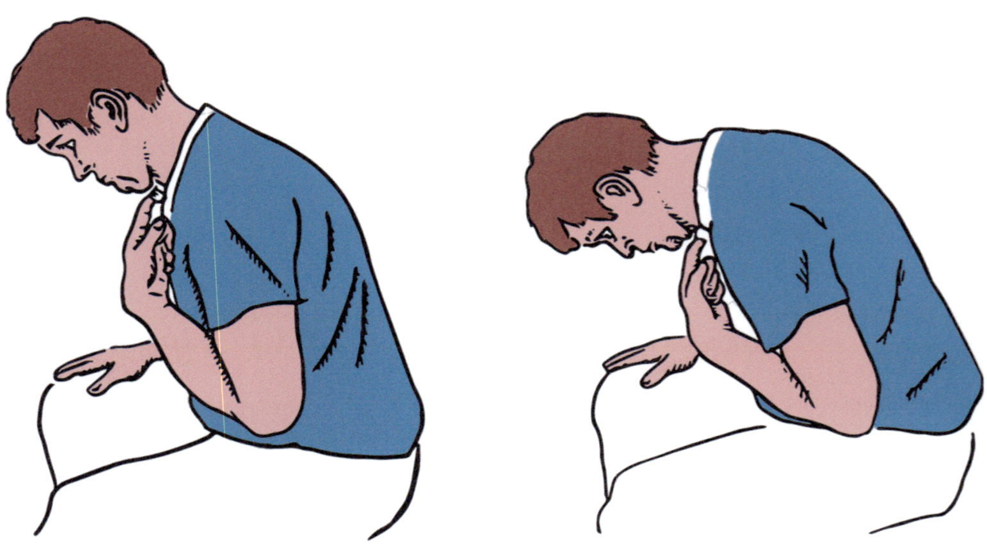

Fig. 9.1 Facilitating postures allow to reinforce the levels of laryngeal closure in order to reduce laryngeal penetrations. The patient tilts the head forward, with the chin close to the sternum. It is sometimes associated with a rotation of the head toward the side of the missing arytenoid in order to protect the respiratory tract, increase the opening of the remaining piriform sinus to receive the food bolus, and promote the ascent of the larynx

9.2.2 Arytenoid Mobilization

Arytenoid mobilization is fundamental to obtain the sphincteric action of neoglottic achieved by approximation of arytenoid cartilage(s) and base of the tongue (together with the epiglottis if preserved). Regarding the sphincteric action, one condition should be mentioned. In OPHL I extended to the base of the tongue (OPHL I + BOT), patients may have more difficulty during swallowing rehabilitation, especially for liquids, due to an imperfect approximation of the structures of the neo-larynx [5]. Therefore, the rehabilitation period could increase and sometimes patients need postoperative injective laryngoplasty to fill this anatomical gap.

Exercises on arytenoid mobilization also play an important role in providing a mucosal source of vibration during airflow passage, useful for phonation.

A couple of exercises that patient should learn are the following [6]:

- Raclage: the patient in sitting position with tracheostomy tube closed by a finger, should perform a slow inspiration followed by a scrape, as loud as possible with mouth open.
- Raclage with vowels: the patient should produce a raclage, followed by a vowel, starting from /a/, then /e/ or /ɛ/ and /o/ or /ɔ/, ultimately, he should try with /i/ and /u/.

9.2.3 Swallowing Rehabilitation

To obtain the best possible functional results, swallowing rehabilitation should be based on 4 key points that enhance each other:

- Facilitating posture.
- Swallowing compensation maneuver.
- Food characteristics.
- Dietary precautions.

9.2.3.1 Facilitating Posture

The facilitating postures are different maneuvers with the aim of promoting laryngeal elevation by shortening neck and facilitate the bolus descent along the digestive tract (Fig. 9.1). Swallowing with the head flexed anteriorly is used when the triggering of the swallowing reflex is delayed; the head flexed laterally promotes the bolus progression along the same side of the flexion; the head rotated, used especially in case of neck dissection and sacrifice of one arytenoid cartilage, determines the closure of ipsilateral piriform sinus and allows the bolus transit contralaterally [6]. Finally, a combination of each posture (head flexed anteriorly and laterally; head rotated and flexed anteriorly; head and chest flexed anteriorly) could be used.

9.2.3.2 Swallowing Compensation Maneuver

Swallowing maneuvers are voluntary behaviors designed to modify the timing and extent of selected phases of oropharyngeal swallowing to minimize the risk of aspiration and protect the airways before, during, and after swallowing. The first facilitating maneuver that is tested by the patient involves the therapist placing one hand behind the patient's neck and the other one on the chin. The patient prepares the bolus, makes an inspiration, and holds the breath; when swallowing begins, the therapist pushes on the head in a postero-anteriorly direction and posteriorly on the chin [7]. In addition, some other maneuvers[1] could be learned by the patient to prevent his/her airway from aspiration/penetration:

(i) *Supraglottic maneuver*. The patient holds his breath lightly, then swallows in apnea, and, at the end of the deglutition act, he coughs.
(ii) *Super-supraglottic maneuver*. The patient holds his breath with more effort than the previous one; then he contracts abdominal muscles, and he proceeds with swallowing action in apnea with abdominal muscles contracted; at the end of the deglutition act, he coughs.
(iii) *Effortful swallow*. The patient applies a great effort with the tongue against the hard palate and maintains the pressure throughout, and a few seconds after the swallowing process.
(iv) *Mendelsohn maneuver*. The laryngeal elevation is prolonged manually for few seconds until the end of swallowing.

The hyoid position is not affected by these breath-holding maneuvers, while the laryngeal elevation depends on contraction of the thyro-hyoid muscle and the cranio-caudal level of the pexy in the neck. In fact, the purpose of these breath-holding maneuvers is an earlier cricopharyngeal opening and a prolonged pharyngeal swallowing which are determined by laryngeal elevation and horizontal traction of the hyoid, responsible for the shortening of the distance between the larynx and hyoid component.

9.2.3.3 Food Characteristic

The first attempts of swallowing are made with saliva, after which first foods are introduced. The choice of the typology of food that could be administered is based on the difficulties highlighted by the patients in swallowing and on the intrinsic characteristics of the food itself [6].

Among them, the most relevant is density (or consistence). Usually, the patients begin with semisolids (i.e., yogurt, mousse, pudding, soft cheese), then semisolids denser (i.e., blended meal), followed by solids (i.e., well-

[1] All these maneuvers are performed closing tracheostomy tube with a finger.

done cooked pasta, boiled vegetables, tender meat—better if steamed—omelet, banana); lastly semi-liquids and liquids (i.e., first fruit smoothies, vegetables soup, then water, tea, infusions). In the case of the latter ones, it could be advisable to start with a teaspoon, then use a tablespoon and only in the end the patients can drink liquids from a glass.

Another aspect to consider is viscosity (or slipperiness). The higher it is, the easier the passage of food will be.

Cohesion and homogeneity are two other food characteristics considered during swallowing rehabilitation; the food needs to remain compact, not to crumble and the bolus needs to be composed by particles of the same size and consistence.

Moreover, food temperature is another feature to consider for improving aero-digestive tract sensitivity of these patients; fresh meals work as a thermoreceptor stimulus.

To enhance the characteristics of food, some additives could be used, such as thickener (i.e., jelly, potato starch, cereal flour), lubricant (i.e., oil, butter, sauces), or thinner (i.e., milk, broth, fruit juice).

9.2.3.4 Dietary Precautions

While taking the meal, it is essential that the patient is in a quiet and silent place, without distractions. He must consume his meal without haste, and he needs to wait until swallowing has taken place before starting the following bite.

The patient is followed by the therapist on a daily basis until he is defined autonomous in swallowing. To define this functional state, it is important to assess if there is or not spillage and piecemeal deglutition. Spillage is defined as bolus falling over the base of the tongue or lower before wash-out; piecemeal deglutition is defined as division of the bolus into two or more swallows successively rather than swallowing the entire bolus in one [8]. These aspects are influenced by a complex sensorimotor integration that coordinates the contraction and inhibition of musculature involved in the swallowing process and determines the sequence of swallowing events. In case of failure of even just one step, swallowing efficiency and safety may be impaired. Efficiency refers to the ability to transfer bolus from the mouth to the stomach without post-swallow pharyngeal residue; inefficient swallowing may lead to nutritional complications. On the other hand, the term safety refers to the ability to transfer the bolus from the mouth to the stomach without penetration or aspiration into the lower airways; the consequences of unsafe swallowing are pulmonary complications, such as aspiration pneumonia.

9.2.4 Voice Rehabilitation

Voice rehabilitation helps to improve also swallowing. It is recommended to perform vocal exercises before the meal to further enhance the arytenoid dynamic. The target of voice rehabilitation is to achieve an arytenoid voice determined by approximation and vibration of structures of the neo-larynx, that is the arytenoid(s) (with or without the epiglottis) with the base of the tongue [9].

It is essential for the patient to learn costodiaphragmatic respiration and to clear aspirated substances; throat clearing (or raclage) is made standing up, with the head slightly bend forward and chin tucked toward the chest to facilitate the retropulsion of the tongue. In the same position, the patient begins setting short and energic vowels using his new voice.

The goal in these patients is to recover a voice as similar as possible to the presurgical one, guaranteeing them the opportunity to converse freely; this result is achieved gradually by making progressively more complex vocal exercises, which need to be done on daily basis.

As mentioned above, the arytenoid voice consists of the vibration of neo-laryngeal structures; therefore, the first phonemes associations include a velar plosive consonant (/k/, /g/), a trill uvular one (/R/), and a vowel (i.e., GRA GRO GRE GRI GRU, KRA KRO KRE KRI KRU). The next step consists of emission of nasal phoneme (/m/) and a vowel such as MA MO ME (MI MU). After that, the patients perform vocal exercises pronouncing dental and labio-dental plosive consonants (/d/), combined to trill one and a vowel. Thereafter, patients try exercises without trill consonants, and eventually, the words are introduced [6]. Firstly, short and energic sounds are produced, and successively exercises with prolonged vowels are performed. The duration of vocalization depends on the patient's phonatory capacity.

References

1. Rizzotto G. Attualità in Oncologia Laringea. XCVII Congresso Nazionale; 2010.
2. Alicandri-Ciufelli M, Piccinini A, Grammatica A, Chiesi A, Bergamini G, Luppi MP, et al. Voice and swallowing after partial laryngectomy: factors influencing outcome. Head Neck. 2013;35(2):214–9.
3. Calcaterra TC, Zwitman DH. Vocal rehabilitation after partial or total laryngectomy. Calif Med. 1972;117(2):12–5.
4. Pizzorni N, Schindler A, Castellari M, Fantini M, Crosetti E, Succo G. Swallowing safety and efficiency after open partial horizontal laryngectomy: a videofluoroscopic study. Cancers. 2019;11(4):549.
5. Webster KT, Samlan RA, Jones B, Bunton K, Tufano RP. Supracricoid partial laryngectomy: swallowing, voice, and speech outcomes. Ann Otol Rhinol Laryngol. 2010;119(1):10–6.
6. Luppi MP, Nizzoli F, Bergamini G, Ghidini A, Palma S. Speech therapy rehabilitation. Acta Italica. 2010;30(5):244–7.
7. Ohmae Y, Logemann JA, Hanson DG, Kaiser P, Kahrilas PJ. Effects of two breath-holding maneuvers on oropharyngeal swallow. Ann Otol Rhinol Laryngol. 1996;105(2):123–31.
8. Schindler A, Pizzorni N, Fantini M, Crosetti E, Bertolin A, Rizzotto G, et al. Long-term functional results after open partial horizontal laryngectomy type IIa and type IIIa: a comparison study: open partial horizontal laryngectomy type IIa and IIIa functional outcomes. Head Neck. 2016;38(S1):E1427–35.
9. Silveira HSL, Simões-Zenari M, Kulcsar MA, Cernea CR, Nemr K. Combined vocal exercises for rehabilitation after supracricoid laryngectomy: evaluation of different execution times. J Voice. 2018;32(6):723–8.

Complication and Dysfunctional Operated Larynx

10

Marco Trebbi, Alfredo Lo Manto, Michael Ghirelli, Aniello Montalbano, and Christopher Fabbri

10.1 Introduction

Open partial horizontal laryngectomies (OPHLs) are a well-established classification system for partial laryngectomies [1].

The decision to perform an OPHL also goes through the knowledge of its complications as well as the possibility of correcting them.

We can divide them into complications related to surgery: hemorrhage, infection, pexy failure, lymphorrhagia, and dysfunctions after surgery: dysphagia, dyspnea, and dysphonia that can impact functional outcomes.

Early postoperative surgical complications of any kind were noted in 11.7% of patients.

10.2 Related to Surgery

10.2.1 Hemorrhage

After laryngeal surgery, the frequency of hemorrhage is around 2%.

The vessels most frequently affected by postoperative hemorrhage are as follows:

- Upper laryngeal pedicles, which are isolated during surgical maneuvers.
- Thyroid vessels mobilized during the suspension of the thyroid gland used to stabilize the pexy anteriorly.
- Internal jugular vein and carotid artery or its principal branches.

The incidence of this complication is greater due to the presence of the following factors: preoperative radiotherapy, infections, necrosis of the skin flap, and salivary fistulas.

Treatment of this complication requires, in most cases, surgical correction.

In case of small bleeding with hematomas, their drainage is recommended to avoid infections and possible skin dehiscences or pexy.

10.2.2 Infection

Post-surgical neck infection was noted in 4.2% of patients, it is the main early postoperative surgical complication. The neck dissection was the only variable that statistically increased the risk for wound infection after OPHL [2].

The risk of wound infection is higher in diabetic patients, in case of poor nutritional status, which must always be assessed before and after surgery.

Prophylactic antibiotic therapy is always performed and continued for at least 3 days postoperatively. This therapy must guarantee an adequate spectrum for GRAM+ and GRAM−.

Isolation of the tracheostomy from the cervical spaces could theoretically reduce the risk of infection; however, studies in this sense do not provide definitive data.

10.2.3 Pexy Failure

The pexy failure is an infrequent complication.

In the literature, the incidence of pexy failure is reported to range from 0.8% to 4.9% [3, 4]. In a large series described by Rizzotto et al., this complication was noted in 4 of 469 cases [5].

Dysphagia, after a partial laryngectomy in a patient without post-operative complications, may indicate detachment of the pexy.

M. Trebbi (✉) · A. Lo Manto · A. Montalbano · C. Fabbri
Otorhinolaryngology Unit, Infermi Hospital of Rimini, Rimini, Italy
e-mail: marco.trebbi@auslromagna.it; aniello.montalbano@auslromagna.it; christopher.fabbri@auslromagna.it

M. Ghirelli
ENT Unit, AUSL Romagna, Ospedale Infermi di Rimini, Rimini, Italy

F. Mattioli et al. (eds.), *Atlas of Open Partial Horizontal Laryngectomy*, https://doi.org/10.1007/978-3-031-48023-2_10

A neck 3D CT scan is a new technology in imaging diagnostics that gives high-definition three-dimensional reconstructions, including multiplanar reformations (MPR) reconstructed from thin axial slices [6]. This technique allows a rupture of the pexy to be confirmed if there is a gap of more than 3 cm between the lower border of the hyoid bone and the cricoid cartilage [7].

Some authors have identified as predisposing factors for detachment of the pexy [8]: Transection of the cricoid arch by sutures, partial resection of the cricoid cartilage, non-ossified cricoid, and the need to relocate a tracheal cannula in an emergency. Other authors have indicated previous laryngeal irradiation as one of the most important risk factors for rupture of the pexy because of osteitis induced on the hyoid bone [3]. To avoid this complication, before doing a pexy, Naudo et al. [2] suggested a mediastinal dissection of the anterior tracheal wall to reduce the tension at the level of the suture line.

Tension-free sutures should be made 1 cm away from the midline at the time of the pexy in the initial surgery to avoid rupture of the pexy [8].

Other factors that can lead to pexy failure are post-surgery bleeding, infections, and poor nutritional status.

10.2.4 Lymphorrhagia

The appearance of a lesion in the lymphatic duct, resulting in a chyle fistula, represents a relatively infrequent complication, mostly the prerogative of neck dissection, where it has an estimated incidence between 1% and 2.5% [1].

Locally, it can lead to delayed wound healing, necrosis, infections, and, above all, it is a predisposing factor for the detachment of pexy or bleeding.

The thoracic duct is sometimes easily seen during dissection, but in other cases, it is smaller or more difficult to isolate. To avoid any possible injury, the surgeon should clamp and ligate all lymphatic vessels. During the dissection of the left IV cervical level, the high-risk region is the distal portion of the internal jugular, always and in any case conducting a careful and bloodless dissection [2].

10.3 Dysfunction

10.3.1 Dysphagia

10.3.1.1 Anatomical Basis of the Swallowing Defect

The swallowing defects after OPHL are correlated to a modification of anatomy and biomechanics of the larynx and its sensitivity.

The anatomical status that most frequently causes dysphagia are as follows [8]:

- Stiffness, reduced motility, or improper movements of the arytenoid/s due to inferior laryngeal nerve damage or a block of the cricoarytenoid joint.
- Reduced pharyngeal sensitivity due to damage to the superior laryngeal nerve [3].
- Mistakes in the pexy construction or pexy detachment: when it occurs, the residual portion of the larynx cannot move upwards and allow satisfactory swallowing.
- Reduced elevation of the neo-larynx (erroneous detachment of the suprahyoid muscles).
- Diffuse idiopathic skeletal hyperostosis syndrome (DISH or Forestier syndrome): elevation of the neo-larynx may be the cause of contact with a previously asymptomatic cervical osteophyte.
- Reduce retropulsion of the lingual base.
- Cicatricial stenosis of the pyriform sinuses.

Causes of dysphagia—Key points
Reduced or no-sensitivity of pharynx and/or neo-larynx
Reduced propulsive efficiency of pharyngeal muscles
Detachment of pexy
Reduced elevation of hyoid bone (deficit of passive opening of upper esophageal sphincter–UES)
Tongue base smoothed out or concave
Reduced motility of arytenoid/s
DISH syndrome
Hypertonic cricopharyngeal muscle
Stenosis/fibrosis of UES

10.3.1.2 Diagnosis of Swallowing Disorders

The instrumental evaluation must allow a diagnostic definition of the symptom by documenting the progression of secretions or bolus in the lower respiratory tract, the presence of signs of penetration (progression up to the vocal cords), or inhalation (progression under the vocal cords). This finding can be used as a clinical severity parameter [4].

Several tools allow the study of swallowing defects:

- **Functional Endoscopic Evaluation of Swallow** (FEES) [5]: It allows evaluation of the morphology, motility, and sensitivity of neo-glottis and the underlying trachea. The endoscopic evaluation also allows identification of the point of penetration in the neoglottic region and comparative evaluation (fundamental is videorecording) of results after revision surgical procedures [6].
  Some authors have defined a dysphagia rating scale in patients with partial laryngectomy [7].
- **Videofluoroscopic:** According to some authors, it is considered the *gold standard* for the evaluation of swallowing disorders allowing an accurate observation of the pharyngolaryngeal and esophageal dynamics [9] (Figs. 10.1, 10.2).
- **3D-Computed Tomography** (3D CT). The CT scan allows a high-resolution three-dimensional reconstruction

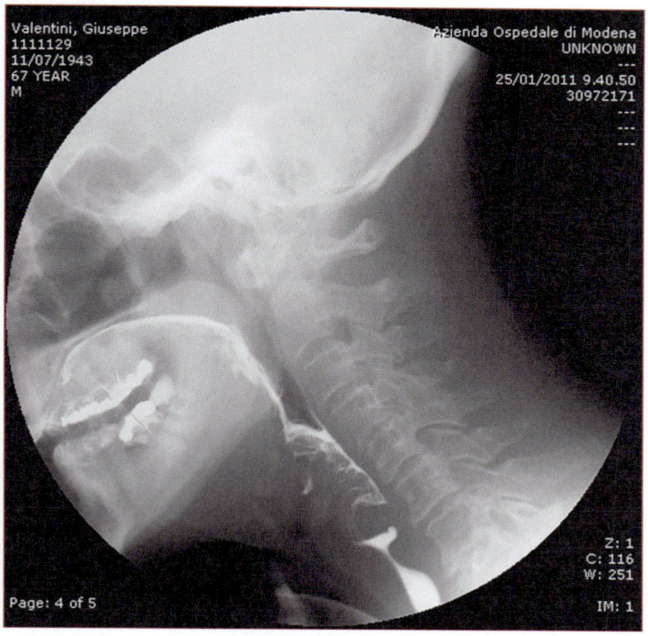

Fig. 10.1 Videofluoroscopy showing cricopharygeal barr meaning a functional upper esophageal dysfuction

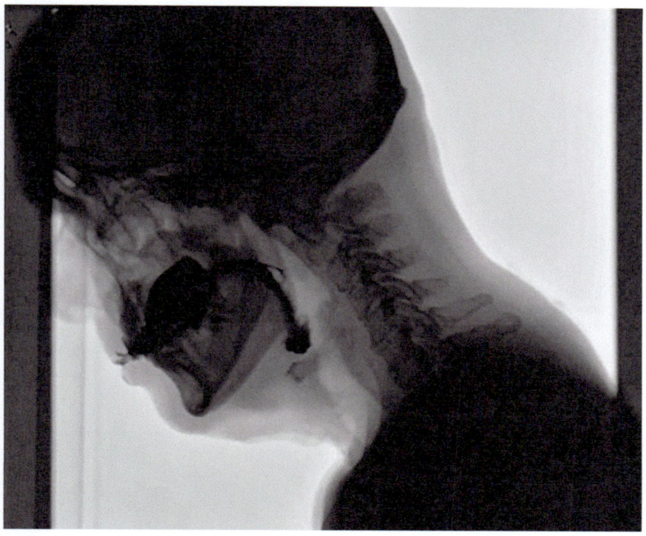

Fig. 10.2 Videofluoroscopy showing an upper esophageal hypertone

from thin-layer sequences of axial sections. In OPHL, the average distance between the body of the hyoid bone and the lower edge of the cricoid cartilage is 11 mm (range between 2 and 30 mm, Fig. 10.3) [10]. Greater distances must suggest a detachment of the pexy.

- **Esophageal manometry.** It allows the evaluation of pressure changes during the progression of the bolus from the oropharynx to the esophagus and any changes in the progression of the sphygmic wave. This biomechanical investigation provides valuable information to study in greater detail the effects of surgical intervention on swallowing, and the results of the therapeutic strategies implemented [11].
- **Subjective evaluations.** Several questionnaires help the clinician in evaluating the discomfort induced by the disorder under examination, including SWAL-QoL [12], MDADI [13], HNPSP [14], UW-QoL [15], and EORTC QLQ [16].

How to diagnose swallowing disorders after OPHL—Key points
Functional endoscopic evaluation of swallow (FEES)
Videofluoroscopic
3D-computed tomography (3D CT)
Esophageal manometry
Subjective evaluations

10.3.1.3 Surgical Rehabilitation of Dysphagia

Cricopharyngeal myotomy (MCF): It is considered useful to reduce the basal tone to speed up the transit of the bolus and shorten the contact time with the laryngeal structures.

Myotomy should be reserved only for patients for whom the presence of gastroesophageal reflux is excluded [1].

MCF can be performed externally or endoscopically with the use of a LASER.

The first LASER myotomy was described in 1994 by Halvorson [17]. The endoscopic approach is the first choice of treatment as it is safe, and efficient, with a low incidence of complications and with an excellent swallowing outcome [18]. The intervention with the traditional technique is performed under general anesthesia and involves a cervicotomy approach, preferably from the left side.

Exposed the posterior wall of the pharynx and cervical esophagus, The myotomy is started superiorly, dividing the inferior constrictor muscle of the pharynx for about 2 centimeters, and then proceeding caudally dividing the muscle fibers of the cricopharyngeal muscle and the cervical esophagus for a length of 4–5 centimeters (Fig. 10.4).

Cricopharyngeal hypertonia can also be corrected by minimally invasive techniques such as botulinum toxin injection, under general anesthesia (endoscopic technique) or local anesthesia, such as percutaneous approach or fibroendoscopic techniques (FEPS–FiberEndoscopic PhonoSurgery). The surgical technique was first described by Schindler [19] in 1994. It consists of the injection of 20–25 units of botulinum toxin into the cricopharyngeal muscle. It is necessary to wait 48 h before obtaining the functional result [20]. Hypertonia should also be revolved using balloon esophageal dilation (Fig. 10.5)

Although the "open" technique predisposes to complications such as recurrent laryngeal nerve injury and pharyngocutaneous fistula, it is indicated in patients with difficult endoscopic exposure or where other surgical procedures are required [21].

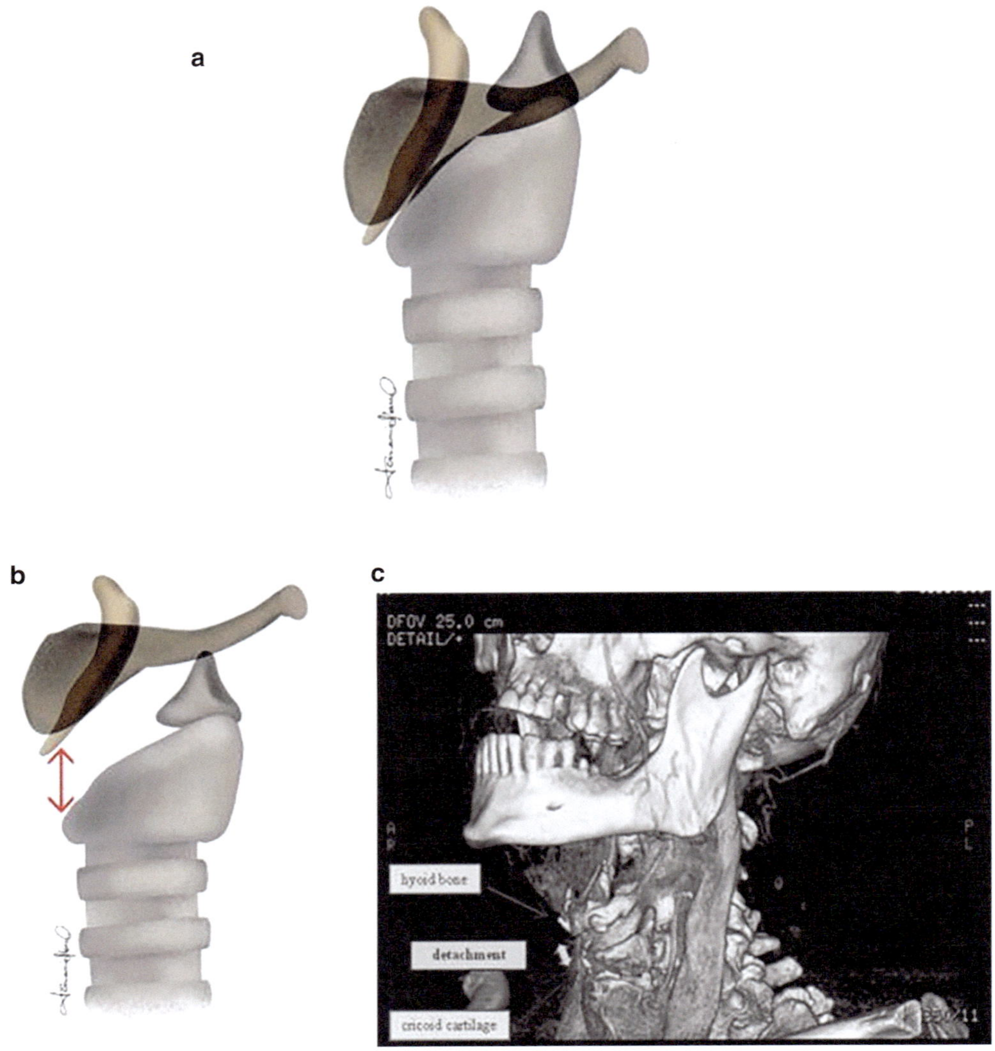

Fig. 10.3 The image shows the correct position of the hyoid bone compared to the cricoid in a case of crycohyoidoepiglottoopexy (CIEP) (**a**); (**b** and **c**) show the pexy failure

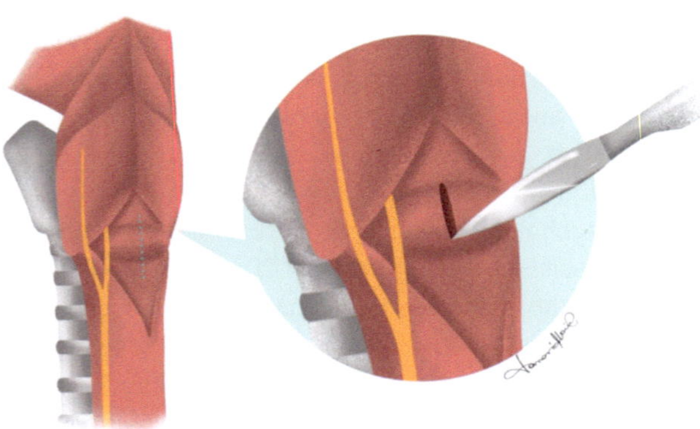

Fig. 10.4 The image shows the point where the myotomy is performed. In the image on the left, the dotted line shows the cranio-caudal extension of the myotomy

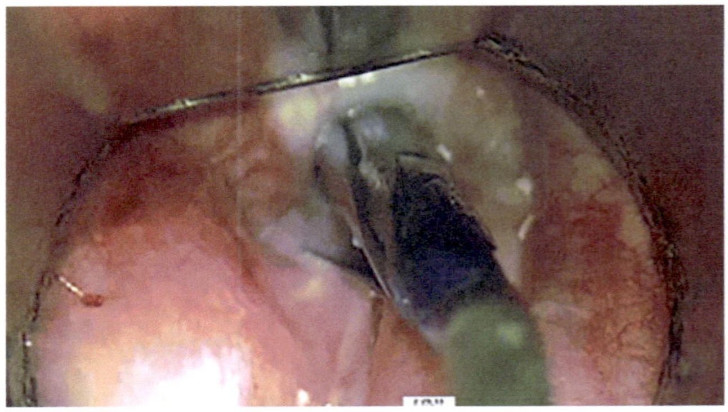

Fig. 10.5 Endoscopica balloon dilation positioning insede a upper esophagea scar tissue related to post ratherpy treatment

Treatment of pharyngoesophageal stenosis: The surgical procedures for the resolution of pharyngoesophageal stenosis include dilation and surgical resections at the level of the stenosis with end-to-end suture of the pharyngeal stumps. However, endoscopic dilation treatment with possible injection of Mitomycin C should be preferred as the invasive surgical approach is at high risk of relapse [21].

Injection laryngoplasty: A neoglottic incompetence can be corrected, first, by injecting material into the neoglottic region, thanks to an injection laryngoplasty [22, 23].

When the ariteno-epiglottic or ariteno-lingual opposition does not allow a complete closure of the neoglottic lumen, there is a neoglottic insufficiency with a variable impact on phonation and swallowing. The most frequently used materials are hyaluronic acid (absorbable) [24], autologous fat (absorbable) [1], calcium hydroxyapatite (Renú® Voice injectable implant) [25], polydimethylsiloxane (Vox-implant®—not resorbable) [26]. The choice of material is not easy. The optimal characteristics to obtain the best functional results are as follows:

- Tolerability.
- Biomechanical and rheological characteristics compatible with the site where the material is infiltrated.
- Durable and resistant to resorption or migration.
- Stability over time adequate for the purposes of the intervention.

The injection points are chosen during the endoscopic diagnostic phase and according to the material chosen (Fig. 10.6) [27]. A preliminary FEES is essential for the site injection plane. It could be a useful picture of the new aditus drawing injection points for planning the surgery.

Vox-implant® is widely used to correct dysphagia problems after partial laryngectomy. It is often a multistep procedure; other corrective laryngoplasty can be performed to progressively correct possible residual defects. Moreover, it can sometimes be associated with open surgery (pexy revision, surgery of cervical osteophytes, and compaction of base of tongue) (Figs. 10.7, 10.8, 10.9, 10.10, 10.11, 10.12). Long-term functional results are described by authors in a long follow-up study to confirm that Vox-implant laryngoplasty is safe and effective treatment in long term (mean follow-up of 8 years) [28].

Several authors report an increased uptake of 2-fluoro-2-deoxy-D-glucose (FDG) in PET-TC: this is important to be remembered in cancer follow-up to exclude a relapse [29].

Pexy revision surgery: Pexy represents a fundamental moment in the reconstruction of the neolarynx. Several authors agree that three separate points (Vycryl II or PDS 1) are required to best achieve a pexy, with the central one surrounding the cricoid cartilage and the hyoid bone and crossing the epiglottis (if present), less than 3 cm away from the base of the tongue (Fig. 10.13). The cricoid ring should be pushed posterior to the hyoid bone in the case of OPHL 2A to ensure patency of the neolarynx and anteriorly in OPHL 2B to better protect the neoglottis [30, 31].

In all cases in which there is a neoglottic insufficiency that cannot be resolved with speech therapy or injection and

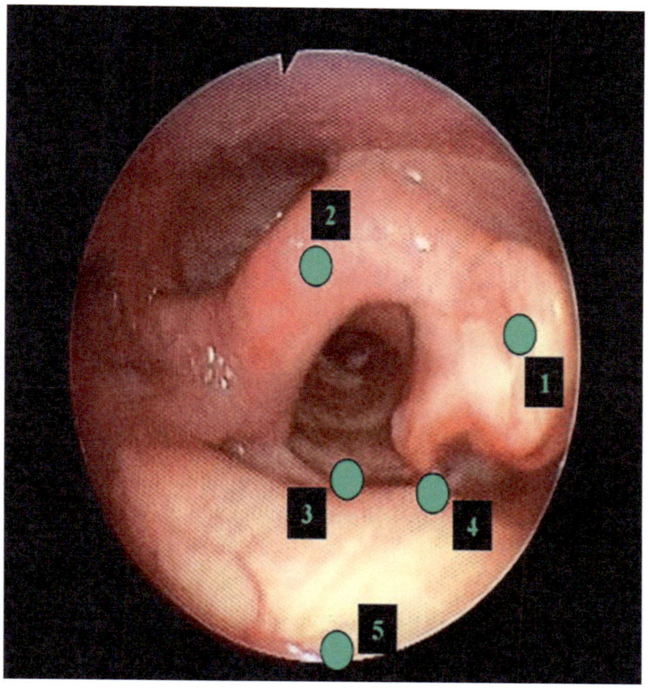

Fig. 10.6 Injection points in the neo-glottis and materials indicated: (1) arytenoid (hyaluronic acid); (2) residual mucous cap upon removal of the arytenoid (hyaluronic acid, Radiesse®, Vox®); (3) anterior part of the cricoid ring (Vox®, Radiesse®); (4) lateral part of the cricoid ring (Vox®, Radiesse®); (5) base of the tongue/pre-epiglottic space (autologous fat, Vox®, Radiesse®)

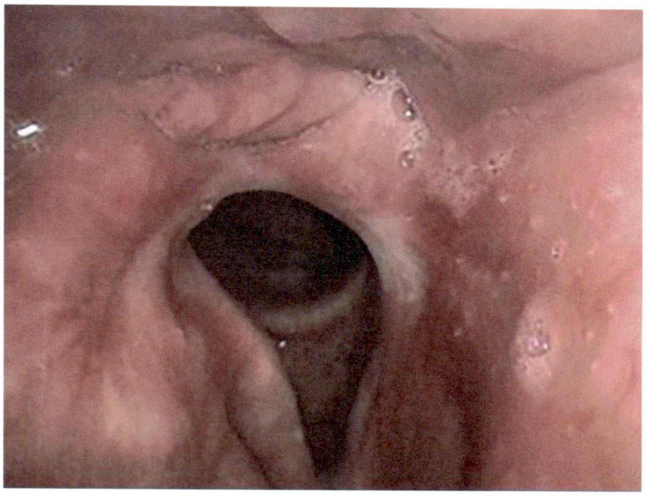

Fig. 10.7 Neoglottis gap; the lack of arytenoid wall cause food penetration in the left side

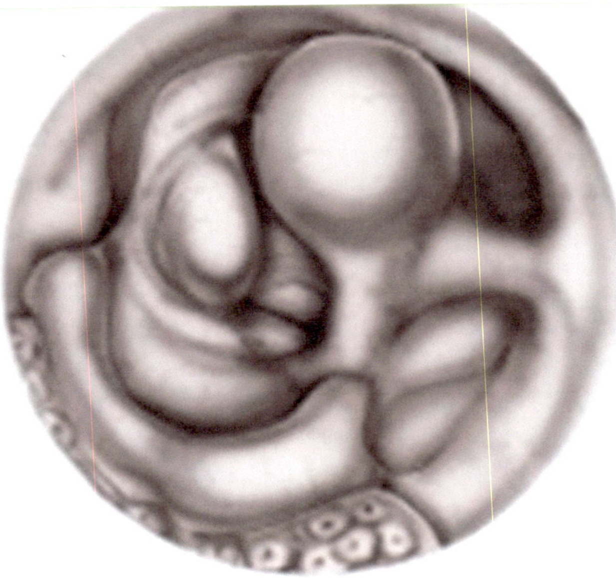

Fig. 10.8 A schematic draw, explaining where inject the material to restore the neoglottic gap

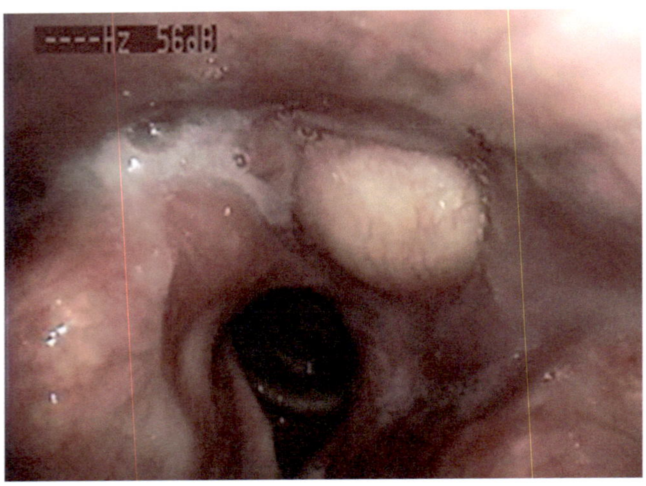

Fig. 10.9 Vov implant injection to restore the aryteoid left wall, helping the food to go through pyriform sinus into the esophagus

when the CT shows the collapse of the cricohyoid suture, revision of the pexy must be considered, possibly using an "8 shaped" suture which favors the correct alignment of the abutments (Fig. 10.14). In our experience, an early revision, allowing the correct repositioning of the hyoid and cricoid, greatly accelerates the recovery of feeding (Fig. 10.15).

How to resolve post OPHL dysphagia—Key points	
A. Open surgery	B. Endoscopic surgery
Reoperation for detachment of pexy	Injection laryngoplasty
Compaction of the base of the tongue	Laser myotomy of cricopharyngeal muscles
Surgery on cervical osteophytes	Botox in cricopharyngeal muscle
Myotomy of cricopharyngeal muscles	Esophageal dilation

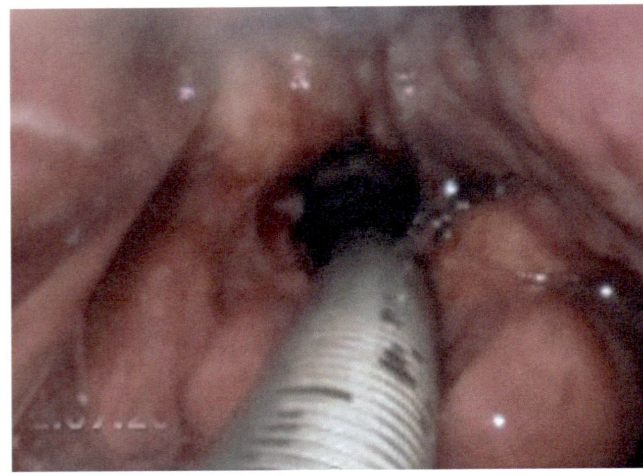

Fig. 10.10 A tongue base concavity after OPHL Type 2b; the distance between base tongue ad arytenois is too far

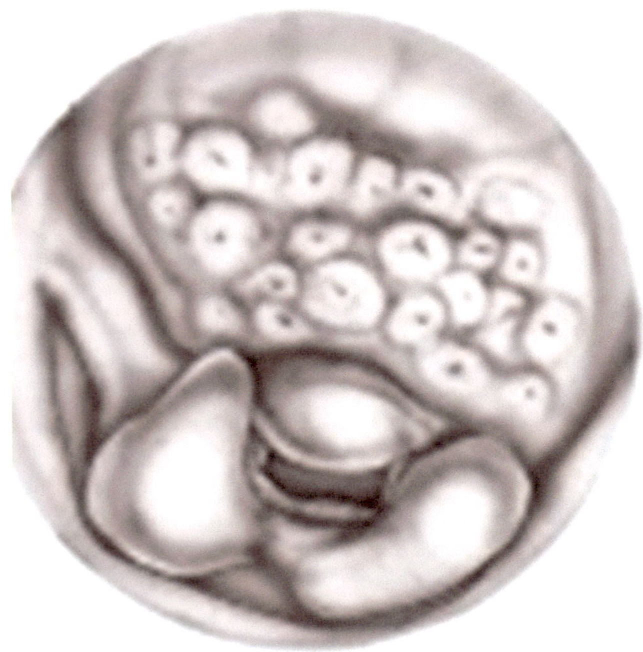

Fig. 10.11 A schematic draw, explain where inject the material to restore the bae of the tongue gap

10.3.2 Dyspnea

Severe dyspnea, however, is rarely reported as a complication following OPHL in the literature. The mean time to decannulation is 7 to 9 days. The risk of stenosis is higher in OPHL 3 due to the lack of the cricoid ring which is of fundamental importance in the maintenance of neoglottic patency [2, 32]. Decannulation failure at this point should prompt further evaluation [33] (Fig. 10.16).

Dehiscence of the epiglottic pexy during OPHL2 without disruption of the cricohyoidopexy is also possible. This com-

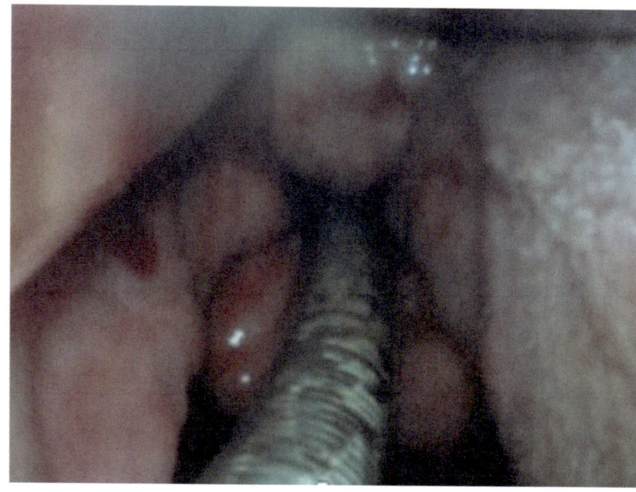

Fig. 10.12 Tongue base concavity filled with vox implant; the distance between tongue and arytenoid is reduced. The presence of orotharcheal tube help the surgeron to understand how much neoglottic space

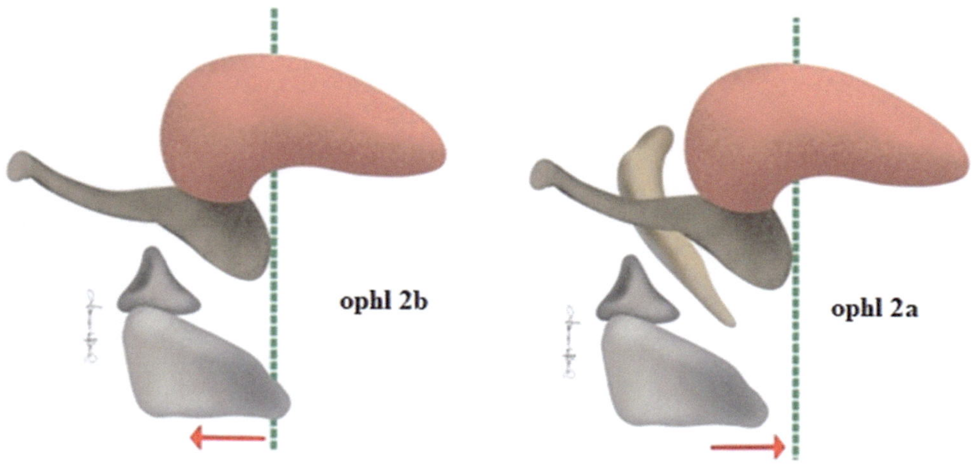

Fig. 10.13 Correct positioning of cricoid and hyoid bone in case of OPHL2a and OPHL2b

plication likely results from the inadequate placement of the sutures through the epiglottis at the time of the pexy (transmucosal way). Dehiscence of the epiglottic pexy will be evident on fiberoptic laryngoscopy, which shows posterior prolapse of the epiglottis that will create airway obstruction with respiration. A possible treatment is surgical revision of the pexy or transoral resection of the epiglottis [31].

Arytenoid edema after OPHL is not uncommon and presents as dyspnea and a delay in decannulation. The usual treatment involves systemic or inhaled steroids. In the absence of anatomic defects, conservative management with steroids should result in edema resolution. Carbon dioxide laser reduction of the edematous area can be employed in selected cases [31, 33].

Airway granulomas after OPHL have long been described in the literature. They occur when chronic inflammation and a foreign body reaction lead to the formation of an organized collection of macrophages. Laryngeal granulomas have been extensively described after prolonged intubation, external laryngeal trauma, and placement of polytetrafluoroethylene implants [28, 34]. We do recommend proton-pump inhibitors (PPIs) in all OPHL cases to prevent inflammation at the reconstruction site.

Tracheal stenosis, with breathing difficulties may require further medical and/or surgical treatments.

10.3.3 Dysphonia

Dysphonia is not a real complication but a consequence of this type of intervention. In OPHL type I, the voice is produced by the vibration of the vocal cords and is analyzed by:

- Objective acoustic evaluation: Jitter—Shimmer—maximum phonatory time (MPT).
- Perceptual evaluation: GRBAS-scale.
- Voice self-assessment: Voice Handicap Index 10.

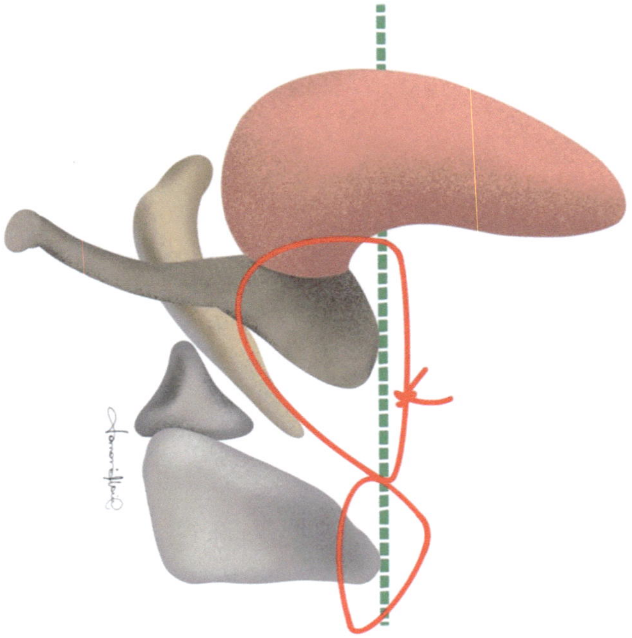

Fig. 10.14 "8 shaped" suture

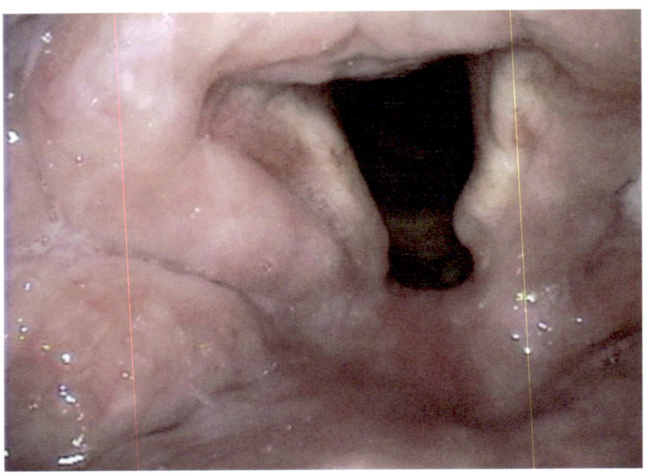

Fig. 10.15 Type 1 ophl showing a huge gap between vocal fold and base of the tongue. This situation cannot be resolved by injection laryngoplasty. A revision of pexy is resquire

In OPHL types II and III, there is a replacement voice that must be rehabilitated through speech therapy. Some authors suggest PROEL as a rehabilitation method. The perceptual evaluation scale is described by Moerman et al. in 2006 [35] . In cases of poor/insufficient voice quality even after rehabilitation therapy, especially when neoglottic insufficiency is diagnosed with an adequate laryngostroboscopic work-up, it is possible to surgically facilitate the neoglottic closure and vibration through injection laryngoplasty through a transoral microscopic or transnasal fiberendoscopic approach.

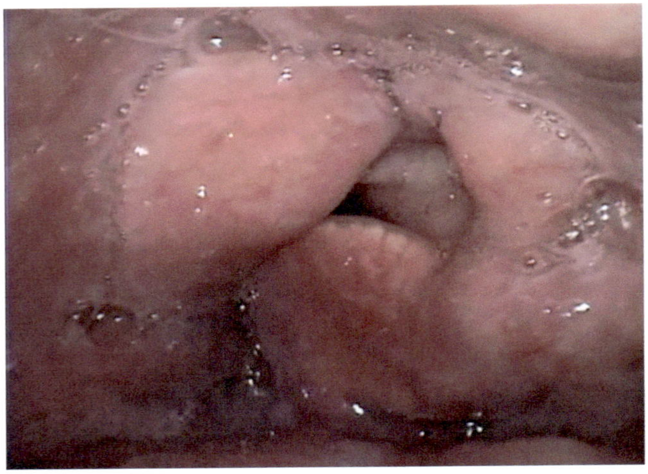

Fig. 10.16 A noglottis stenosis caused by an epliglottis slipping inside the lumen

10.4 Conclusions

Open partial horizontal laryngectomy (OPHL) is a well-known organ-preserving surgery technique used for the treatment of early or locally advanced laryngeal tumors. The most frequent complications are dysphagia and aspiration pneumonia. FEES and videofluoroscopy are useful tools to address the diagnosis.

A rigorous surgical technique represents the best way to prevent complications, and the surgeon who performs this type of surgery must be able to manage any complications.

References

1. De Gier HHW, Bruning PF, Theo Gregor R, et al. Systematicapproach to the treatment of chylous leakage after neck dissection. Head Neck. 1996;18(4):347–51.
2. Gunnlaugsson CB, Iannettoni MD, Yu B, et al. Management of chyle fistula utilizing thoracoscopic ligation of the thoracic duct. ORL. 2004;66(3):148–54.
3. Bastian RW, Riggs LC. Role of sensation in swallow function. Laringoscope. 1999;109(12):1974–7.
4. Logemann JA. Swallowing disorders. Best Pract Res Clin Gastroenterol. 2007;21(4):563–73.
5. ASHA Special interest division 13, Swallowing and swallowing disorders. 1998.
6. Pizzorni N, Schindler A, Castellari M, et al. Swallowing safety and efficiency after open partial horizontal laryngectomy: a videofluoroscopic study. Cancer. 2019;11(4):549.
7. Pizzorni N, Crosetti E, Santambrogio E, et al. The penetratior-aspiration scale: adaptation to open partial laryngectomy and reliability analysis. Dysphagia. 2020;358(2):261–71.
8. Ricci Maccarini A, Stacchini M, Salsi D, et al. Surgical rehabilitation of dysphagia after partial laryngectomy. Act Otorhinolarigol Ital. 2007;27:294–8.
9. Martin-Harris B, Jones B. The videofluorographic swallowing study. Phys Med Rehabil Clin N Am. 2008;19(4):769–8.

10. Bely-Toueg N, Halimi P, Laccourreye O, et al. Normal Laryngeal CT Findings after Supracricoid Partial Laryngectomy. Am J Neuroradiol. 2001;22(10):1872–80.
11. Cock C, Omari T. Diagnosis of swallowing disorders: how we interpret pharyngeal manometry. Curr Gastroenterol Rep. 2017;19(3):11.
12. McHorney CA, Robbins J, Lomax K, et al. The SWAL-QOL and SWAL-CARE outcomes tool for oropharyngeal dysphagia in adults: III. Documentation of reliability and validity. Dysphagia. 2002;17(2):97–11.
13. Chen AY, Frankowski R, Bishop-Leone J, et al. The development and validation of a dysphagia-specific quality-of-life questionnaire for patients with head and neck cancer: the M. D. Anderson dysphagia inventory. Arch Otolaryngol Head Neck Surg. 2001;127(7):870–6.
14. List MA, D'Antonio LL, Cella DF, et al. The Performance Status Scale for Head and Neck Cancer Patients and the Functional Assessment of Cancer Therapy-Head and Neck Scale. A study of utility and validity. Cancer. 1996;77(11):2294–301.
15. Weymuller EA Jr, Alsarraf R, Yueh B, et al. Analysis of the performance characteristics of the University of Washington Quality of Life instrument and its modification (UW-QOL-R). Arch Otolaryngol Head Neck Surg. 2001;127(5):489–93.
16. Wójtowicz JG, Wierzbicka M, Szyfter W. Usefulness of questionnaire EORTC QLQ C-30 and EORTC QLQ H&N C-35 in assessment of quality of life before surgical treatment in patients with head and neck cancer. Otolaryngol Pol. 2001;55(6):627–34.
17. Halvorson DJ, Kuhn FA. Transmucosal cricopharyngeal myotomy with the potassium-titanyl-phosphate laser in the treatment of cricopharyngeal dysmotility. Ann Otol Rhinol Laryngol. 1994;103(3):173–7.
18. Dale OT, Mackeith S, Burgess CA, et al. Functional outcomes following endoscopic lasercricopharyngeal myotomy with mucosal repair. Eur Arch Otorrinolaringol. 2014;271(6):1631–4.
19. Schneider I, Thumfart WF, Pototschnig C, et al. Treatment of dysfunction of the cricopharyngeal muscle with botulinum A toxin: introduction of a new, non-invasive method. Ann Otol Rhinol Laryngol. 1994;103:31–5.
20. Moerman MBJ. Cricopharyngeal Botox injection: indications and techniques. Curr Opin Otolaryngol Head Neck. 2006;14:431–43.
21. Duvillard C, Ballester M, Romanet P. Pharyngeal stenosis: treatment by resection end to end anastomosis. Ann Otolaryngol Chir Cervicofac. 2003;120(1):45–8.
22. Bergamini G, Presutti L, Molteni G. Injection Layngoplasty. Springer; 2015.
23. Bergamini G, Alicandri-Ciufelli M, Molteni G, et al. Therapy of unilateral vocal fold paralysis with polydimethylsiloxane injection laryngoplasty: our experience. J Voice. 2010;24(1):119–25.
24. Alaskarov E, Öztürk Ö, Batıoğlu-Karaaltın A, et al. Functional outcomes of the hyaluronic acid injections in patients who underwent partial laryngectomy. J Voice. 2020:S0892-1997(20)30240-X.
25. Bryant L, Peak W. Use of injectable hydroxyapatite in the secondary setting to restore glottic competence after partial laryngectomy with arytenoidectomy. Ann Otol Rhinol Laryngol. 2004;113(8):618–22.
26. Mattioli F, Fernandez IJ, Bassano E, et al. Surgical rehabilitation of swallowing with polydimethylsiloxane injections after open partial horizontal laryngectomy: long-term functional results and quality of life. Head Neck. 2021;43(4):1161–73.
27. Ricci Maccarini A, Stacchini M, Salsi D, et al. Surgical rehabilitation of dysphagia after partial laryngectomy. Acta ORL Ital. 2007;27:294–8.
28. Levitan N, Dowlati A, Remick SC. Rates of initial and recurrent thromboembolic disease among patients with malignancy versus those without malignancy. Risk analysis using Medicare claims data. Medicine (Baltimore). 1999;78:285–91.
29. Piccinini A, Alicandri-Ciuffelli M, Ghidini A, et al. FDG-PET/TC appearance of injected silicone particles (VOX Implants®) in head and neck tissues. Acta Biomed. 2015;86(3):283–9.
30. Laudadio P, Presutti L, Dall'olio D, et al. Supracricoid larygectomiesa: long-term oncological and functional results. Acta Otolaryngol. 2006;126:640–9.
31. Rombaux P, Hamoir M, Plouin-Gaudon I, et al. Obstructive sleep apnea syndrome after reconstructive laryngectomy for glottic carcinoma. Eur Arch Otorrinolaringol. 2000;257:502–6.
32. Laccourreye H, Laccourreye O, Weistein G, et al. Supracricoid laryngectomy with cricohyoidopexy: a partial laryngeal procedure for selected supraglottic and transglottic carcinomas. Laryngoscope. 1990;100:735–41.
33. Loyo M, Espinoza S, Giraud P, et al. Early and severe dyspnea after supracricoid partial laryngectomy. Ann Otol Rhinol Laryngol. 2014;123(1):53–7.
34. Rivera-Serrano CM, Smit LJ. Laryngeal Teflon granuloma: endoscopy, laryngeal videostroboscopy, and CT imaging. Ear Nose Throat J. 2011;90:E25–6.
35. Moerman M, Martens JP, Crevier-Buchman L, et al. The INFVo perceptual rating scale for substitution voicing: development and reliability. Eur Arch Otorrinolaringol. 2006;263(5):435–9.

Salvage OPHL After Transoral LASER Microsurgery/(Chemo)Radiotherapy

11

Erika Crosetti, Martina Tascone, Giulia Arrigoni, and Giovanni Succo

The widespread use of primary organ-preservation protocols for the treatment of early-stage malignant laryngeal tumors (LSCC) made salvage surgery a controversial topic.

The recurrence rates after the failure of primary non-surgical treatments have been reported to range between 9% and 21% in T1 glottic squamous cell carcinoma (SCC) and 28–37% in T2 glottic carcinomas [1, 2], whereas for supraglottic cancer, the failure rates are 24–30% and 25–45% for T1 and T2 lesions, respectively [3, 4]. Disease recurrence after primary non-surgical therapy usually occurs within 2 years from treatment, presenting more frequently as advanced tumors.

Recurrent LSCC treatment represents a challenge for surgeons. The early endoscopic diagnosis of the recurrence is sometimes difficult for the presence of chronic laryngeal inflammation and fibrosis, resulting in a high number of false negative biopsies [5]. Recurrent and persistent LSCC after radiotherapy is generally undifferentiated, characterized by more aggressive growth patterns (infiltrative with multiple foci), a tendency to extra laryngeal extension, and more frequently present intravascular and perineural invasion than primary tumors [5].

The superficial recurrences are easily diagnosed with the endoscopic work-up, whose sensitivity is enhanced using bio-endoscopic tools (NBI, Autofluorescence endoscopy, HD SPIES endoscopy). On the contrary, submucosal recurrences are more difficult to identify, because the tumor could grow submucosally within the laryngeal deep spaces, without endoscopic signs, masked by post-treatment scar tissue.

Moreover, the radiological exams available (CT-scan and MRI) are characterized by a low specificity after treatment, especially radiotherapy [6].

MRI, due to its high tissue contrast resolution, could be considered a valuable tool in the radiological follow-up of pre-treated patients (TLM: transoral laser microsurgery or RT), especially if surface coils are used, providing a very high signal over a small field of view (limited to 5 cm), but sufficient to include the larynx.

Moreover, the enhancement does not provide valuable information about the malignancy of the lesions, because a variable grade of enhancement is present in scars, inflammatory edema, and granulation tissue. Furthermore, the enhancement strongly depends on the type of sequence and the scan timing after the contrast media administration, as shown by dynamic contrast enhancement MRI studies [7].

These aspects make difficult the correct re-staging of these tumors.

For these reasons, the standard treatment for recurrent LSCC after the failure of primary non-surgical protocols/primary transoral laser microsurgery is the total laryngectomy (TL).

While the role of salvage open partial laryngectomies after non-surgical primary approaches to LSCC have failed is well documented, it has yet to be established in cases of failed TLM. This is presumably due to the lack of oncological studies on large cohorts of patients with LSCC recurring after primary TLM. From the data in Literature, many Authors suggest a second TLM or RT for early-stage recurrences, reserving TL in advanced cases [4, 8–10].

In Literature, salvage TL for early-stage LSCC (T1/T2) has been reported to ensure cancer control in 75% of patients [11], with a 5-year OS rate of 43% to 55% if considering all stages combined [12].

In 1950, Hofmann-Saguez [13], first reported a "subtotal conservative laryngectomy," in a patient with recurrent laryngeal carcinoma after RT who refused TL.

E. Crosetti (✉)
ENT Department Head and Neck Cancer Unit, San Giovanni Bosco Hospital, Torino, Italy

M. Tascone · G. Arrigoni
Otorhinolaryngology Department—Head Neck Cancer Unit, San Giovanni Bosco Hospital, Turin, Italy

G. Succo
ENT Department Head Neck Cancer Unit, San Giovanni Bosco Hospital, Torino, Italy

Oncology Department, University of Turin, Turin, Italy

F. Mattioli et al. (eds.), *Atlas of Open Partial Horizontal Laryngectomy*, https://doi.org/10.1007/978-3-031-48023-2_11

11.1 Oncological Outcomes

Several studies have reported the clinical significance of salvage OPHLs (in most cases, however, the salvage procedure consisted of supracricoid partial laryngectomy) for early recurrences (yrcT1–2) of LSCC and selected cases of yrcT3 tumors after RT failure [14].

Considering recurrences after RT, Piazza et al. [12] reported a DSS at 5 years of 95% and an LPR of 75%, for endoscopic surgery in early cases, and of 100% and 83%, respectively, for open partial laryngectomy.

Pellini et al. [15], reported a multi-institutional retrospective analysis in 78 consecutive patients treated by OPHLs for the recurrence of glottic-supraglottic cancer after RT, which demonstrated an OS at 3 and 5 years of 85.2% and 81.8%, respectively, and a DFS at 3 and 5 years of 95.5%.

Similarly, Holsinger et al. [16] reported that in recurrent LSCCs after RT, loco-regional control was obtained in 86.7% of patients with TL and 84.4% of patients after conservation surgery.

In 2019, Bertolin et al. [17] reviewed the clinical charts of 70 recurrent LSCC patients after primary RT failure undergoing salvage OPHL; the final LC, OS, DSS, and LFS were 87%, 75%, 87%, and 91%, respectively. Their results revealed similar DSS between OPHL type II and III, although the latter had worse OS. The Authors concluded that the advanced T stage (yrcT3-4a) and the neck status (yrcN+) were negatively related to prognosis and could be considered the most informative pre-operative parameters to predict the success of salvage OPHL. Moreover, in the present series, only in 19 cases (27%), a pathologically extra laryngeal tumor extension (yrpT4a) was proven, and a significantly low rate of regional recurrences (none with extranodal extension) was reported (2 cases, 2%).

From the data in the Literature [17, 18], it emerges that younger patients (< 65 years old) showed a trend toward a worse prognosis if compared with elderly patients, probably due to the more aggressive behavior of the tumor.

Regarding the use of OPHLs for recurrences after TLM, the data in Literature are poor and in very small samples of patients [18–20]. The most important experience is the one of Lucioni et al. (62 patients) [21]. The Authors found an OS and DSS both of 82% and a loco-regional control rate and an ultimate organ preservation rate of 82% and 70%, respectively. The patient's age and the recurrence's T classification did not correlate with the second recurrence rate (SRR), DFS, or laryngeal preservation rate (LPR). In this study, the statistical analysis showed that patients who had primary bilateral cordectomy in two stages tended to have a significantly higher SRR and shorter DFS.

Although a planned two-stage cordectomy is considered a safe approach, there is a paucity of Literature on the prognostic relevance of a bilateral cordectomy scheduled in two stages. The present results suggest that two-stage primary bilateral cordectomy may represent a negative prognostic factor (in terms of SRR) for salvage OPHL after the failure of primary TLM, so TL as a first salvage approach should be considered in such cases.

Regarding the involvement of surgical margins, many studies have shown that this aspect represents a negative prognostic factor [22–24]. For this reason, when performing salvage OPHL, it is mandatory to carry out frozen sections of resection margins, as well as primary surgery, although it could be more problematic than in naive patients [25]. The status of surgical margins and the perineural and vascular invasions should be kept in mind during follow-up to identify those patients with higher risk who may benefit from a closer follow-up to recognize further recurrences soon after surgery that still could be managed with TL.

11.2 Functional Outcomes

Regarding functional outcomes after salvage OPHLs, the post-operative complications rate ranges from 15% to 67% [11–13, 17, 25], whereas the perioperative mortality ranges from 0% to 13% [11, 12, 15, 17, 26–28]. Moreover, the incidence of major postoperative complications seems comparable with that of salvage TL (41.2% for previous chemoradiotherapy, 29.4% for previous RT) [29].

The most frequently reported complications include delayed wound healing, infections, fistula formation, and aspiration pneumonia (that can lead to the need for TL) occurring in up to 25% of cases.

Other less common complications cited include granuloma formation, perichondritis, and surgical emphysema or laryngeal stenosis/edema, with the need for a second transoral laser revision [16, 17, 29, 30].

The reported rate of TL for functional failure ranges between 0% and 10% [11, 27, 31–34].

The correct indications for a conservative surgery for salvage, however, still represent a matter of debate. A correct re-staging of the recurrence is an essential pre-requisite for the success of the salvage treatment.

OPHLs can be considered for salvage after RT/TLM failure in selected patients when proper selection criteria are adopted. Indications and contraindications are the same as partial laryngectomies performed for primary LSCC.

In the choice of the therapeutic option (between OPHL and TL), we must keep in mind not only tumor-related factors (clinical stage) but also the patient's general conditions, medical comorbidities, and acceptable pulmonary and swallowing functions.

Salvage surgical options should be discussed with the patient, and the willingness to accept a potentially lengthy rehabilitation must be considered before performing an OPHL.

In general, the trend is toward clinical understaging of the recurrence after RT, which could be related to the previously mentioned unpredictable patterns of local relapse. An integrated diagnostic work-up with the use of state-of-the-art imaging is mandatory in these cases.

Nevertheless, the patient should be prepared for a TL and the surgical staff should have obtained informed consent for the procedure.

It would be helpful for the surgeon, however, to identify some clinical or pathological factors that could predict a higher risk of failure for salvage OPHL to recognize those patients who may, respectively, benefit from TL as first-line salvage treatment or a closer follow-up to early detect further recurrences.

References

1. Jose B, Calhoun DL, Mohammed A. Recurrences after irradiation in early vocal cord cancer with literature review. J Surg Oncol. 1984;27:224–7.
2. DeSchyver A. Radiotherapy of laryngeal cancer. General principles and results in T1 and T2 cases. Acta Otolrhinolaryngol Belg. 1992;46:187–95.
3. Greisen O, Carl J, Pedersen MA. Consecutive series of patients with laryngeal carcinoma treated by primary irradiation. Acta Oncol. 1997;36:279–82.
4. Bataini JP, Brumin F. Early and moderately advanced cancers of supraglottic larynx and their management by radiotherapy. In: Kagan AR, Miles J, editors. Head and neck oncology: clinical management. New York, NY: Pergamon; 1989. p. 69–82.
5. Zbären P, Nuyens M, Curschmann J, Stauffer E. Histologic characteristics and tumor spread of recurrent glottis carcinoma: analysis on whole-organ sections and comparison with tumor spread of primary glottic carcinomas. Head Neck. 2007;29:26–32.
6. Goodwin WJ Jr. Salvage surgery for patients with recurrent squamous cell carcinoma of the upper aerodigestive tract: when do the ends justify the means? Laryngoscope. 2000;110:1–18.
7. Ravanelli M, Farina D, Rizzardi P, Botturi E, Prandolini P, Mangili S, Peretti G, Nicolai P, Maroldi R. MR with surface coils in the follow-up after endoscopic laser resection for glottic squamous cell carcinoma: feasibility and diagnostic accuracy. Neuroradiology. 2013;55(2):225–32. https://doi.org/10.1007/s00234-012-1128-3.
8. Roedel RM, Matthias C, Wolff HA, Christiansen H. Repeated transoral laser microsurgery for early and advanced recurrence of early glottic cancer after primary laser resection. Auris Nasus Larynx. 2010;37(3):340–6.
9. Canis M, Ihler F, Martin A, Matthias C, Steiner W. Transoral laser microsurgery for T1a glottic cancer: review of 404 cases. Head Neck. 2015;37(6):889–95.
10. Ansarin M, Santoro L, Cattaneo A, et al. Laser surgery for early glottic cancer: impact of margin status on local control and organ preservation. Arch Otolaryngol Head Neck Surg. 2009;135(4):385–90.
11. Schwaab G, Mamelle G, Lartigau E, et al. Surgical salvage treatment of T1/T2 glottic carcinoma after failure of radiotherapy. Am J Surg. 1994;168:474–5.
12. Philippe Y, Espitalier F, Durand N, Ferron C, Bardet E, Malard O. Partial laryngectomy as salvage surgery after radiotherapy: oncological and functional outcomes and impact on quality of life. A retrospective study of 20 cases. Eur Ann Otorhinolaryngol Head Neck Dis. 2014;131:15–9.
13. Hofmann-Saguez MR. Conservative subtotal laryngectomy. Ann Otolaryngol. 1950;67:811–6.
14. Laccourreye O, Weinstein G, Naudo P, Cauchois R, Laccourreye H, Brasnu D. Supracricoid partial laryngectomy after failed laryngeal radiation therapy. Laryngoscope. 1996;106:495–8.
15. Piazza C, Peretti G, Cattaneo A, Garrubba F, De Zinis LO, Nicolai P. Salvage surgery after radiotherapy for laryngeal cancer: from endoscopic resections to open-neck partial and total laryngectomies. Arch Otolaryngol Head Neck Surg. 2007;133:1037–43.
16. Pellini R, Pichi B, Ruscito P, et al. Supracricoid partial laryngectomies after radiation failure: a multi-institutional series. Head Neck. 2008;30:372–9.
17. Holsinger FC, Funk E, Roberts DB, Diaz DM. Conservation laryngeal surgery versus total laryngectomy for radiation failure in laryngeal cancer. Head Neck. 2006;28:779–84.
18. Mortuaire G, Francois J, Wiel E, Chevalier D. Local recurrence after CO_2 laser cordectomy for early glottic carcinoma. Laryngoscope. 2006;116(1):101–5.
19. Huang J, Yu Z, Fang J, Chen X, Chen X, Huang Z. Salvage transoral laser microsurgery for early recurrent glottic carcinoma after primary laser treatment. Acta Otolaryngol. 2013;133(5):531–7.
20. Bertino G, Degiorgi G, Tinelli C, Cacciola S, Occhini A, Benazzo M. CO_2 laser cordectomy for T1–T2 glottic cancer: oncological and functional long-term results. Eur Arch Otorrinolaringol. 2015;272(9):2389–95.
21. Lucioni M, Bertolin A, Lionello M, Giacomelli L, Rizzotto G, Marioni G. Open partial horizontal laryngectomy for salvage after failure of CO_2 laser-assisted surgery for glottic carcinoma. Eur Arch Otorrinolaringol. 2016;273(1):169–75. https://doi.org/10.1007/s00405-015-3734-2.
22. Bertolin A, Lionello M, Zanotti C, Franz L, Giacomelli L, Rizzotto G, Marioni G. Oncological and functional outcomes of primary and salvage total laryngectomy. Laryngoscope. 2021;131(2):E569–75. https://doi.org/10.1002/lary.28955.
23. Lucioni M, Bertolin A, Lionello M, Giacomelli L, Rizzotto G, Marioni G. Salvage transoral laser microsurgery for recurrent glottic carcinoma after primary laser-assisted treatment: analysis of prognostic factors. Head Neck. 2016;38:1043–9.
24. Tucker HM. Conservation laryngeal surgery in the elderly patient. Laryngoscope. 1977;87:1995–9.
25. Nichols RD, Stine PH, Greenawald KJ. Partial laryngectomy after radiation failure. Laryngoscope. 1980;90:571–5.
26. Nakayama M, Okamoto M, Hayakawa K, et al. Clinical outcome of supracricoid laryngectomy with cricohyoidoepiglottopexy: radiation failure versus previously untreated patients. Auris Nasus Larynx. 2013;40:207–10.
27. Marchese-Ragona R, Marioni G, Chiarello G, Staffieri A, Pastore A. Supracricoid laryngectomy with cricohyoidopexy for recurrence of early-stage glottis carcinoma after irradiation. Long-term oncological and functional results. Acta Otolaryngol. 2005;125:91–5.
28. Leon X, Lopez M, Garcia J, Viza I, Orus C, Quer M. Supracricoid laryngectomy as salvage surgery after failure of radiation therapy. Eur Arch Otorrinolaringol. 2007;264:809–14.
29. Rizzotto G, Crosetti E, Lucioni M, Succo G. Subtotal laryngectomy: outcomes of 469 patients and proposal of a comprehensive and simplified classification of surgical procedures. Eur Arch Otorrinolaringol. 2012;269:1635–46.

30. Naudo P, Laccourreye O, Weinstein G, et al. Complications and functional outcome after supracricoid partial laryngectomy with cricohyoidoepiglottopexy. Otolaryngol Head Neck Surg. 1998;118:124–9.
31. Furuta Y, Homma A, Oridate N, et al. Surgical complications of salvage total laryngectomy following concurrent chemoradiotherapy. Int J Clin Oncol. 2008;13:521–7.
32. Motamed M, Laccourreye O, Bradley PJ. Salvage conservation laryngeal surgery after irradiation failure for early laryngeal cancer. Laryngoscope. 2006;116:451–5.
33. Ganly I, Patel SG, Matsuo J, et al. Results of surgical salvage after failure of definitive radiation therapy for early-stage squamous cell carcinoma of the glottic larynx. Arch Otolaryngol Head Neck Surg. 2006;132:59–66.
34. de Vincentiis M, De Virgilio A, Bussu F, et al. Oncologic results of the surgical salvage of recurrent laryngeal squamous cell carcinoma in a multicentric retrospective series: emerging role of supracricoid partial laryngectomy. Head Neck. 2015;37:84–91.

Anatomy and Physiology of the Operated Larynx

12

Marco Stacchini, Tiziano Perrone, Giuseppe Di Prinzio, Fabio Buzzi, Luca Burgio, Federica Morolli, and Massimo Magnani

12.1 Introduction

As already mentioned in the previous chapters, open partial horizontal laryngectomy (OPHL) is the most suitable solution in the conservative approach of advanced laryngeal cancer. The OPHLs represent the step before total laryngectomy [1, 2], and they have also established an important oncological role in the management of radio-resistant laryngeal carcinoma [3, 4].

The strength of the OPHLs is their modularity; the surgeon can decide the most appropriate upper and lower limit of excision during surgery, based on the local extension of the tumor, up to a total laryngectomy.

We recall that the current classification identifies three types of surgical procedures based on the lower limit of resection:

Type I Supraglottic laryngectomies (Fig. 12.1);
Type II Supracricoid laryngectomies (Figs. 12.2, 12.3);
Type III Supratracheal laryngectomies (Fig. 12.4);

For type II and III OPHLs, the suffixes "a" and "b" are used to identify, respectively, the saving or removal of the suprahyoid portion of the epiglottis.

Each type may include the excision of other nearby structures indicated by the following abbreviations (specifying the side of resection):

+ARY → one arytenoid (Figs. 12.5, 12.6);
+PIR → one pyriform sinus;
+CAU → one cricoarytenoid unit composed by arytenoid, cricoarytenoid joint, and underlying hemicricoid plate (Fig. 12.7);
+BOT → the base of the tongue (Fig. 12.8).

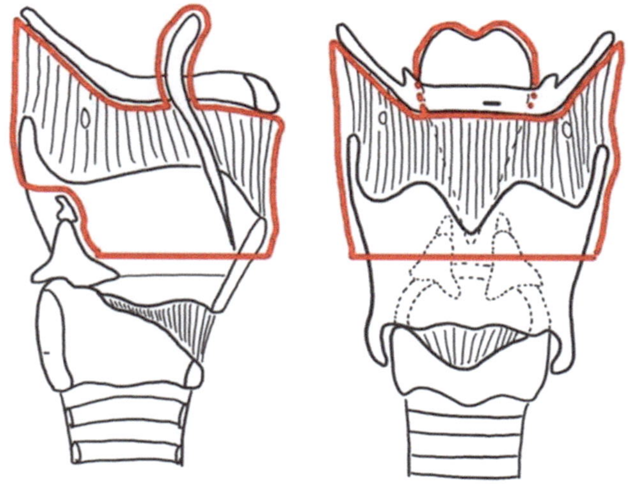

Fig. 12.1 OPHL type I

M. Stacchini (✉) · L. Burgio · F. Morolli · M. Magnani
Department of ENT, M. Bufalini Hospital, Cesena, Italy
e-mail: marco.stacchini@aulsromagna.it; luca.burgio@ausl.bologna.it; federica.morolli3@auslromagna.it; massimo.magnani@auslromagna.it

T. Perrone · G. Di Prinzio · F. Buzzi
Department of ENT & Audiology, University of Ferrara, Ferrara, Italy
e-mail: prrtzn@unife.it; giuseppe.diprinzio@ospfe.it; fabio.buzzi@edu.unife.it

F. Mattioli et al. (eds.), *Atlas of Open Partial Horizontal Laryngectomy*, https://doi.org/10.1007/978-3-031-48023-2_12

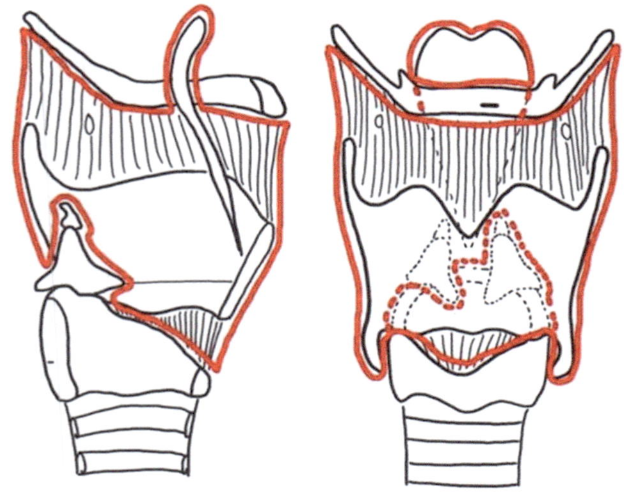

Fig. 12.2 OPHL type II (The image herein illustrates an OPHL IIb + ARY dx)

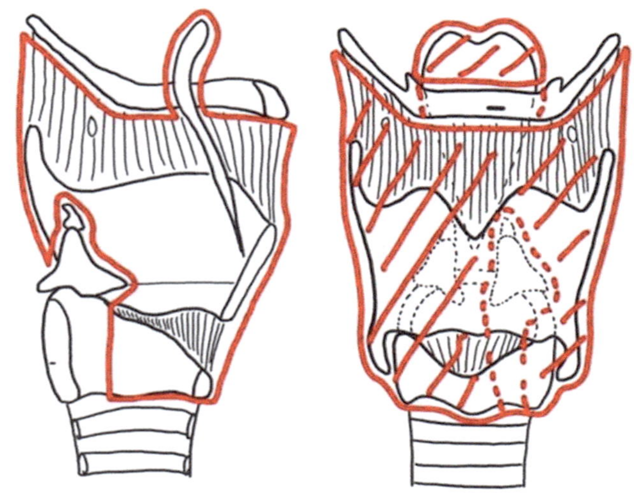

Fig. 12.3 OPHL TYPE 3b + CAU

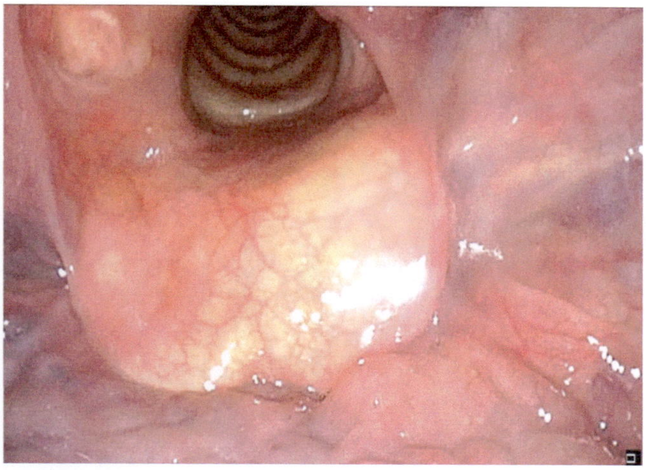

Fig. 12.4 OPHL type III

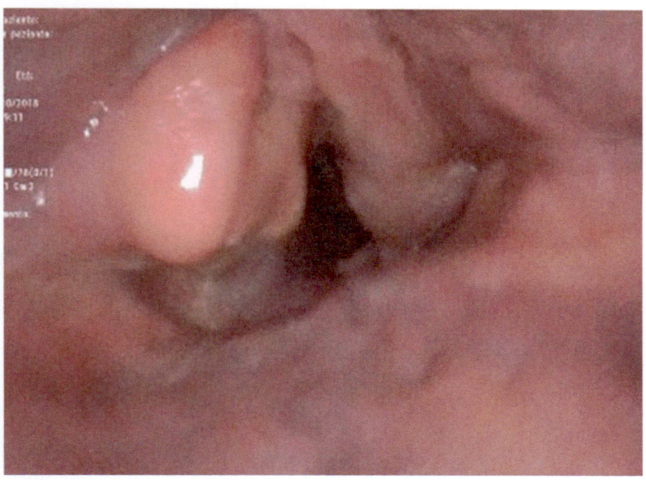

Fig. 12.5 OPHL TYPE 2A + ARY

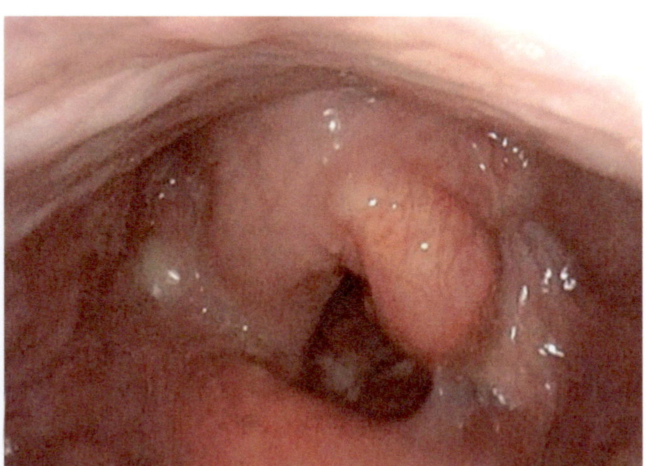

Fig. 12.6 OPHL TYPE 2B + ARY

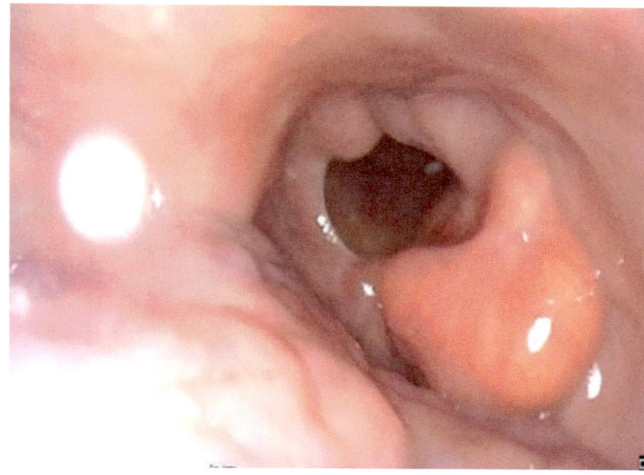

Fig. 12.7 OPHL TYPE 3b + CAU

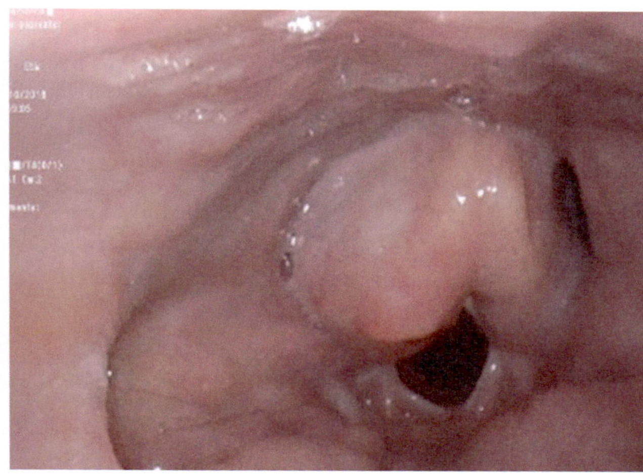

Fig. 12.8 OPHL type 2B

12.2 The Neolarynx

The role of OPHLs is to provide a surgical solution that is oncologically radical, while preserving the three basic functions of the larynx: breathing, swallowing, and phonating.

Naturally, after OPHL such as type II and type III, it is no longer possible to call "glottis" the residual anatomical structures, therefore it is preferable to define the new sphincter as neoglottis.

The original description by Piquet of neoglottis sphincter basically includes an anterior and a posterior part:

- **Anteriorly**, there is the tongue-base muscular part plus an eventual residual epiglottis.
- **Posteriorly**, the sphincter is composed of one or two cricoarytenoid units (CAUs), depending on the extension of the surgery.

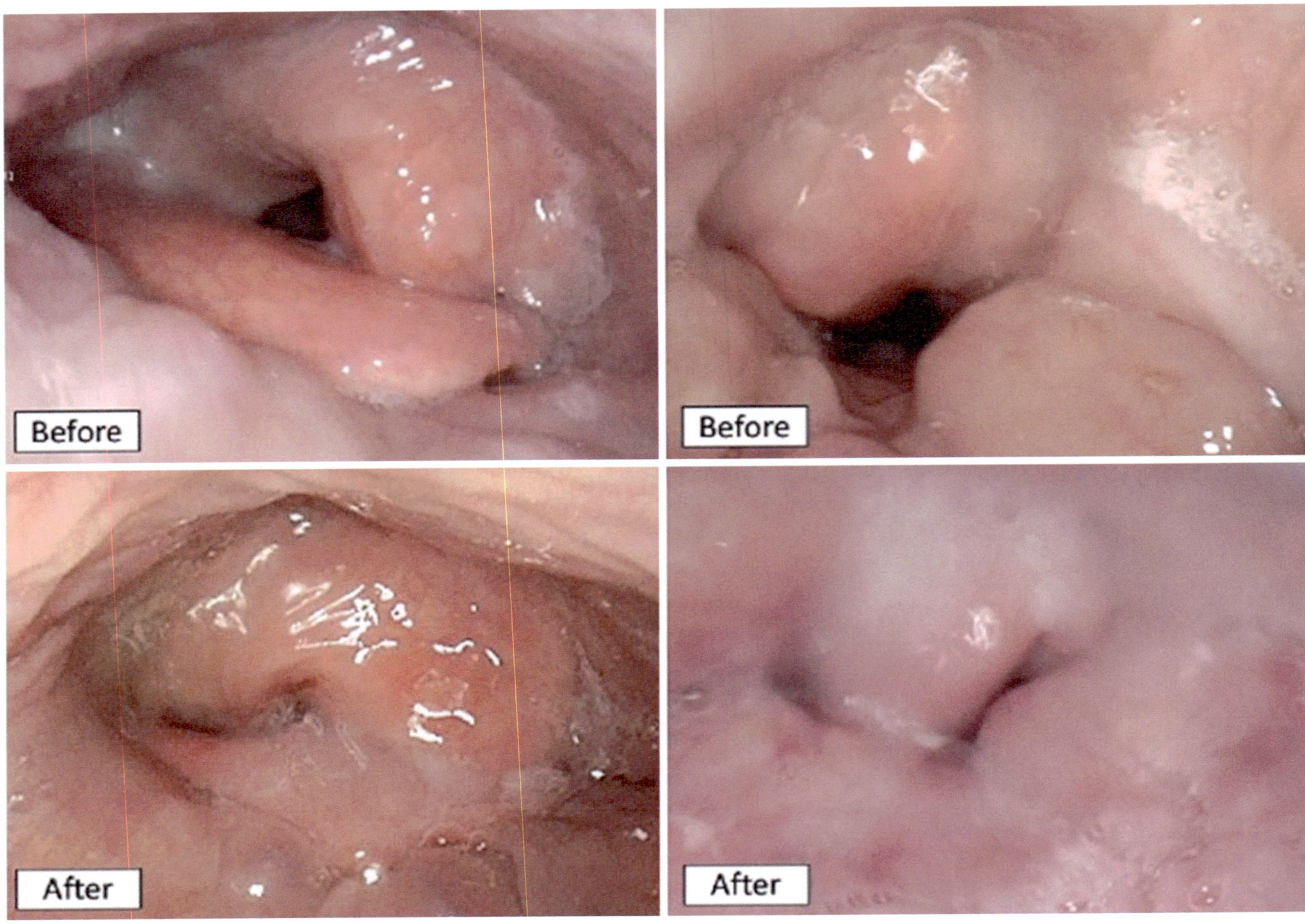

Fig. 12.9 Neoglottis behaviour

This convergence of two normally separated structures is possible, thanks to the OPHL, which overlaps the two anatomical residual parts, creating a new sphincter. In fact, to preserve the larynx functions, it is essential to create an optimal vertical connection between the spared structures during the pexy and to establish a good spatial relationship between the residual moving arytenoid/s and the frontal structures of the neolarynx. The residual epiglottis, when present and if positioned correctly, helps the closure of the sphincter by following the base of the tongue movement, without representing an obstacle for the respiratory lumen [5] (Fig. 12.9).

12.3 Essential Anatomical and Functional Structures of the Neolarynx

12.3.1 At Least One Cricoarytenoid Unit (CAU)

According to Piquet's original definition, the CAU is composed by a fibro-cartilaginous skeleton, made by part of cricoid cartilage plus one arytenoid. The arytenoid and the cricoid are joined in a single unit. This articulation is functional only if lateral and posterior cricoarytenoid muscles plus interarytenoid muscles are preserved, as well as their innervation and vascularization with a mucosal flap covering the cartilage [6].

A more recent definition by Rizzotto et al. (2006) simply defines the CAU as "half posterior cricoid plate and one arytenoid" [7]. In case of OPHL type III in fact, the cricoid cartilage is partially removed and only the posterior portion of the plate to which the arytenoid articulates is spared.

As mentioned, the CAU is the posterior essential element for the competence of the neoglottis, thanks to the contraction of the cricoarytenoid muscles (posterior and lateral) and, only if present both CAUs, of the interarytenoid muscle.

More in detail:

- Lateral cricoarytenoid muscle pulls the muscular apophysis downwards and forwards, moving the vocal apophysis and the arytenoid body forwards, inwards, and downwards.
- Simultaneously, the posterior cricoarytenoid muscles relax, tilting forwards the arytenoid body.
- When both CAUs are preserved, the simultaneous contraction of the interarytenoid muscle is possible, and it produces a stronger action of the posterior sphincter, while also closing more tightly the arytenoids anteriorly [5].

12.3.2 Innervation

As well as the sensitive neurons, each muscle needs its motor innervation to be preserved in order to move properly, voluntarily, and involuntarily. Both reflex arches and voluntary cortical commands require an intact neuronal pathway. So, it is mandatory for the surgeon to preserve the innervation during the surgical demolition phase.

The larynx is innervated by the superior laryngeal nerve, recurrent laryngeal nerve, and sympathetic fibers [8–11]:

- *The superior laryngeal nerve* (*SLN*) branches from the vagus approximately 2.5 cm below the base of the skull. The SLN has an internal and external branch:
  - *The internal branch* supplies sensory and autonomic innervation to the superior mucosa of the larynx. This includes general sensory innervation to the superior portion of the laryngeal cavity, including the epiglottis and superior surface of the vocal folds. Visceral afferents to the epiglottis also assist in taste. Preganglionic parasympathetic fibers also travel via the internal laryngeal nerve.
  - *The external branch* supplies motor innervation and visceral efferent to the cricothyroid muscle.

  Preserving the SLN is crucial to maintaining the swallowing reflex arc for the subsequent rehabilitation phase. During the OPHL surgery, the time of the superior laryngeal vascular pedicle ligature represents an important phase, because of its proximity to the SLN. The superior laryngeal pedicle runs close to the superior horn of the thyroid cartilage. After its identification, it is necessary to identify and isolate the superior laryngeal vascular pedicle and the SLN. The vascular pedicle is then ligated and sectioned. The SLN should be spared until the lateral ramus of the internal branch. That ramus must be preserved, because it gives the sensory innervation to the pyriform sinus. At this time of the surgery, it could be useful to perform a manual medial rotation maneuver of the thyroid cartilage, in order to move the SLN superiorly to the superior horn of the thyroid cartilage. This surgical tip moves the SLN away from the vascular pedicle, to better protect the nerve during the ligature of the vessels.
- The *Recurrent laryngeal nerve* (RLN) gives the motor innervation to all intrinsic muscles of the larynx (except the cricothyroid muscle), to the cricopharyngeus muscles, and to the inferior constrictor. Besides, it carries the visceral sensory fibers from the inferior region of the glottis.

  The RLN runs behind the inferior horn of the thyroid cartilage to reach the inferior margin of the cricoid cartilage. Preserving the RLN is crucial for the movement of the residual CAU and therefore for the subsequent recovery of the neolarynx functions. To protect from injury of the RLN during the surgery, in the previous chapters, it has been described the technique of resection of the lower horn of the thyroid cartilage.

12.3.3 Motor Central Area

The neuronal plasticity of the brain motor central area is essential to acquire again the control of the neolarynx after surgery. The great importance of the brain area involving the tongue and pharynx sensitivity and movements has been known for over a century, proven by the size of these structures in the "cortical homunculus." Therefore, during the preoperative patient selection phase, it is crucial to assess the patient's general condition, with a particular attention to the brain functions and to the attitude of the patient to perform coordination exercises aimed at swallowing recovery after surgery. The residual neuronal plasticity of patients that undergo reconstructive surgery of the larynx is a key element to the following creation of a functional myomucosal speaking and swallowing shunt. In the rehabilitation phase, after any type of near-total laryngectomy, early speech exercises are essential to promote an adaptation of the brain cells connections to control and coordinate the movements of the neolarynx. Moreover, it is essential to reduce the time in which the patient, after surgery, remains inactive in order to facilitate an early recovery of the laryngeal functions [12–16].

12.3.4 Mucosa

A large amount of residual mucosa that covers the neolarynx cartilages is essential to produce a valid voice after OPHL surgery. In fact, the mucosa must vibrate during the contact between the spare structures of the larynx to obtain an effective sound. Therefore, redundant, flexible, and elastic mucosa will favor sound production. On the other hand, fibrotic areas will be an obstacle to it. In fact, mucosal vibration might be impeached by factors such as radiotherapy, due to the increase of scar tissues, worsening the neovoice as a result.

The vibration of the mucosa covering the epiglottis (E), arytenoid (A), and pyriform sinus (S) are involved in the process. Depending on which combination of these anatomical mucosal structures produces speech, Saito et al. [17] defined various vibratory patterns: Type A, Type S, type AS, Type AE, and Type AES.

It is commonly found that the various mucous areas involved in voice production after surgery change even among patients going through the same type of OPHL. The result is that patients could present different neovoice patterns, although identical surgery, due to different mucosal vibration sites. Performing several laryngostroboscopy in the assessment of the OPHLs voice, we noticed that in some patients, it is not the mucosa of the spared CAU that produces the vibration, but the arytenoid caps mucosa left (on the side of the sacrificed arytenoid). It is therefore essential to spare as much mucosa as we can during surgery, because the following site of voice production is not always predictable.

12.3.5 Pyriform Sinus

The valleculae and the pyriform sinuses are known as the pharyngeal recesses or side pockets, into which food may fall and reside before or after the swallowing reflex triggers. Preserving the pyriform sinus and its innervation, during the demolition surgical phase, is crucial to recover the swallowing function of the neolarynx. During the swallowing, the alimentary bolus is pushed by the tongue from the oral cavity into the pyriform sinus, which promotes the deglutition reflex. This mechanism is possible only if its mucosa and nerves have been spared during surgery. Furthermore, part of the mucosa of the pyriform sinus is put into vibration for producing sounds in some OPHL patients, as previously mentioned [18].

12.3.6 Laryngeal Framework

In order to obtain good functional results, the spared laryngeal structures of the OPHL have to be stable and well aligned. As we mentioned before, there must be at least one CAU (with its motility preserved) that has to be uplifted to the tongue base and well linked to it, during the neolarynx closure in phonation and swallowing. The relative positions of each component are essential to conserve all the three physiological functions. The stability of the neolarynx is obtained by overlapping and positioning the concave portion of the hyoid body on top of the residual lower part of the larynx (cricoid cartilage or tracheal ring) [5].

12.4 Physiology of the Neolarynx (Figs. 12.10, 12.11, 12.12)

12.4.1 Speech

With regard to vocal production, it is necessary to separate OPHL I from OPHL II and III. In type I, the glottic plane is spared and the voice continues to be produced by the vibration of the vocal cords. On the contrary, in the type II and III, both vocal folds are removed and therefore the vocal production is guaranteed by the spared structures.

To produce sounds, in these patients undergoing OPHL II and III, it is essential to promote, with the speech therapy, two movements of the CAUs spared: vertical and horizontal. These two movements are respectively called "Le salut aryténoidienne" and "Le Rideau de scène" by Piquet in the very first description of the subtotal laryngectomy technique [19]. The CAU gets close and touches the tongue base (and possibly the portion of epiglottis spared in Type A) to determine an increase of pressure under the neoglottis that therefore puts into vibration the residual mucosae. The resulting sound produces generally an effective neovoice that is defined as "substitution voice."

According to the European Laryngological Society (ELS), there are two main assessment systems used to evalu-

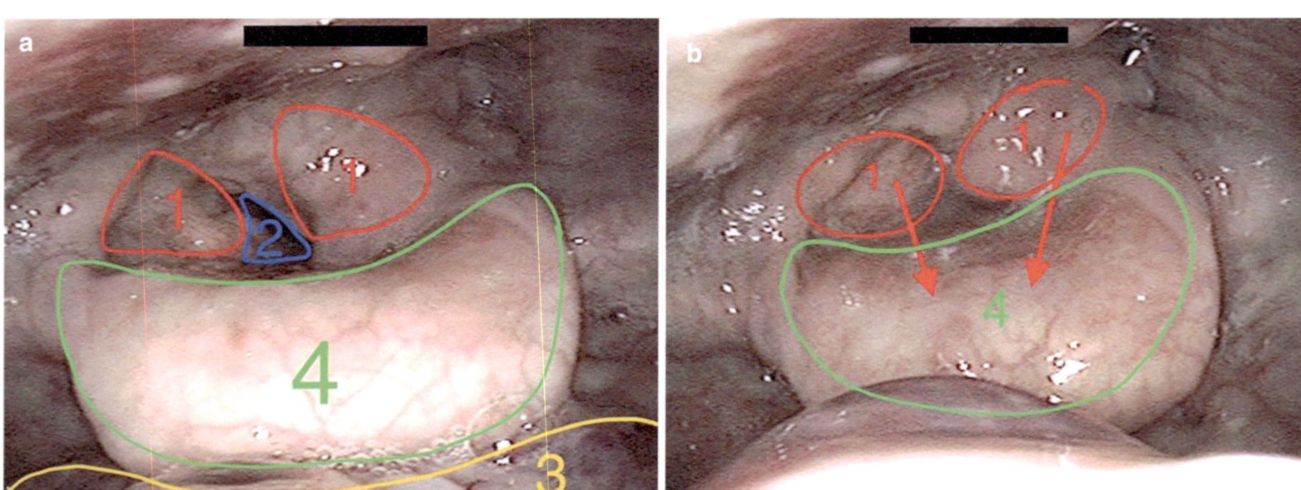

Fig. 12.10 (**a**) endoscopic view of OPHL IIa during breathing; (**b**) same patient during phonation: notice how the CAU gets close to the epiglottis and the base of the tongue (BOT). The contact between the spared structures produces the mucosal vibration and therefore the voice. 1.CAU (red), 2. Trachea (blue), 3. Base of tongue (yellow), 4. Epiglottis (green)

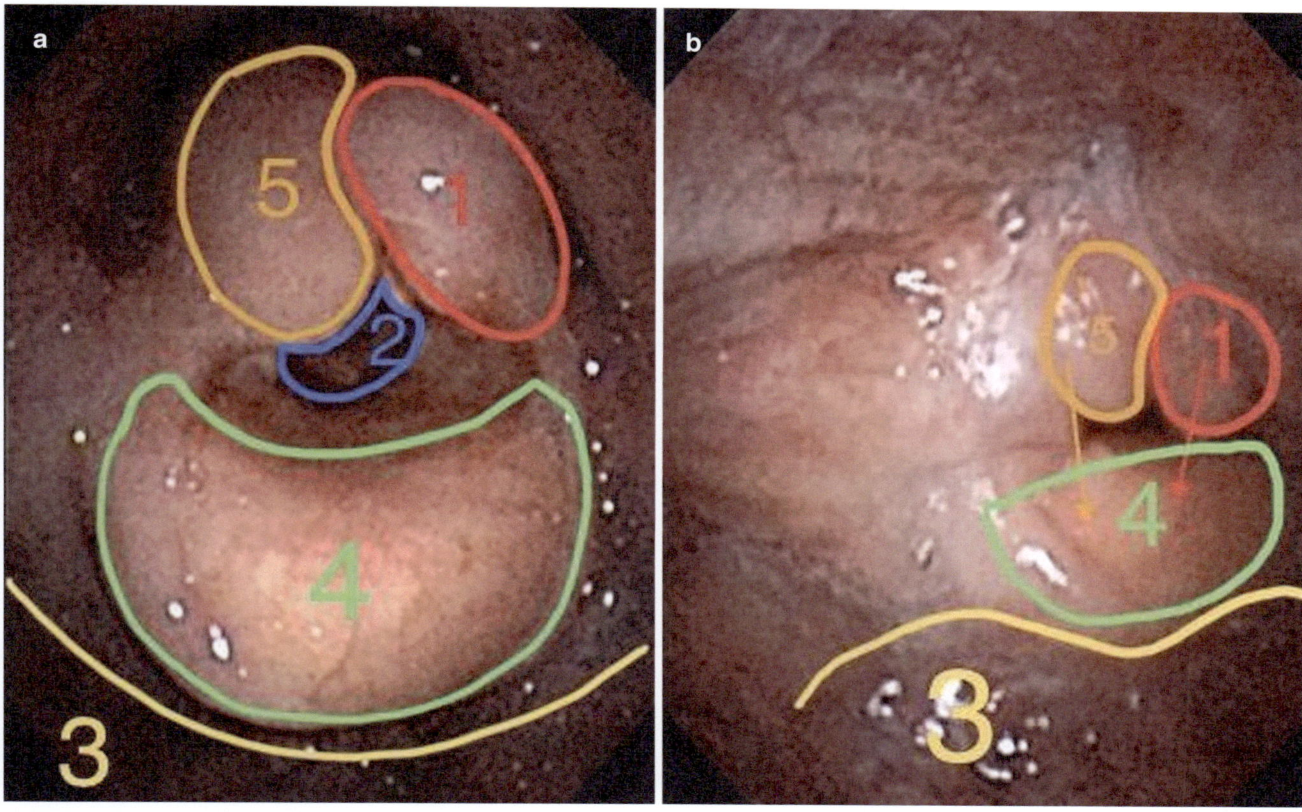

Fig. 12.11 (**a**) OPHL type IIa + ARY dx during breathing; (**b**) same patient during phonation. In this case, the laryngostroboscopy shows the vibration of the mucosa covering the arytenoid cap, at the side of arytenoid resection. 1.CAU (red), 2. Trachea (blue), 3. Base of tongue (yellow), 4. Epiglottis (green), 5. arytenoid cap mucosa (orange)

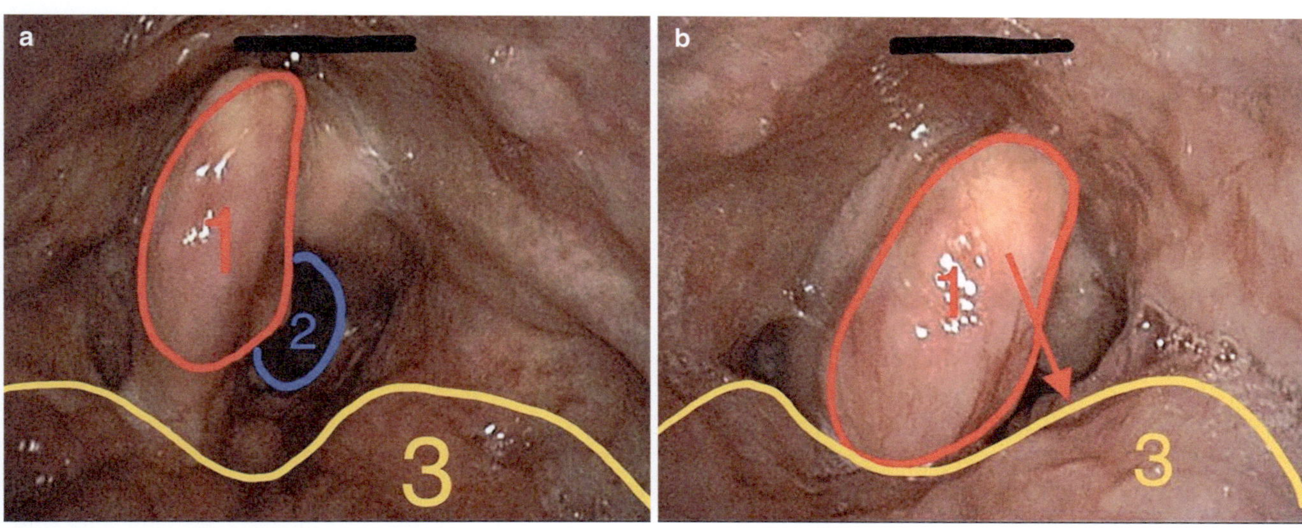

Fig. 12.12 (**a**) OPHL type IIIb + ARY sn during breathing; (**b**) same patient during phonation. The CAU dx moves forward to get in touch with the BOT. 1.CAU (red), 2. Trachea (blue), 3. Base of tongue (orange)

ate the severity of a vocal disorder: VHI-10 (voice handicap index-10) that is a voice self-assessment questionnaire and GRBAS (G: grade of dysphonia, R: roughness, B: breathiness, A: asthenic, S: strain) that represent the primary perceptual evaluation scale of voice quality (Hirano). Both systems, however, can be used for patients who maintain the anatomical integrity of the vocal folds (VF).

It is clear, therefore, that these cannot be adopted for the evaluation of voice quality in patients undergoing OPHL II and III, but only in case of OPHL I, in which the VF is spared.

In OPHL II and III, the neovoice can be assessed through the SECEL (Self-Evaluation of Communication Experiences after Laryngeal Cancer) or with its Italian version I-SECEL [20], which have been developed specifically for substitution voice. It represents a self-report instrument that measures the perceived adjustment to substitution voice through 35 items in three subscales (General, Environment, Attitude). Patients have to rate each statement on a 4-point categorical scale. A total score from 0 to 102 and three subscores can be obtained. A score $\geq$ 60 suggests the need for specific psychological intervention for acceptance of the new voice.

One of the proper scales that has been proposed for the assessment of the perceptual evaluation of the voice after OPHLs type II and III is the INFV0 rating scale [21]. This scale is a standard for rating substitution voices used in speech therapy. The INFV0 includes overall impression (I), amount of unintended additive noise (N), fluency (F), and quality of voicing (Vo). For each parameter, the score can vary from 0 to 10. The higher the score, the better is the perceived voice quality.

A recent study has shown that there are no significant differences in voice production ability between Type II and Type III OPHLs. The only difference was found in the quality perceived by the patient [22].

12.4.2 Swallowing

Swallowing is initiated by sensory impulses transmitted as a result of stimulation of receptors on the fauces, tonsils, soft palate, base of the tongue, and posterior pharyngeal wall. Sensory impulses reach the brain stem primarily through the seventh, ninth, and 10 cranial nerves, while the efferent (motor) function is mediated through the ninth, 10th, and 12th cranial nerves. The opening of the cricopharyngeal sphincter is a reflex, a relaxation that occurs when the bolus reaches the posterior pharyngeal wall.

After OPHL surgery, patients progressively begin to eat through the natural digestive ways, initially with difficulties and then improving thanks to the rehabilitation exercises. The time required for the complete rehabilitation is variable and it depends on the type of OPHL performed and the capacity of the patient to learn how to manage the bolus in the new anatomical condition. Usually, the patients reach almost full recovery after the first 6 postoperative months [23–25], achieving a free diet by the end of the first year in most cases [24, 26–30].

To complete the swallowing recovery, the base of the tongue (BOT) has a main active role in pushing behind the alimentary bolus, to facilitate its entrance into the pyriform sinus and then in the esophagus, with a backward and downward movement, and tightly closing the upper respiratory airways in order to protect them from penetration. Moreover, the BOT has to move in concert and coordinate with the spare(s) arytenoid(s). The closure of the new anatomical sphincter is so determined by the movement of these structures together with the elevation of the neolarynx.

At the same time, the expansion of the pyriform sinus is necessary to convey the bolus into the esophagus. To maintain this important function, during the OPHL surgery, a suture can be placed between the inferior constrictor muscles of the pharynx. The muscles, previously separated by the lateral margin of the thyroid cartilage, are sutured together in front of the neolarynx, in order to bring both muscles to a more anterior position. This surgical trick facilitates the expansion of the piriform sinus during the pharyngeal reflex phase of swallowing, triggered by the passage of the bolus from the oral cavity into the pharynx [31].

Normally in this phase, the protection of the respiratory tract is realized by the elevation and closure of the larynx at all three sphincters (epiglottis/aryepiglottic folds, false vocal folds, and true vocal folds). This movement prevents material from entering the airway. After OPHL, part of these anatomical structures is obviously lacking, so the remaining functional parts of the larynx have to compensate for the closure of the neolarynx. The remaining arytenoid(s) have to accomplish the closure, by the movement of intra rotation and anteriorization, until reaching the BOT or part of the epiglottis (if spared). At the same time, the elevation of the larynx is considered a key moment for the recovery of swallowing function.

Swallowing impairment is an important cause of disability and in a very few cases of death in patients with head and neck cancers because of aspiration pneumonia [25, 26]. Postoperative deglutition failure could be therefore a cause of surgical revision, up to total laryngectomy. Although swallowing evaluation is a basic item for the rehabilitation of these patients, up to date there are no standard tests for assessing the presence and the degree of penetration and aspiration after OPHL. So generally, the clinicians commonly use the same assessment that is adopted for patients with a normal larynx. Various centers use different methods to evaluate deglutition after surgery. Several non-validated scales exist nowadays, thus most centers use the Fiberoptic Endoscopic Evaluation of Swallowing (FEES), widely spread, but difficult to standardize in patient underwent

OPHL [32]. Therefore, it is challenging to compare the results among hospitals to assess swallowing after surgery.

To overcome this issue, it has been recently proposed a modification of the Penetration Aspiration Scale (PAS) [33], a validated deglutition assessment test for normal anatomy, commonly used during FEES. The authors propose a new PAS adapted to the new morphology and anatomy of the patients after surgery and they named it OPHL-PAS [34]. If this scale would be accepted and largely adopted, in the future it could be easier to compare the swallowing results after surgery in different clinical trials.

12.4.3 Breathing

To keep an adequate breathing function, it is essential to create a sufficiently large lumen in the neolarynx, while trying to maintain an efficient closing movement by the neoglottis, to ensure a good deglutition and phonation. The first requisite to obtain this balance between breathing space and neo-glottic sphincter closure is to achieve a stable and aligned position of the spared structures of the larynx during the pexy. The vertical positioning of the residual laryngeal cartilages (half thyroid cartilage in OPHL I, cricoid in OPHL II, tracheal ring plus CAU in the OPHL III), of the hyoid bone and of the BOT must guarantee enough space for the air fluxes among every segment of the neolarynx. If we perform an OPHL type a, sparing part of the epiglottis, it is crucial to suture the residual cartilage portion together with BOT. The suture has to permit a certain residual movement of the epiglottis during the retropulsion of the bolus while swallowing, but at the same time, it has to avoid the epiglottic retroflexion, that could reduce the breathing space (see previous chapter on surgery).

As we mentioned in the previous paragraph about swallowing, another important item is to preserve a wide movement of the spare(s) CAU(s), especially (talking about breathing) in the abduction phase. When the neolarynx is relaxed, the CAU should be in a postero-lateral position without covering the tracheal lumen.

Another key point to preserve the breathing function is to avoid excessive mucosal redundancy. The presence of an adequate amount of mucosa over the spared structures of the larynx is essential to preserve a good voice after surgery. However, the surgeon has to maintain a balance between vibrating soft tissue and excessive amount of spared tissue that could reduce the breathing space. In case of postoperative laryngeal obstruction after OPHL, Lucioni proposed different techniques of tissue resection by transoral laser microsurgery, in order to remove the redundancy of tissue covering the lumen [35].

Up to date, to evaluate the breathing results after OPHL, we only differentiate patients with or without tracheostomy tube. The possibility to close the tracheostomy depends on the diameters of the neolarynx, on the air fluxes and pressure among the lumen, but also on the overall health status of the patient. An objective and accepted evaluation scale for breathing in OPHL patients is not yet available.

References

1. Lefebvre JL. What is the role of primary surgery in the treatment of laryngeal and hypopharyngeal cancer? Hayes Martin lecture. Arch Otolaryngol Head Neck Surg. 2000;126:285–8.
2. Thomas L, Drinnan M, Natesh B, Mehanna H, Jones T, Paleri V. Open conservation partial laryngectomy for laryngeal cancer: a systematic review of English language literature. Cancer Treat Rev. 2012;38:203–11.
3. Pellini R, Pichi B, Ruscito P, Ceroni AR, Caliceti U, Rizzotto G, Pazzaia A, Laudadio P, Piazza C, Peretti G, Giannarelli D, Spriano G. Supracricoid partial laryngectomies after radiation failure: a multi institutional series. Head Neck. 2008;30:372–9.
4. Piazza C, Peretti G, Cattaneo A, Garrubba F, de Zinis LO, Nicolai P. Salvage surgery after radiotherapy for laryngeal cancer: from endoscopic resections to open-neck partial and total laryngectomies. Arch Otolaryngol Head Neck Surg. 2007;133:1037–43.
5. Cunsolo EM. Anatomy and physiology of the operated larynx. Acta Otorhinolaryngol Ital. 2010;30(5)
6. Pinar E, Imre A, Calli C, Oncel S, Katilmis H. Supracricoid partial laryngectomy: analyses of oncologic and functional outcomes. Otolaryngol Head Neck Surg. 2012;147:1093–8.
7. Rizzotto G, Crosetti E, Lucioni M, Succo G. Subtotal laryngectomy: outcomes of 469 patients and proposal of a comprehensive and simplified classification of surgical procedures. Eur Arch Othorinolaryngol. 2012;269:1635–46.
8. Williamson AJ, Shermetaro C. Unilateral vocal cord paralysis. Treasure Island (FL): StatPearls Publishing; 2021.
9. Espinosa MC, Ongkasuwan J. Recurrent laryngeal nerve reinnervation: is this the standard of care for pediatric unilateral vocal cord paralysis? Curr Opin Otolaryngol Head Neck Surg. 2018;26(6):431–6.
10. Mahabadi N, Goizueta AA, Bordoni B. Anatomy, thorax, lung pleura and mediastinum. Treasure Island (FL): StatPearls Publishing; 2021.
11. Daggumati S, Panossian MDH, Sataloff RT. Vocal fold paresis: incidence, and the relationship between voice handicap index and laryngeal EMG findings. J Voice. 2019;33(6):940–4.
12. Martin RU, Goodyear BG, Gati J, et al. Cerebral cortical representation of automatic and volitional swallowing in humans. J Neurophysiol. 2001;85:938–50.
13. Bomeli SR, Desai SC, Johnson JT, et al. Management of salivary flow in head and neck cancer patients—a systematic review. Oral Oncol. 2008;44:1000–8.
14. Michou E, Hamdy S. Cortical input in control of swallowing. Curr Opin Otolaryngol Head Neck Surg. 2009;17:166–71.
15. Palmer JB, Hiiemae KM, Matsuo K, et al. Volitional control of food transport and bolus formation during feeding. Physiol Behav. 2007;91:66–70.
16. Ludlow CL, Hoit J, Kent R, et al. Translating principles of neural plasticity into research on speech motor control recovery and rehabilitation. J Speech Lang Hear Res. 2008;51:S240–58.
17. Saito K, Araki K, Ogawa K, Shiotani A. Laryngeal function after supracricoid laryngectomy. Otolaryngol Head Neck Surg. 2009;140(4):487–92.
18. Sprecher A, Olszewski A, Jiang JJ, Zhang Y. Updating signal typing in voice: addition of type 4 signals. J Acoust Soc Am. 2010;127:3710–6.

19. Decroix G, Piquet JJ, Desaulty A, Hequet B, Bossut MY, Lacroix D. Etude de la phonation après laryngectomie reconstructive [Phonation following reconstructive laryngectomy]. Ann Otolaryngol Chir Cervicofac. 1976;93(3):129–48.
20. Schindler A, Mozzanica F, Brignoli F, Maruzzi P, Evitts P, Ottaviani F. Reliability and validity of the Italian self-evaluation of communication experiences after laryngeal cancer questionnaire. Head Neck. 2013;35(11):1606–15.
21. Moerman MBJ, Martens JP, Van der Borgt MJ, Peleman M, Gillis M, Dejonckere PH. Perceptual evaluation of substitution voices: development and evaluation of the (I)INFVo rating scale. Eur Arch Otorrinolaringol. 2006;
22. Schindler A, Pizzorni N, Fantini M, Crosetti E, Bertolin A, Rizzotto G, Succo G. Long-term functional results after open partial horizontal laryngectomy type IIa and Type IIIa: a comparison study. Head Neck. 2015;263(2):183–7.
23. Woisard V, Serrano E, Yardeni E, Puech M, Pessey JJ. Deglutition after supra-glottic laryngectomy. J Otolaryngol. 1993;22:278–83.
24. Naudo P, Laccourreye O, Weinstein G, Jouffre V, Laccourreye H, Brasnu D. Complications and functional outcome after supracricoid partial laryngectomy with cricohyoidoepiglottopexy. Otolaryngol Head Neck Surg. 1998;118:124–9.
25. Benito J, Holsinger FC, Pérez Martín A, Garcia D, Weinstein GS, Laccoureye O. Aspiration after supracricoid partial laryngectomy: incidence, risk factors, management, and outcomes. Head Neck. 2011;33:679–85.
26. Webster KT, Samlan RA, Jones B, Bunton K, Tufano RP. Supracricoid partial laryngectomy: swallowing, voice, and speech outcomes. Ann Otol Rhinol Laryngol. 2010;119:10–6.
27. Bron L, Pasche P, Brossard E, Monnier P, Schweizer V. Functional analysis after supracricoid partial laryngectomy with cricohyoidoepiglottopexy. Laryngoscope. 2002;122:1289–93.
28. Goeleven A, Dejaeger E, Vander Poorten V, Delaere P. Swallowing and functional outcome after partial laryngectomy: a literature review. B-ENT. 2005;1:165–72.
29. Schindler A, Favero E, Nudo S, Albera R, Schindler O, Cavalot AL. Long-term voice and swallowing modifications after supracricoid laryngectomy: objective, subjective and self-assessment data. Am J Otolaryngol. 2006;27:378–83.
30. Schindler A, Fantini M, Pizzorni N, Crosetti E, Mozzanica F, Bertolin A, Ottaviani F, Rizzotto G, Succo G. Swallowing, voice and quality of life after supratracheal laryngectomy: preliminary long-term results. Head Neck. 2015;37:557–66.
31. Holsinger FC, Laccourreye O, Weinstein GS, Diaz E, McWhorter AJ. Technical refinements in the supracricoid partial laryngectomy to optimize functional outcomes. J Am Coll Surg. 2005;201(5):809–20.
32. Colodny N. Interjudge and intrajudge reliabilities in fiberoptic endoscopic evaluation of swallowing (fees) using the penetration-aspiration scale: a replication study. Dysphagia. 2002;17:308–15.
33. Farneti D. Pooling score: an endoscopic model for evaluating severity of dysphagia. Acta Otorhinolaryngol Ital. 2008;28:135–40.
34. Pizzorni N, Crosetti E, Santambrogio E, de Cillis G, Bertolin A, Rizzotto G, Fantini M, Succo G, Schindler A. The penetration-aspiration scale: adaptation to open partial laryngectomy and reliability analysis. Dysphagia. 2020;35(2):261–71.
35. Lucioni M, Bertolin A, Lionello M, Giacomelli L, Ghirardo G, Rizzotto G, Marioni G. Transoral laser microsurgery for managing laryngeal stenosis after reconstructive partial laryngectomies. Laryngoscope. 2017;127(2):359–65.

13 Surgical Training on Animal Model for Open Laryngeal Surgery

Francesco Maccarrone, Matteo Fermi, Michael Ghirelli, Andrea Martone, Costanza Galloni, and Edoardo Bassano

13.1 Introduction

Surgical training represents an essential part of the learning process of a surgeon [1]. Technical skill acquisition is a cornerstone of surgical competence that can be achieved only through constant training.

This is true for both novice surgeons first approaching surgery and expert practitioners, to refine practical skills, increase surgical confidence and speed, and perform new procedures.

Fresh human cadaver models are the gold standard for surgical training. Nevertheless, they are inevitably hard to obtain and expensive.

The animal cadaver model constitutes therefore a valid alternative in terms of ease of finding and cost, even though they are not free from disadvantages. Using animal specimens, for example, might raise ethical and religious problems, which could be overcome by using only animals whose welfare and slaughtering observe regular veterinary permissions and regulations.

Animal models might be a vehicle for infections. The Q fever, for instance, is a zoonosis caused by *Coxiella burnetii*, a bacterium that resides in the amniotic fluid and placental tissue of pregnant animals [2]. Therefore, it is of paramount importance that complete veterinarian health certificates are provided. It would be preferable the use male or prepubescent female beasts to reduce the risk of infection. The use of personal protective clothing and equipment, such as disposable gloves, face masks, head covers, gowns, and shoe covers is mandatory.

Several animal models have been used for head and neck surgical training. It is in the authors opinion that ovine specimens are the most suitable animal model for head and neck surgery.

The sheep larynx has an intermediate dimension between the human male and female larynx. The most significant differences are as follows:

- The arytenoid cartilages are bigger.
- There is no thyroid cartilage notch.
- The laryngeal ventricle is absent, and the upper part of the larynx is narrower [3].

Anyway, all these differences are marginal in terms of suitability for surgical training, therefore it is possible to affirm that open laryngeal procedures can be accurately performed on sheep larynx since both lifelike, anatomy, and reproducibility score are rated high [4]. Ovine models represent an excellent model not only for larynx surgery but for most head and neck surgical training [4]. Sheep have been used in training of ear, facial nerve, and sinonasal and tracheal surgery [5–7].

Pigs and horses have also been used as models in several head and neck surgical training studies with satisfactory outcomes [8–10], whereas rabbits have been reported to be less appropriate [11]. On the other hand, bovine specimens find a

F. Maccarrone (✉)
Department of Otolaryngology, Ospedale "B. Ramazzini" di Carpi, AUSL Modena, Carpi, Italy

Department of Otorhinolaryngology, AUSL Romagna, Infermi Hospital, Rimini, Italy

M. Fermi
Otorhinolaryngology Head and Neck Surgery, Azienda Ospedaliero Universitaria di Bologna IRCCS, Bologna, Italy

Alma Mater Studiorum, Università di Bologna, Bologna, Italy

M. Ghirelli
ENT Unit, AUSL Romagna, Ospedale Infermi di Rimini, Rimini, Italy

A. Martone
Department of Otorhinolaryngology—Head and Neck Surgery, IRCCS Azienda Ospedaliero-Universitaria di Bologna, Bologna, Italy

C. Galloni
Department of Otolaryngology—Head and Neck Surgery, Azienda Ospedaliero Universitaria di Modena, Modena, Italy

E. Bassano
Otolaryngology Unit, Azienda USL-IRCCS di Reggio Emilia, Reggio Emilia, Italy

F. Mattioli et al. (eds.), *Atlas of Open Partial Horizontal Laryngectomy*, https://doi.org/10.1007/978-3-031-48023-2_13

wilder application as models in other surgical fields, such as gynecology or orthopedics [12, 13].

Finally, open surgical training may be executed with the aid of exoscopes (possibly with 3D technology) [14] positioned above the surgical field to project the image to a high-definition monitor. Video-aided training is particularly useful in free flap surgery since both microvascular anastomoses and flap harvesting and in setting are procedures for which optimal depth and spatial perception are crucial.

13.2 Ovine Model

13.2.1 Preparation of the Specimen

A 6-months old lamb's larynx has the most similar dimensions to the human larynx. The specimen should include the whole neck up to the thoracic inlet so that most of the trachea is included. The specimen must be prepared and stored at −18° and then thawed 24 h before the dissection. The neck of the ovine should be sheared up to the mandible to have clean skin, more suitable for surgical dissection. The necessary instruments to perform the training should include surgical knives, surgical scissors, forceps, needle holders, threads, and gauzes [4] (Fig. 13.1).

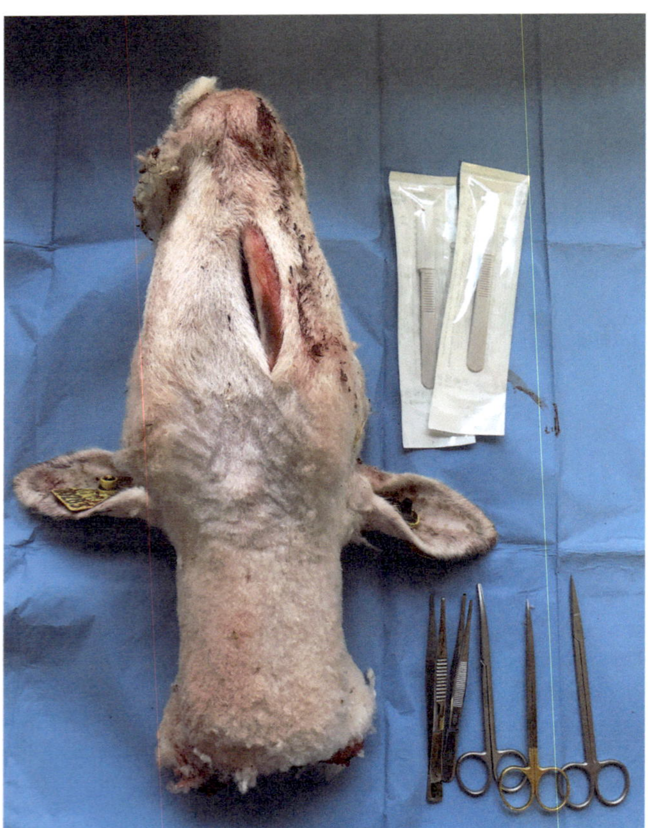

Fig. 13.1 Animal model preparation and surgical instruments

13.2.2 Surgical Steps of Dissection

13.2.2.1 Specimen Positioning

The sheep sample lies on the table with the head slightly extended. Surgeons must be positioned on the sides of the table.

13.2.2.2 Skin Incision

A standard apron incision is performed following the anatomical surface landmarks (i.e., thyroid cartilage, cricoid cartilage, and trachea) from both the angles of the mandible up to the level of the cricothyroid membrane.

13.2.2.3 Subplatysmal Flap and Laryngotracheal Framework Dissection

The subplatysmal flap is raised to obtain full exposure of the laryngotracheal framework, the hyoid bone, and the submandibular glands. Strap muscles and cricothyroid muscles are identified. Sternohyoid and thyrohyoid muscles are separated by the submandibular glands, detached from their cranial insertions onto the inferior ridge of the hyoid bone, and then reflected inferiorly (Fig. 13.2). Detachment of the caudal insertions of suprahyoid muscles onto the superior ridge of hyoid bone should be avoided when performing partial laryngectomies. Greater horns of ovine hyoid bone extend more laterally and superiorly than human ones [5].

13.2.2.4 Inferior Constrictor Muscles Dissection and Pyriform Sinus Isolation

Once the laryngeal framework has been freed from its connections with infrahyoid muscles and submandibular glands, the thyroid cartilage can be manually rotated medially and inferiorly to ease the section of the constrictor muscles at the posterior edge of the thyroid cartilage (Fig. 13.3). The superior laryngeal pedicle, formed by the homonym artery, vein, and nerve, is identified. The vascular structures are sectioned. In the ovine model, the superior laryngeal pedicle always lies lateral to the superior horn of the thyroid cartilage; thus, it is safer to approach this region after retracting the larynx medially and downward, letting the nerve overstep the cartilage (Fig. 13.4). The thyrohyoid ligaments are dissected, and the inner perichondrium of the pyriform fossa is detached from the thyroid lamina to preserve the pyriform sinus mucosa. At this level, the sensitive branch of the superior laryngeal nerve for the pyriform sinus is visible (Fig. 13.5).

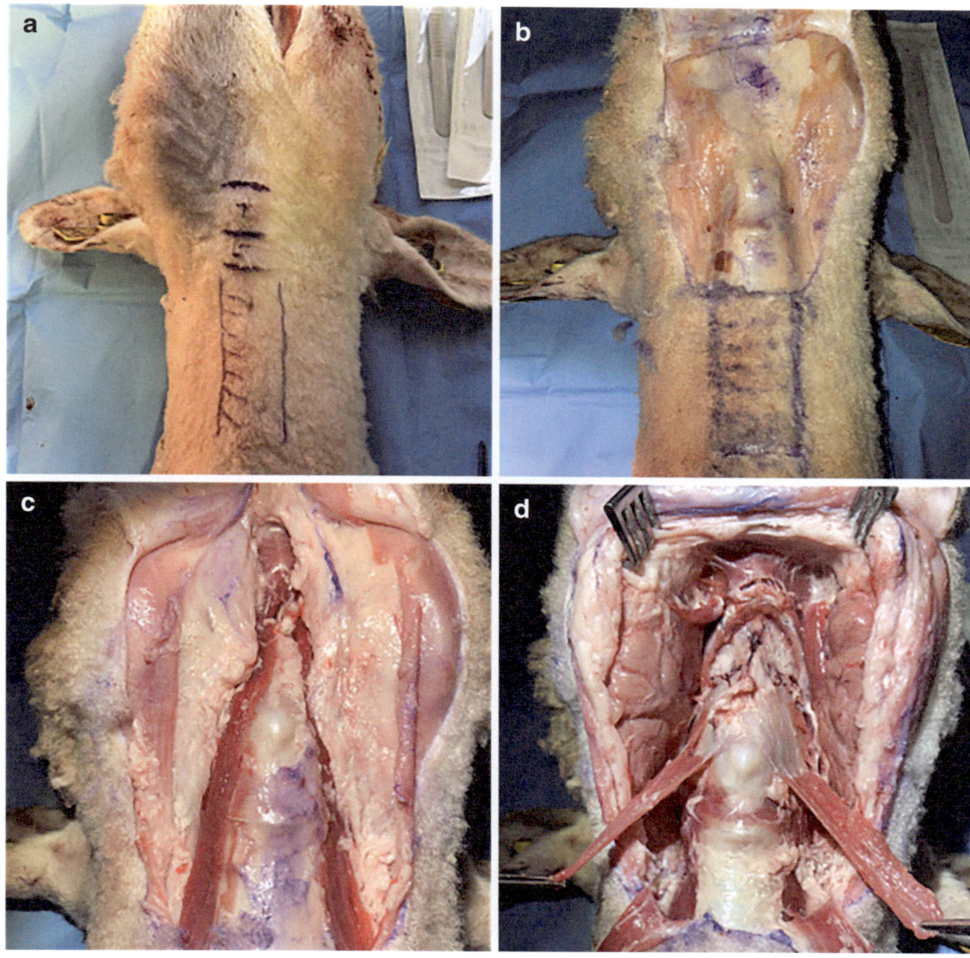

Fig. 13.2 (Panel **a**) Anatomical landmarks: hyoid bone, thyroid, and cricoid cartilages, trachea; (Panel **b**) Superior sub-platysmal flap elevation; (Panel **c**) Strap muscles and laryngotracheal framework identification; (Panel **d**) Detachment of the sternohyoid and thyrohyoid muscles from the hyoid bone and submandibular glands. Strap muscles reflected inferiorly

The fundamental prerequisite is the preservation of at least one functional cricoarytenoid unit.

13.2.2.5 OPHL I

Firstly, a dissection of the pre-epiglottic space, bounded by the thyrohyoid membrane and by the thyroepiglottic ligament, is performed (Fig. 13.6). The pre-epiglottic content is detached from its upper and posterior attachments up to the epiglottis foot, then the thyrohyoid membrane is incised just below the hyoid bone. This step is mandatory for OPHL I. Thyroid cartilage is incised immediately superiorly to the external projection of the anterior commissure and prolonged laterally, just over the glottic plane (Fig. 13.7). Once pharyngotomy and laryngotomy have been performed, supraglottic resection is obtained by cutting the aryepiglottic folds (Figs. 13.8 and 13.9). This step is usually performed by positioning behind the head of the model. Lines of resection are herein resumed:

- Inferiorly: horizontal incision of thyroid cartilage immediately superior to the anterior commissure.
- Superiorly: sub-hyoid incision, at the level of the mucosa of glossoepiglottic valleculas.
- Laterally: constrictor muscle incision, at the level of lateral pyriform sinus mucosa.

It is possible to extend the resection superiorly to the base of the tongue, laterally to a pyriform sinus, and inferiorly to an arytenoid.

Successively, a thyro-hyoido-pexy is made connecting the residual thyroid cartilage and hyoid bone with 3 or 5 Vicryl 1.0 stitches, which should be passed inferiorly through the thyroid cartilage in an extra-mucosal plane and superiorly through the base of the tongue, surrounding the hyoid bone; it is advisable to start from the midline and to continue 5–10 mm away from it on each side. The central stitch is generally placed at least 1 cm over the hyoid bone (to impact thyroid cartilage to hyoid bone), while the lateral ones are placed immediately over it, to not injure the lingual artery or hypoglossal nerve.

In the case of extension of resection, also reconstruction steps will be different (see also Sect. 6.3.2).

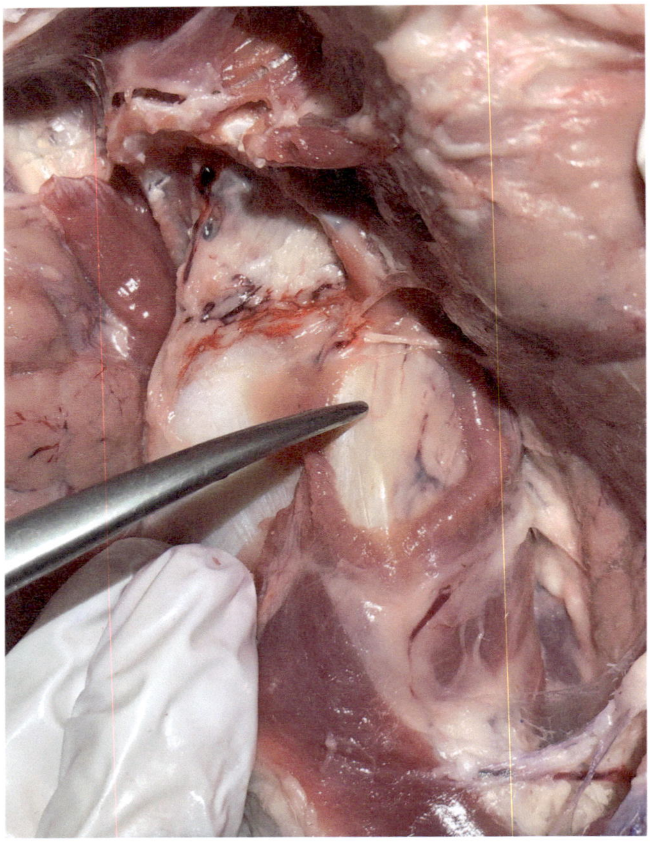

Fig. 13.3 Left side. Thyroid cartilage rotated medially and inferiorly, and constrictor muscles were sectioned along its posterior edge. Identification of the superior laryngeal nerve and vascular pedicle

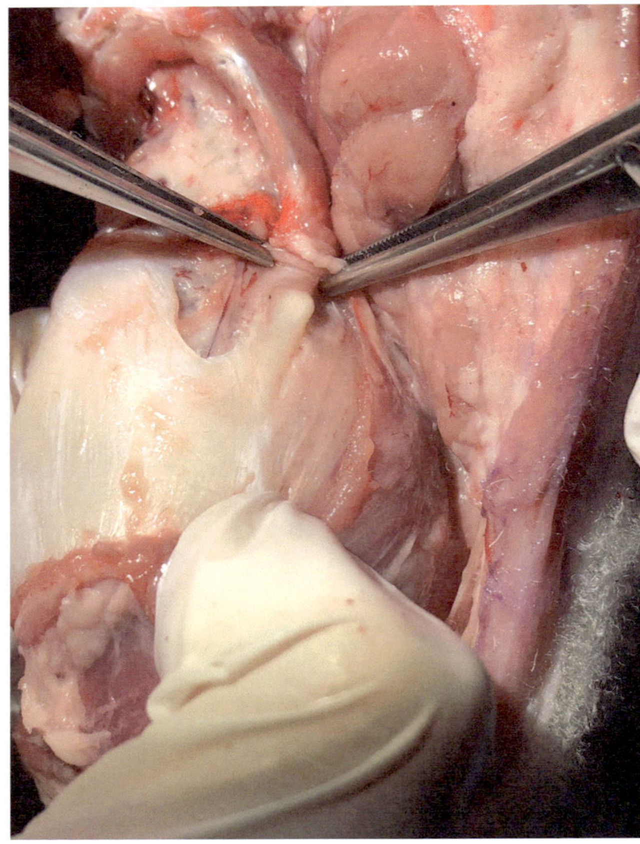

Fig. 13.4 Superior laryngeal nerve displacement over the thyroid cartilage superior horn

Fig. 13.5 (Panel **a**) Left side, skeletonization of the superior horn of the thyroid cartilage; (Panel **b**, **c**) Identification of the superior laryngeal nerve peripheral branches; (Panel **d**) Frontal view of the released thyroid cartilage

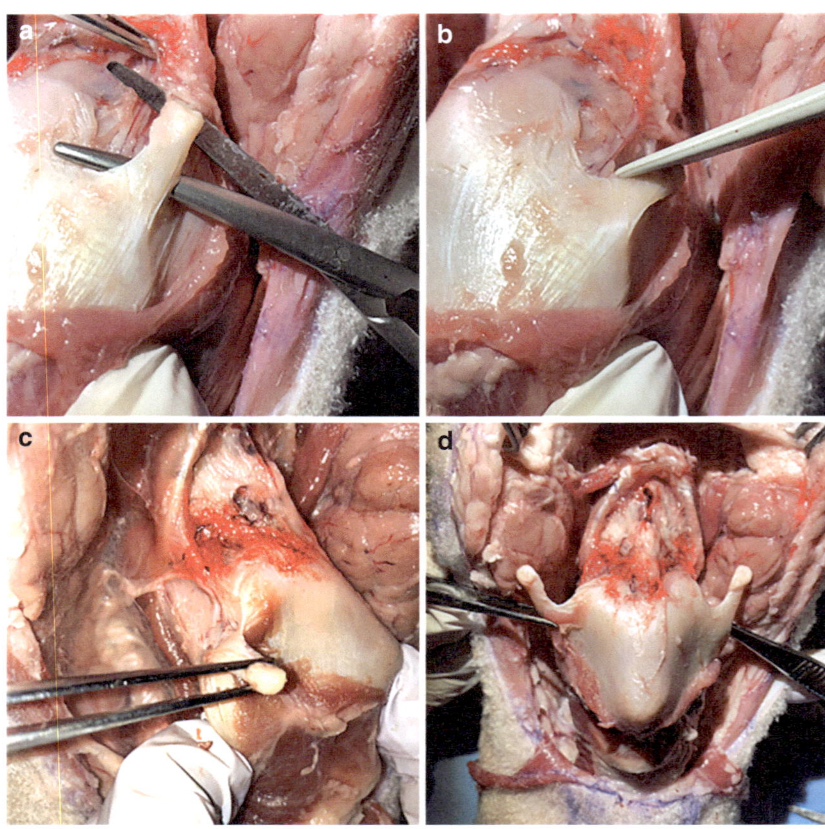

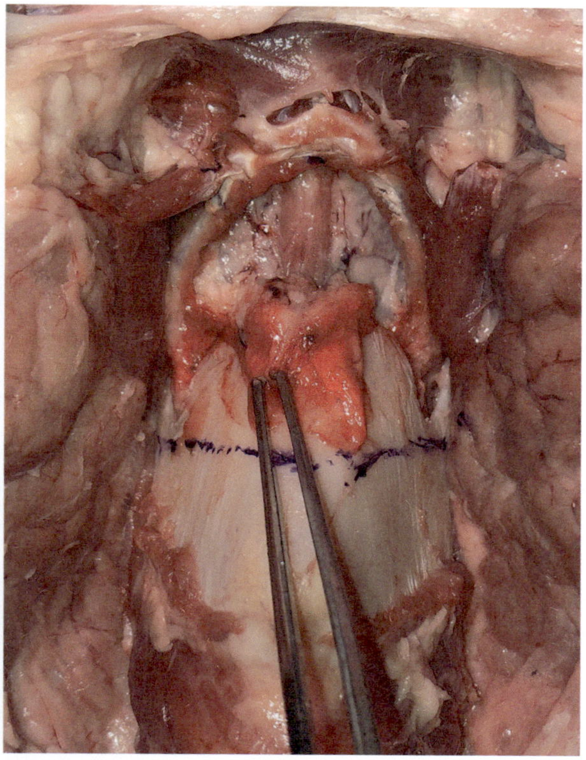

Fig. 13.6 Pre-epiglottic space dissection

13.2.2.6 OPHL II

This technique can be executed ex-novo on the ovine's model, or after some steps of the OPHL I. To exploit at most one sample and to train in the different techniques, it is advisable to perform OPHL II after having completed the monolateral thyrotomy step of OPHL I.

A horizontal incision to the cricothyroid space is made (Fig. 13.10). The isolation of the pyriform sinus must be completed caudally. The inferior horn of the thyroid cartilage can be sectioned to protect the inferior laryngeal nerve, which must be preserved to maintain a functional ipsilateral cricoarytenoid unit (Fig. 13.11).

Successively, if the surgeon chooses to perform an OPHL IIA, the upper limit of the resection is represented by a transepiglottic pharyngotomy, which is carried out perpendicularly to the superior aspect of the thyroid cartilage, to maintain a portion of the epiglottis (Fig. 13.12). Nonetheless, in the author's opinion, it is advisable to include in the resection the pre-epiglottic space, which could be separated by the hyoid bone and pulled down. Conversely, in the case of an OPHL IIB, the thyrohyoid membrane is incised just below the hyoid bone, to excise the epiglottis *en bloc* with the specimen. The upper pharyngeal incision is extended downward through the aryepiglottic fold and the false vocal folds, just anterior to the body of the arytenoids, pointing the scissors to

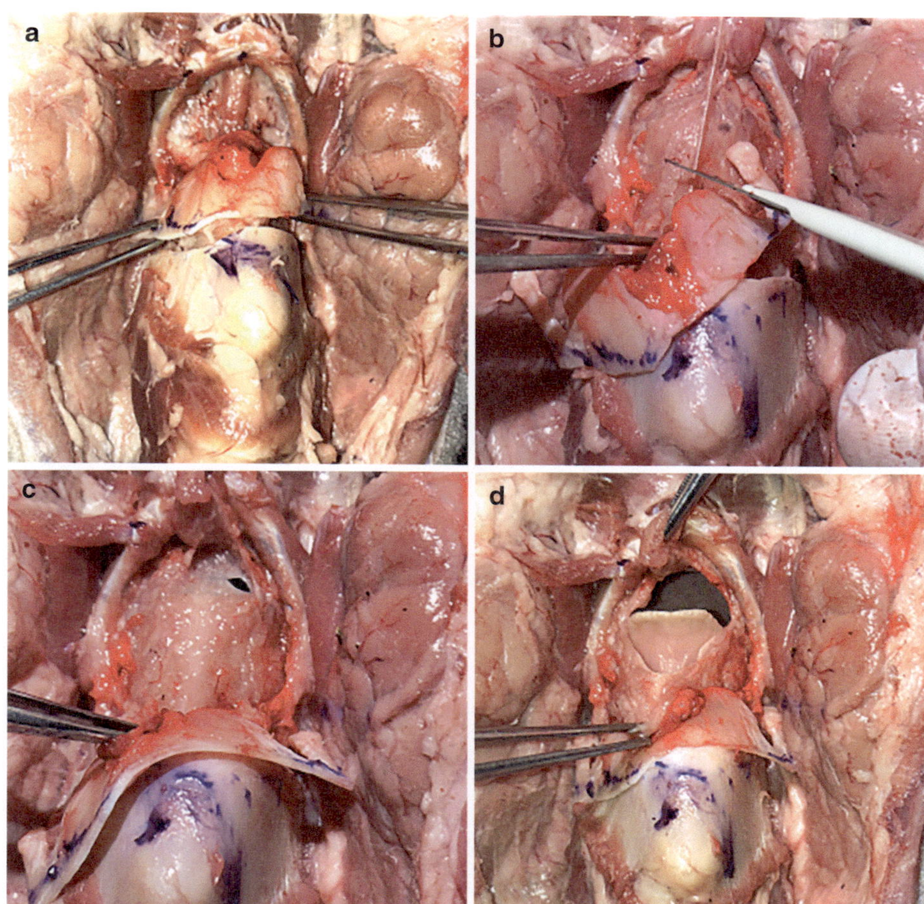

Fig. 13.7 (Panel **a**) Thyroid cartilage incision just above the external projection of the anterior commissure and prolonged laterally over the glottic plane; (Panel **b**) Thyrohyoid membrane incision just below the hyoid bone; (Panel **c**) Anterior pharyngotomy; (Panel **d**) Epiglottis exposure

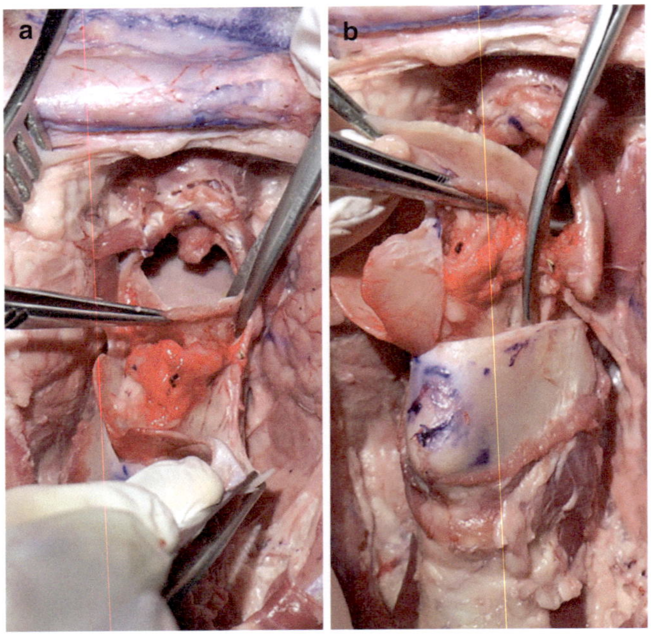

Fig. 13.8 Incision of the aryepiglottic folds. (Panel **a**) frontal view; (Panel **b**) lateral view

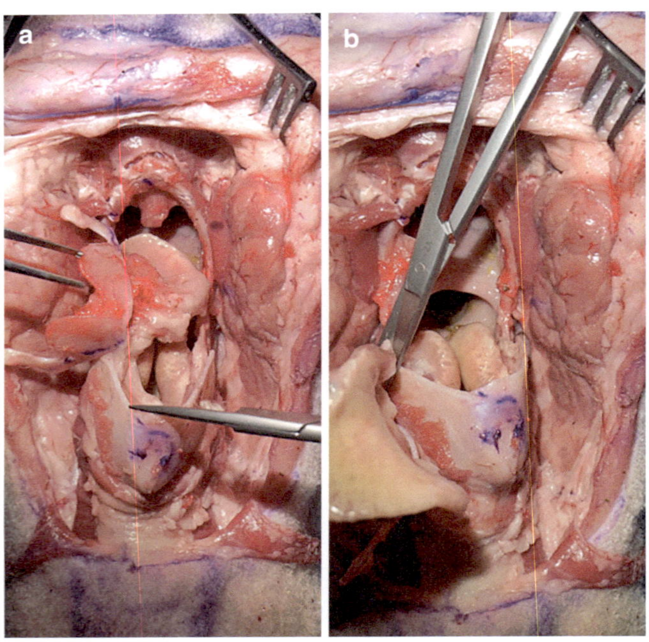

Fig. 13.9 (**a**–**b**) Final steps of supraglottic laryngectomy

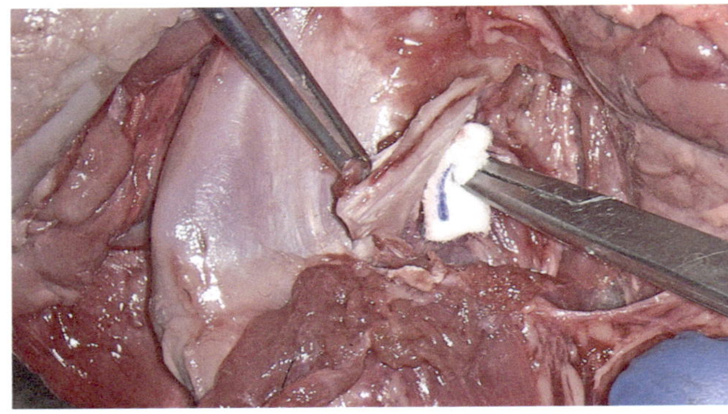

Fig. 13.10 Left side. Subperichondrial detachment of pyriform sinus from thyroid cartilage ala

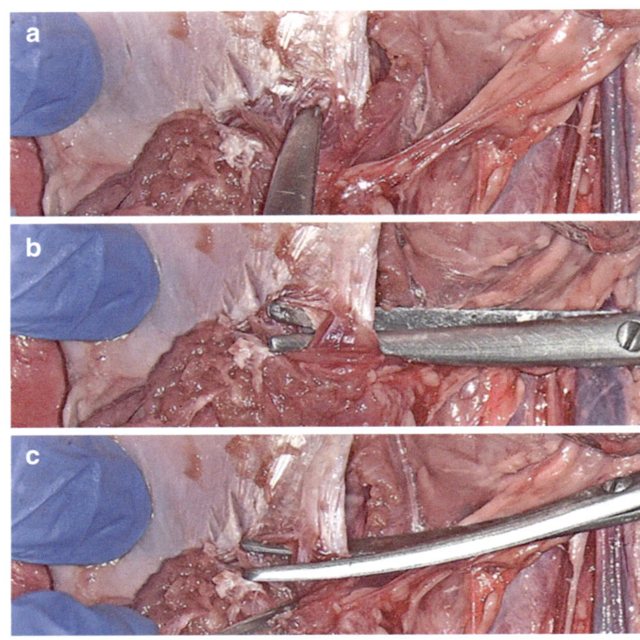

Fig. 13.11 Left side. (Panel **a**) Identification of the inferior horn of the thyroid cartilage; (Panel **b**) Dissection of the inferior horn of the thyroid cartilage; (Panel **c**) Section of the inferior horn of the thyroid cartilage

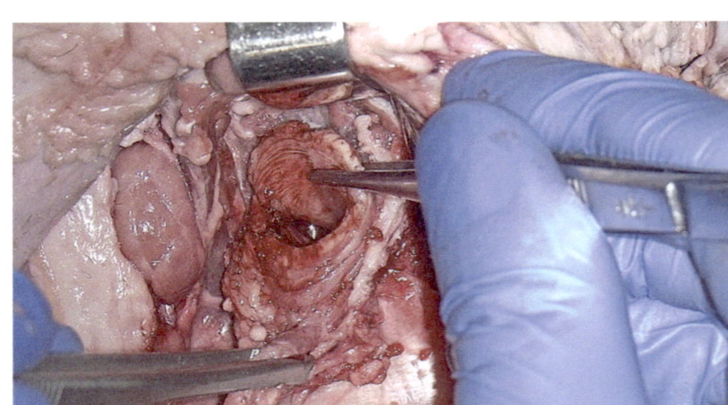

Fig. 13.12 Trans-epiglottic pharyngotomy

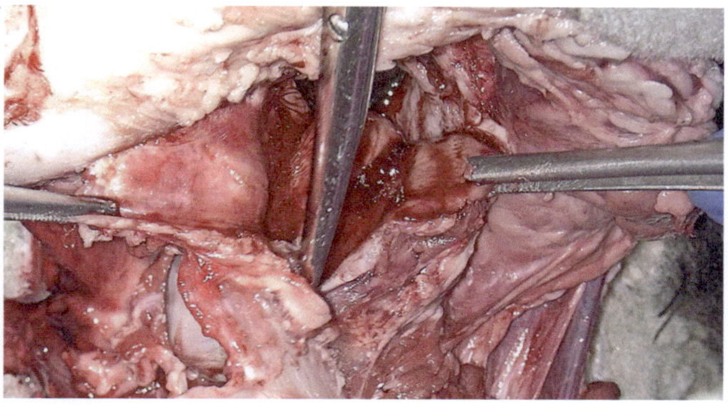

Fig. 13.13 Frontal view. An incision in front of the left arytenoid process encompassing the false and true vocal fold extended up to the cricoid ring surface is performed

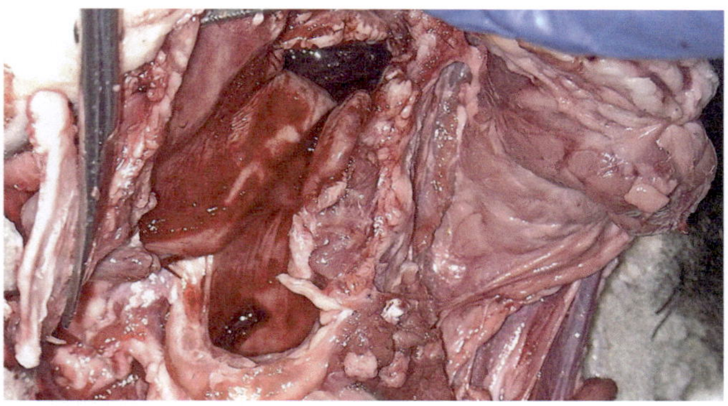

Fig. 13.14 Frontal view. Supracricoid laryngectomy on the left side. The same surgical step should be performed on the right side to complete the surgical resection

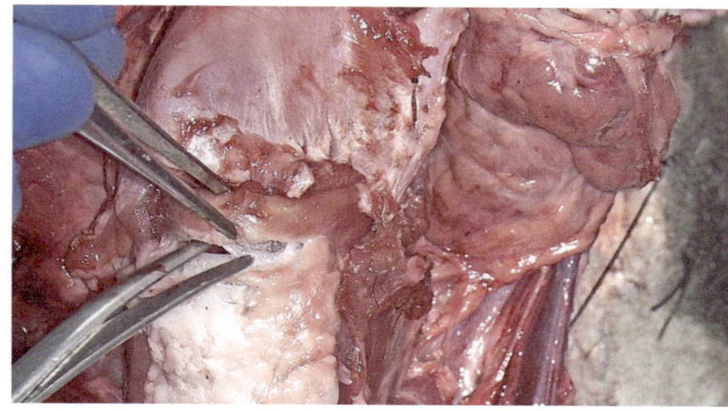

Fig. 13.15 Incision above the first tracheal ring

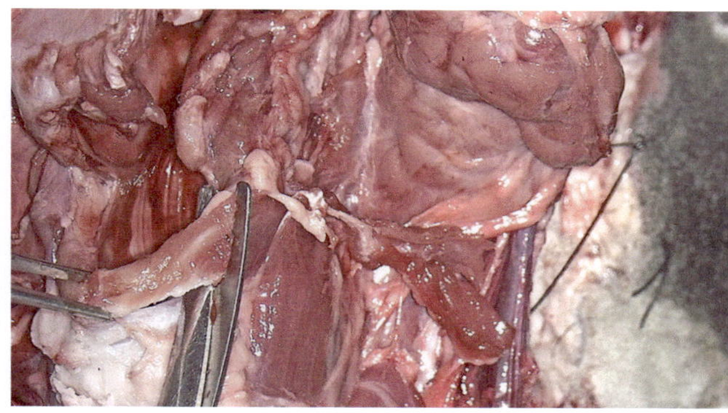

Fig. 13.16 Left cricoid ring incision performed in front of the crico-arytenoid unit

the vocal process of the arytenoid (Fig. 13.13). It is possible to extend the resection to a pyriform sinus or an arytenoid (Fig. 13.14). If the arytenoid is removed, a Vicryl 3.0 stitch is placed through the anterior edge of the remaining arytenoid mucosa and then tied to the cricoid cartilage to enlarge the pyriform sinus opening. In the case of OPHL IIb, the resection can be extended to the base of the tongue.

The reconstruction time consists of the crico-hyoido-epiglottopexy for OPHL IIa and crico-hyoido-pexy for OPHL IIb. Similarly to the OPHL I, the pexy is made with 3 or 5 Vicryl 1.0 stitches; these one should be passed submucosally, inferior to superior, around the cricoid ring and the hyoid bone. For the OPHL IIa reconstruction, the epiglottis should be transfixed by the stitches about 5 mm above the inferior edge to avoid retroflection of the cartilage which may determine further neoglottis stenosis. The same technical advices of thyroid-hyoido-pexy (see Sect. 13.2.2.5) stand valuable for crico-hyoido-epiglottopexy and crico-hyoido-pexy.

13.2.2.7 OPHL III

When an OPHL III is performed, the inferior horizontal incision is made between the cricoid ring and the first or second tracheal ring (Fig. 13.15); the resection should be extended at the junction between the cricoid plate and the cricoid ring bilaterally (Fig. 13.16). This maneuver protects the inferior laryngeal nerve close to its entry point into the larynx. The lateral and superior limits and resection technique are the same as OPHL II. It is possible to include in the resection a cricoarytenoid unit, extending the inferior incision posteriorly until the midline, then completing the dissection with a vertical inter-cricoarytenoids incision; pharyngeal retrocricoid mucosa must be preserved (Fig. 13.17). In order not to damage the mucosa of these hypopharyngeal subsites, it is useful to digitally stretch the pyriform sinus allowing a safer dissection along a submucosal plane (Fig. 13.18). Moreover, when the cricoarytenoid unit is removed, the ipsilateral pyriform sinus should be remodeled as for OPHL I/II with arytenoid sacrifice (Fig. 13.19). This step is mandatory to avoid postoperative dysphagia and inhalation.

The reconstruction time consists of tracheo-hyoido-pexy or tracheo-hyoido-epiglotto-pexy, which follow the same

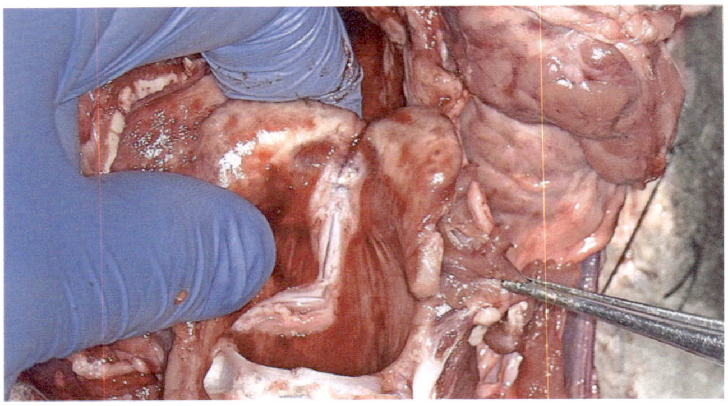

Fig. 13.17 Right cricoarytenoid unit resection. The mucosa of the inner aspect of the larynx is incised together with the underlying cricoid cartilage

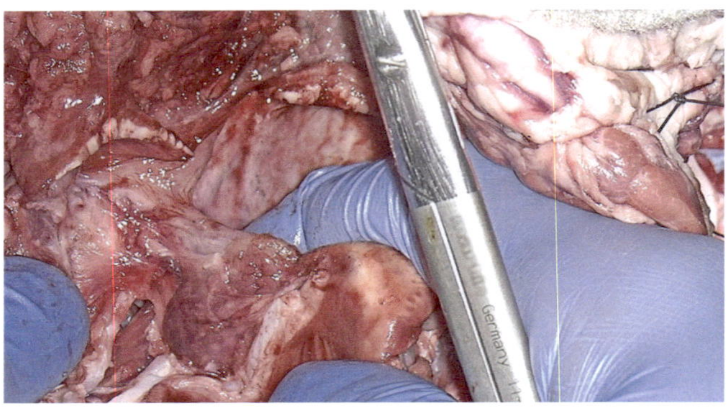

Fig. 13.18 Right cricoarytenoid unit resection. The mucosa of the right pyriform sinus is preserved for further reconstruction

steps as other OPHL II reconstructions. In this instance, 5 stitches will be passed inferiorly between the first and second tracheal ring, superiorly through the base of tongue mucosa, surrounding the hyoid bone as for the other reconstructive procedures described in this chapter (Fig. 13.20). The lateral limits of the reconstruction are the two points of junction between the cricoid plate and the cricoid ring. If a cricoarytenoid unit is sacrificed, the most lateral stitch will seal the hypopharyngeal mucosa. The same technical advices of thyroid-hyoido-pexy (see Sect. 13.2.2.5) stand valuable for tracheo-hyoido-pexy or tracheo-hyoido-epiglotto-pexy.

Box 13.1
In vivo it is wise to perform the access to the endolarynx starting from the side not involved or less involved by the tumor to obtain a wider view of the affected area.

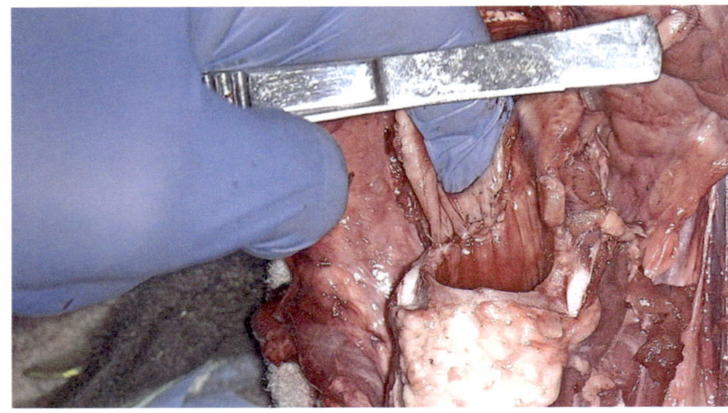

Fig. 13.19 Right pyriform sinus reconstruction suturing the superior edges of the pyriform sinus to the mucosa of the left cricoarytenoid unit and the trachea

13.2.2.8 Final Steps

The sternohyoid muscles can be sutured to the suprahyoid muscles to protect the pexy, as well as inferior constrictor muscles can be sutured to the lateral edges of the sternohyoid muscle. The restoration of the physiologic position of the constrictor muscles might improve swallowing function. Tracheotomy or tracheostomy is optional in training and can be done as one of the final step. The platysma is reapproximated followed by the closure of the skin.

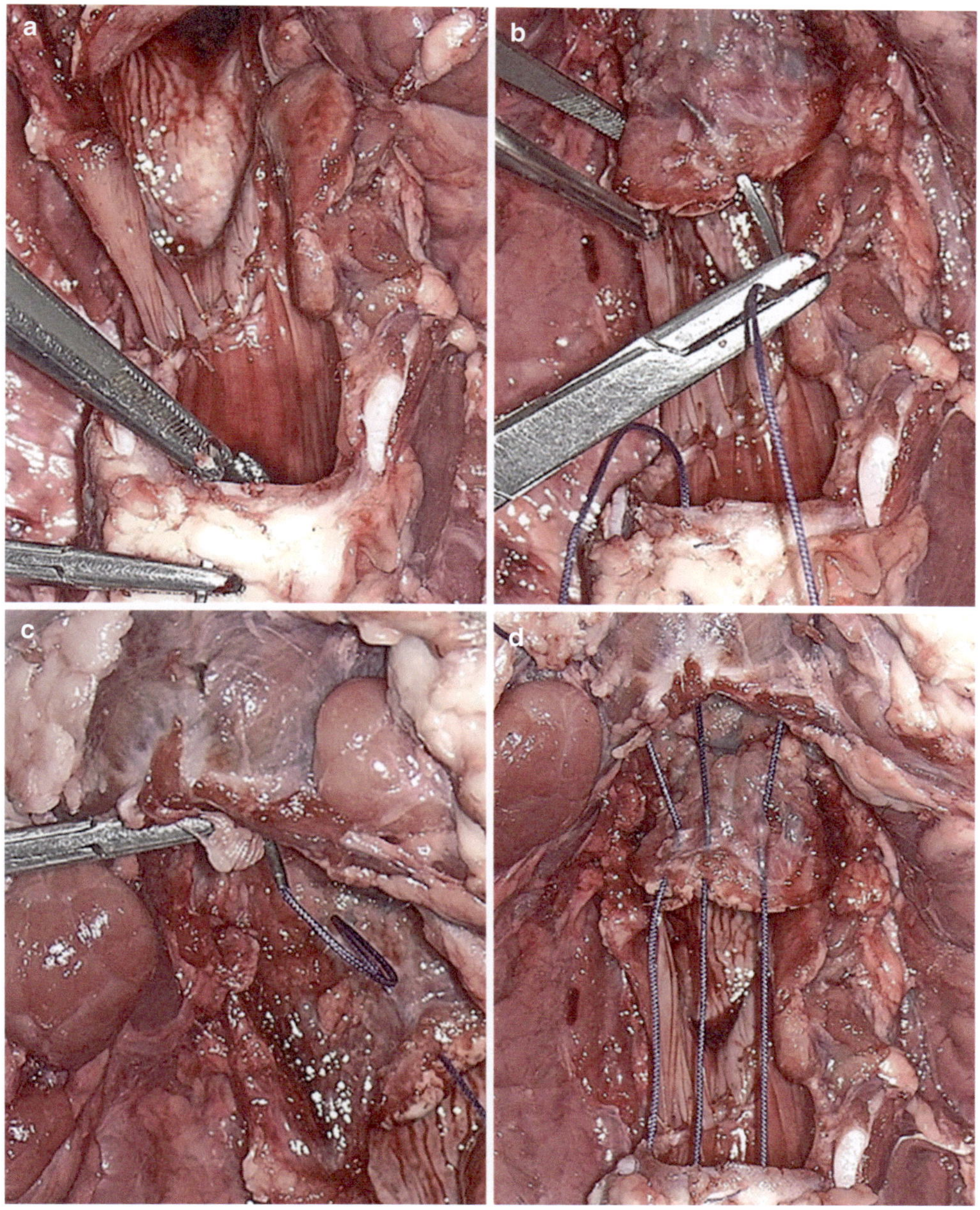

Fig. 13.20 Tracheo-hyoido-epiglotto-pexy. (Panel **a**) stitches are passed through the cartilage rings submucosally; (Panel **b**) central stitch is passed through the lingual surface of the epiglottis in its subperichondrial aspect; (Panel **c**) central stitch is then passed through the base of the tongue encompassing 1–2 cm of lingual tissue and the hyoid bone; (Panel **d**) lateral stitches are passed through the base of the tongue encompassing the hyoid bone and passing close to it

References

1. Gardner AK, Scott DJ, Hebert JC, Mellinger JD, Frey-Vogel A, Ten Eyck RP, Davis BR, Sillin LF 3rd, Sachdeva AK. Gearing up for milestones in surgery: will simulation play a role? Surgery. 2015;158(5):1421–7. https://doi.org/10.1016/j.surg.2015.03.039.
2. Ianacone DC, Gnadt BJ, Isaacson G. Ex vivo ovine model for head and neck surgical simulation. Am J Otolaryngol. 2016;37(3):272–8. https://doi.org/10.1016/j.amjoto.2016.01.015.
3. Zrunek M, Happak W, Hermann M, Streinzer W. Comparative anatomy of human and sheep laryngeal skeleton. Acta Otolaryngol. 1988;105(1–2):155–62. https://doi.org/10.3109/00016488809119460.
4. Fermi M, Mattioli F, Ghirelli M, Maccarrone F, Molteni G, Presutti L, Alicandri-Ciufelli M. Open laryngeal surgery training on ex-vivo ovine model: development and dissection experience. Auris Nasus Larynx. 2021;48(6):1150–6. https://doi.org/10.1016/j.anl.2021.04.001.
5. Nisa L, Teiga P, da Cunha GB, Roy B, Gunaydin RO, Sandu K. Refashioned lamb tissue as an animal model for training complex techniques of laryngotracheal stenosis surgery. Eur Arch Otorrinolaringol. 2017;274(12):4169–81. https://doi.org/10.1007/s00405-017-4775-5.
6. Anschuetz L, Bonali M, Ghirelli M, Mattioli F, Villari D, Caversaccio M, Presutti L. An Ovine model for exclusive endoscopic ear surgery. JAMA Otolaryngol Head Neck Surg. 2017;143(3):247–52. https://doi.org/10.1001/jamaoto.2016.3315.
7. Ghirelli M, Federici G, Melchiorri C, Malagoli A, Presutti L, Fernandez IJ. Ex vivo ovine model for surgical and microsurgical training on parotidectomy and facial nerve reanimation: proposal of structured training program. J Reconstr Microsurg. 2021;37(3):292–9. https://doi.org/10.1055/s-0040-1721122.

8. Ghirelli M, Mattioli F, Federici G, Ferri G, Malagoli A, Trebbi M, Presutti L. Ex vivo porcine larynx model for microlaryngoscopy laryngeal surgery: proposal for a structured surgical training. J Voice. 2020;34(4):629–35. https://doi.org/10.1016/j.jvoice.2019.02.007.
9. Rohlfing ML, Kuperstock JE, Friedman D, Spiegel JH. An ex vivo porcine model of the anterior glottoplasty for voice feminization surgery. Laryngoscope. 2020;130(4):E206–12. https://doi.org/10.1002/lary.28204.
10. Tucker ML, Sumner D, Reinink SK, Wilson DG, Carmalt JL. Ex vivo evaluation of arytenoid corniculectomy, compared with three other airway interventions, performed on cadaveric equine larynges with simulated recurrent laryngeal neuropathy. Am J Vet Res. 2019;80(12):1136–43. https://doi.org/10.2460/ajvr.80.12.1136.
11. Okhovat S, Milner TD, Clement WA, Wynne DM, Kunanandam T. Validation of animal models for simulation training in pediatric laryngotracheal reconstruction. Ann Otol Rhinol Laryngol. 2020;129(1):46–54. https://doi.org/10.1177/0003489419870820.
12. Ewies AA, Khan ZR. Cattle uterus: a novel animal laboratory model for advanced hysteroscopic surgery training. Obstet Gynecol Int. 2015;2015:967693. https://doi.org/10.1155/2015/967693.
13. Rocha de Faria JL, Pavão DM, de Sousa EB, Mozella AP, Leal AC, Guimarães JAM, Salim R, Villardi AM, Valente PAM, Miranda V, Mandarino M. How to create an arthroscopy training laboratory using a bovine knee model. Arthrosc Tech. 2021;10(7):e1865–71. https://doi.org/10.1016/j.eats.2021.04.007.
14. Molteni G, Nocini R, Ghirelli M, Molinari G, Fior A, Veneri A, Nocini PF, Marchioni D. Free flap head and neck microsurgery with VITOM® 3D: surgical outcomes and surgeon's perspective. Auris Nasus Larynx. 2021;48(3):464–70. https://doi.org/10.1016/j.anl.2020.09.010.

14 Histopathologic Workup for Laryngeal Cancers

Elena Maldi and Davide Balmativola

14.1 Introduction

This appendix aims to provide a schematic but comprehensive guide to handling OPHL surgical specimens from the pathological point of view, histologically recognize important anatomical structures both on macroscopic and microscopic examination, compare them with clinical and radiological findings, and formulate a complete histological report.

14.2 Intraoperative Examination

Intraoperative examination/frozen sections should be required by surgeons only if the diagnosis formulated at the extemporary examination would change the intraoperative approach.

In OPHL surgery, frozen sections are mainly requested to assess surgical margins and more rarely to confirm the neoplastic nature of the lesion, since a diagnostic biopsy should be routinely performed in the pre-operatory workup. Due to technical reasons, bone and cartilage tissue samples are not suitable for intraoperative examination.

Some techniques can improve the quality of the intraoperative frozen section, such as ultra-rapid freezing technology, thus preventing artifacts induced by ice crystals.

14.3 Specimen Handling and Orientation

- **Fresh specimen orientation**
  Surgical specimens are sent to the pathology lab fresh or submerged in buffered formalin, depending on local protocols. To maintain orientation and reduce tissue shrinkage/alteration due to formalin fixation, specimens should be orientated on a rigid support (e.g., polystyrene) before fixation.
  - **OPHL** specimens are relatively easy to orientate due to the presence of the horns of the thyroid cartilage, however, fixing the specimen to rigid support will reduce tissue shrinkage and facilitate subsequent tissue sampling (Fig. 14.1).
  - **Neck dissection** specimens oriented on rigid supports allow a more precise attribution of lymph nodes to anatomical levels, consequently guiding radiotherapy, if necessary (Fig. 14.2).
- **Pre-grossing and fixation**
  To preserve tissue integrity, fresh specimens should be promptly submerged in an adequate volume of buffered formalin, since cold ischemia time (time interval between the end of surgical procedure and the start of fixation) has been proven to directly affect morphology and thus interpretation and diagnosis. Due to the safety concerns/limitations related to the use of formalin, this step is frequently impossible to be performed in the operatory theater, and delivering specimens to the pathology lab immediately after removal may be logistically overwhelming.
  Tissue vacuum sealing followed by immediate preservation at 4 °C has been proven to be a safe and cost-effective procedure and guarantees optimal tissue preservation and even molecular analysis [1, 2]
  Room temperature formalin has a relatively low tissue penetration: 1 mm per hour for the first hour, then 1 mm in the subsequent 3 h. To avoid autolysis in the central part of the organs, pathologists can perform "pre-grossing" cuts on the specimen to facilitate fixation. OPHL specimens, due to their dimensions, normally do not require a pre-grossing step. However parallel cuts can be performed on bulky metastatic cervical nodes.

E. Maldi (✉) · D. Balmativola
Unit of Pathology, Candiolo Cancer Institute, FPO—IRCCS, Candiolo, Italy

F. Mattioli et al. (eds.), *Atlas of Open Partial Horizontal Laryngectomy*, https://doi.org/10.1007/978-3-031-48023-2_14

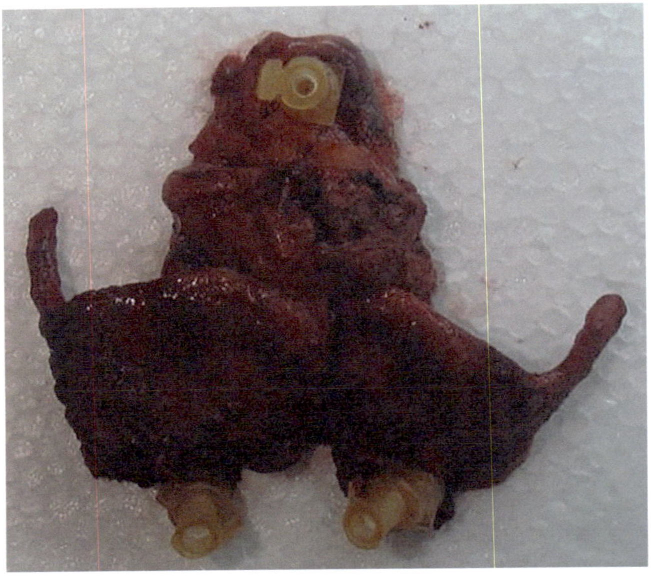

Fig. 14.1 Fresh OPHL specimen oriented on a rigid support

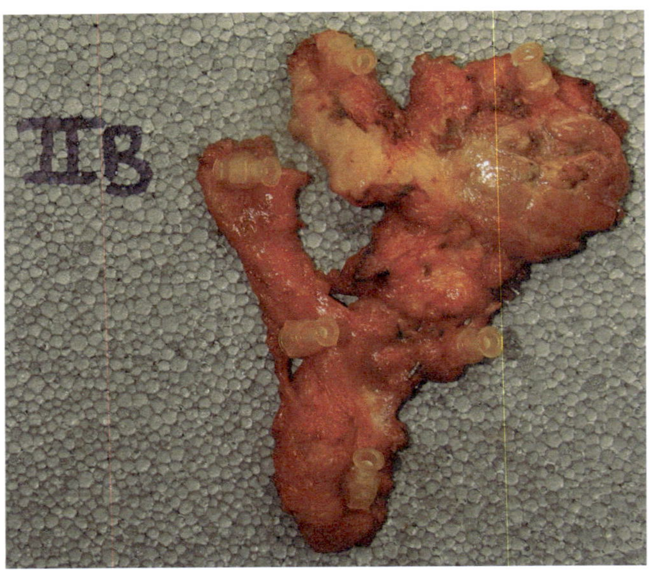

Fig. 14.2 Fresh RND specimen oriented on a rigid support

14.4 Specimen Grossing and Processing

- **Macroscopic examination and margins evaluation**
  Macroscopic examination of surgical specimens represents a crucial step of histological examination in H&N pathology. An accurate description of anatomical structures detected in OPHL surgical specimens (e.g., thyroid cartilage, arytenoid cartilage, and paraglottic space), including dimensions and axial orientation about the glottic plane, is very important, as well as a gross description of the neoplastic lesion: a three-dimensional evaluation, including maximum diameters (cranial-caudal and lateral-lateral) and depth of invasion, is pivotal to be made to compare macroscopic dimensions with microscopic findings, and to integrate the tumor description in cases in which it is not possible to measure a tumoral dimension on the histological slides—maybe as a consequence of the sectioning approach (see "Diagnosis and staging" paragraph).
  Resection margins need to be carefully evaluated: at the gross examination, the surgical specimen has to be inked to mark the surgical margins (ink will be identified on microscopic evaluation). Distance of the neoplastic lesion from the margins has to be recorded, considering fixations artifacts (like the shrinking of the surgical specimen) when dimensions are measured after formalin fixation (Fig. 14.3).
- **Decalcification**
  OPHL surgical specimens usually need to undergo a decalcification process to allow cartilaginous tissue to be sectioned, both macroscopically (when sampling) and microscopically (at the microtome, cutting 4 μm-thick sections to be put on the histological slides). Any specimen has to be properly fixed in formalin before decalcification, to protect tissue from the hydrolytic action of the decalcifying solutions. Later, it will be important to accurately determine the end point of decalcification. Prolonged exposure to decalcifying agents damages the tissues, inducing artifacts potentially compromising micro-histological evaluation. On the opposite, incomplete decalcification, evident when trimming a paraffin block, can result in damaging to the microtome knife, thus jeopardizing the soft tissue surrounding the calcified tissue. The average decalcification turnaround time is about 7–10 days for OPHL specimens. Considering that decalcifying solutions are effective on soft tissues surrounding the cartilage as well and that this could create, again, massive artifacts, it is important to provide *at least* one sample of the neoplastic tissue before decalcification, to preserve the histological morphology and to allow ancillary evaluations (immunohistochemistry and molecular analyses), if necessary.
- **Sagittal vs coronal sampling approach**
  When sampling OPHL specimens different sampling approaches can be used, based on the possibility of better evaluating specific anatomical structures.
  - The "**axial**" sectioning is useful to evaluate neoplastic extension to different anatomical structures, evaluating a specific horizontal plane; to reconstruct craniocaudal extension, the parallel grossing section should be performed at 5mm intervals, clearly stating the anatomical structures involved (e.g., supraglottic, glottic or subglottic region) (Fig. 14.4a).
  - The "**sagittal**" sectioning offers the opportunity to study the craniocaudal neoplastic extension and subglottic

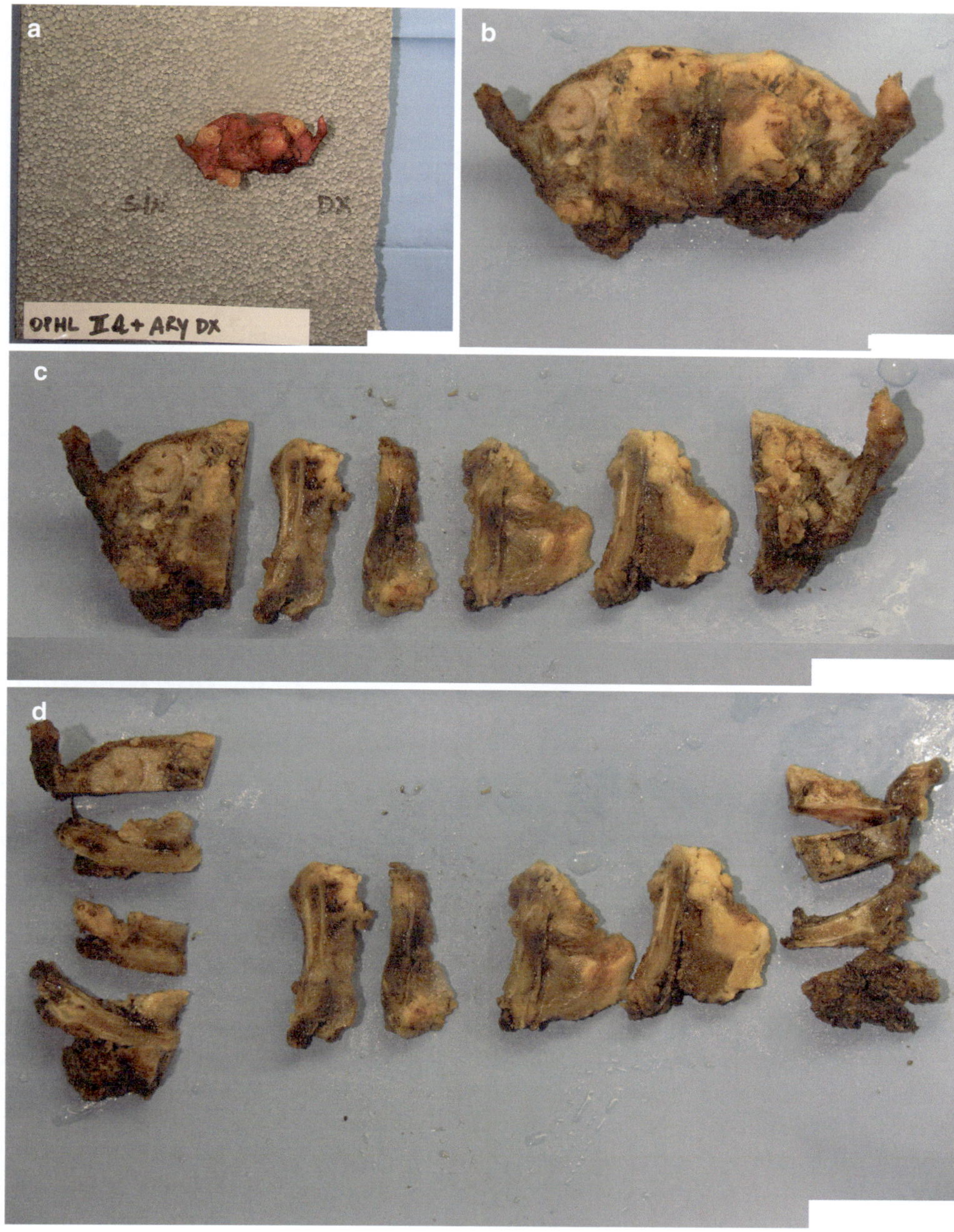

Fig. 14.3 Comparison between the macroscopic appearance of an OPHL specimen before formalin fixation oriented on a rigid support (**a**) and the same specimen after fixation (**b**). Central sections were obtained using the sagittal approach (**c**); sampling of lateral margins was finally performed perpendicularly to the sagittal slices (**d**)

involvement. To reconstruct lateral-lateral extension, the parallel grossing section should be performed at 5 mm intervals, clearly stating the laterality and the structures involved (e.g., anterior commissure) (Fig. 14.4b).

The decision on using the sagittal or the axial approach should be eventually discussed for any case depending on the staging, imaging, and the proximity of the neoplastic lesion to a specific resection margin.

A comprehensive method for efficiently studying the relationship between the tumor and both the margins and the anatomical structures in OPHL surgical specimens may consist of a sagittal approach for slicing the specimen (using macrosections, if possible), then extensively sampling lateral margins perpendicularly to the sagittal slices (the so-called T sampling of resection margins) (Fig. 14.3).

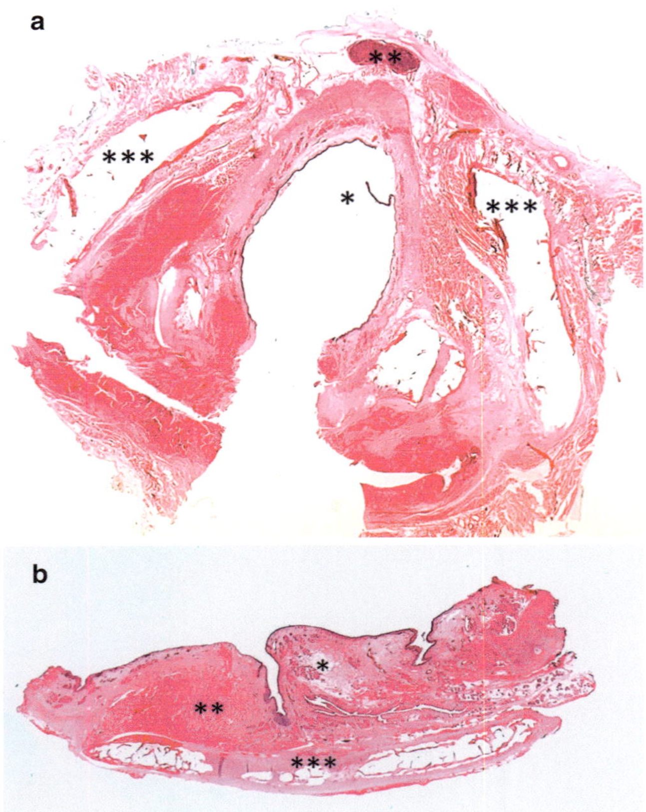

Fig. 14.4 Axial (**a**) vs sagittal (**b**) sections of OPHL specimens. (**a**) Axial macrosection: *larynx lumen; **Delphic lymph node; ***thyroid cartilage. (**b**) Sagittal macro section: *Supraglottis and superior paraglottic space, **Hypoglottis and inferior paraglottic space, ***thyroid cartilage

14.5 Macrosections: Pros and Cons

The use of large format sections (LS), also known as macrosections, consists of processing large samples utilizing large paraffin blocks, a large format microtome, and a large glass slide to accommodate an entire histological section of the organ under study.

In daily practice, LS are potentially useful to understand, diagnose, and manage pathological lesions from all organs. They have been first introduced in surgical pathology more than a century ago for studying breast specimens [3]. Slootweg and Grot applied LS to stage neoplastic lesions of the head and neck district, comprising the different areas of the larynx [4].

In H&N pathology, LS is useful to correlate radiological and histological findings, as their use is simple to compare radiological images to the large histological sections as well as three-dimensional reconstructions [5, 6]. Neoplastic extent and tissue involvement, especially in this district, are of crucial importance to perform a correct staging. LS allows to include bony and cartilaginous tissues together with the surrounding soft tissues, easily and unequivocally demonstrating the type and extension of neoplastic growth.

H&N specimens should be sliced with a large blade, into sections of 5 mm thick. Dedicated LS protocols for automatic processing should be used. Specimens are embedded using the same procedure employed for prostatectomies [7]. After embedding, paraffin blocks thus obtained are then cut with a dedicated macrotome, and eventually, hematoxylin-eosin large slides are obtained. If immunohistochemistry or molecular studies are needed, areas of interest are selected from the LS and cut to obtain small conventional blocks.

As M.P. Foschini and colleagues stated, "… despite their utility in diagnostic pathology, LS are still used in a relatively few laboratories, mainly as a consequence of the fact that their preparation is perceived as more time consuming and expensive than conventional blocks. This difference is only apparent as in LS a large portion of tissue is examined that is far superior to the conventional small blocks…." [5]. It has currently been demonstrated the cost-effectiveness of the use of LS, and the turnaround time in the pathology laboratory is no longer than 24 h.

14.6 How to Recognize…

The aim of this paragraph is not to describe in detail anatomical structures of the larynx, since plenty of more prestigious publications are already available, but to provide a short list of pivotal structures that should be known by the pathologist reporting an OPHL specimen, as well as some information and landmarks suggestion on how to recognize them and their involvement on microscopic examination. The author's suggestion is, however, to always approach an OPHL specimen after studying the pre-operative imaging and to discuss any discrepancy or doubt with the radiologists and the surgeons: cooperation is a crucial aspect not only for the patient's interest but will enrich all the specialists involved.

- **Pre-epiglottic Space (PES)**
  On the sagittal approach is the space, composed of soft tissues, between epiglottic cartilage and thyroid cartilage. It may not be straightforwardly recognized when massively infiltrated by carcinoma: in this case, we suggest following the epiglottis profile and projecting an imaginary line to connect epiglottis and thyroid cartilage, this will help to identify the space. However, a frank PES involvement should at least be suspected by the radiologist, whereas a focal infiltration will only be evident on histology slides (Fig. 14.5).
- **Superior and Inferior Paraglottic Space (SPS and IPS)**
  The definition of these entities changed several times during the past decades. On a practical approach, the paraglottic space consists of the soft tissues (mainly composed of adipose tissue with interspersed small sero-mucinous glands) interposed between the mucosa and the thyroid

cartilage, and it is divided into *SUPERIOR* (supraglottic region) and *INFERIOR* (glottic and hypoglottic region). SPS or IPS neoplastic involvement is present when the tumor penetrates connective tissues (Fig. 14.5). Please consider that exophytic neoplasm may radiologically mimic paraglottic space infiltration as well as a supraglottic extension on imaging.

- **Arytenoid**
  It is a pyramid-shaped cartilaginous tissue in the posterior third of the vocal cord, which is included in the OPHL specimen if imaging and pre-operatory workup suggest its neoplastic involvement. To demonstrate infiltration, particular attention is necessary when sampling this structure since it will be found close to lateral /posterior margins. Depending on the specimen, it can be sampled as part of the "T" shaped inked margin or with the aid of LS.
- **Thyroid Cartilage**
  If macroscopically recognizing thyroid cartilage is not an issue, microscopically examination cannot be as simple. It should be sampled *in toto* at least on the side of the tumor and in correspondence with the anterior commissure, but the authors' suggestion is to microscopically examine both sides. In advanced tumors, it can be sampled together with the mucosal/soft tissue counterpart, after performing a neoplasm sample before decalcification. In earlier stages, mucosa and soft tissues can be sampled *in toto* before decalcification and whereas cartilage sampling can be done after. Different inks can be used to help recognize the exterior and interior surface of the cartilage (Fig. 14.6).

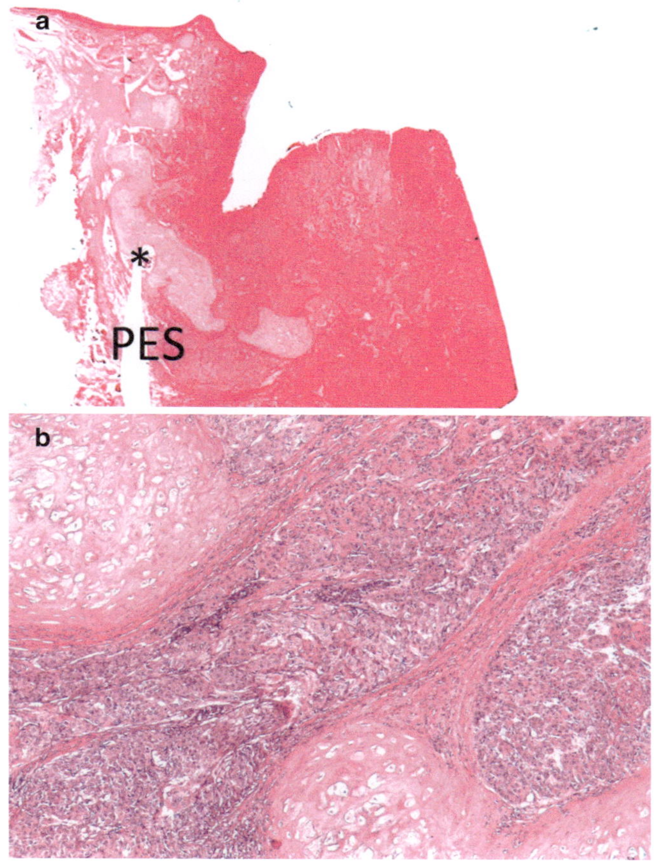

Fig. 14.5 Pre-epiglottic space invasion by squamous cell carcinoma

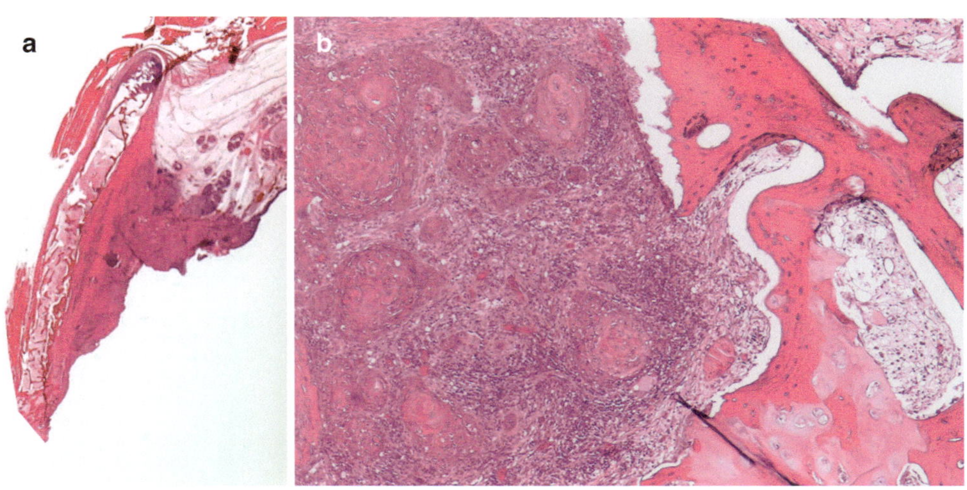

Fig. 14.6 Neoplastic invasion of inferior paraglottic space and through outer cortex of thyroid cartilage

References

1. Annaratone L, Marchiò C, Sapino A. Tissues under-vacuum to overcome suboptimal preservation. N Biotechnol. 2019;52:104–9. https://doi.org/10.1016/j.nbt.2019.05.007.
2. Berrino E, Annaratone L, Miglio U, Maldi E, Piccinelli C, Peano E, Balmativola D, Cassoni P, Pisacane A, Sarotto I, Venesio T, Sapino A, Marchiò C. Cold formalin fixation guarantees DNA integrity in formalin fixed paraffin embedded tissues: premises for a better quality of diagnostic and experimental pathology with a specific impact on breast cancer. Front Oncol. 2020;10:173. https://doi.org/10.3389/fonc.2020.00173.
3. Cheatle GL. Early recognition of cancer of the breast. Br Med J. 1906;1906(1):1205–10.
4. Slootweg PJ, de Grot JAM. Surgical pathological anatomy oh head and neck specimens. Springer; 1999.
5. Foschini MP, Baldovini C, Ishikawa Y, Eusebi V. The value of large sections in surgical pathology. Int J Breast Cancer. 2012;2012:785947. https://doi.org/10.1155/2012/785947.
6. Foschini MP, Righi A, Cucchi MC, et al. The impact of large sections and 3D technique on the study of lobular in situ and invasive carcinoma of the breast. Virchows Arch. 2006;448(3):256–61.
7. Montironi R, Lopez BA, Mazzucchelli R, Cheng L, Scarpelli M. Handling of radical prostatectomy specimens: total embedding with large-format histology. Int J Breast Cancer. 2012;2012:932784. 6 pages

A Modular Form of Informed Consent for the OPHL Surgeries

15

Leone Giordano, Davide Di Santo, Andrea Galli, and Mario Bussi

15.1 Introduction

Open Partial Horizontal Laryngectomies (OPHLs) are nowadays well-accepted procedures for the treatment of selected cases of laryngeal cancer [1, 2]. According to the classification system proposed by the European Laryngological Society [3], three types of OPHLs are defined: type I (supraglottic), type II (supracricoid), and type III (supratracheal). Each type may be extended to adjacent laryngeal and/or pharyngeal sites: OPHL type I to one arytenoid, the base of the tongue, or one pyriform sinus; OPHL type II to one arytenoid; OPHL type III to one crico-arytenoid unit. Moreover, OPHL types II and III are further distinguished by the suffix "a" or "b" depending on the sparing or the removal of the suprahyoid epiglottis. This classification allows to clearly define all possible variations in terms of the extent of resection.

A main advantage of OPHLs, provided by the wide range of variability of the procedures, is the possibility to tailor the surgery to the specific extent of the patient's disease.

The surgeon preoperatively selects the appropriate procedure according to the extension of the tumor, but has the possibility to intraoperatively extend the procedure or shift to the next OPHL type in case safe margins cannot be clearly achieved with the scheduled surgery.

L. Giordano
Department of Otolaryngology-Head and Neck Surgery, Scientific Institutes of Hospitalization and Care San Raffaele Hospital, Milan, Italy

D. Di Santo (✉)
Otorhinolaryngology Unit, IRCCS Humanitas Research Hospital, Rozzano, Milan, Italy
e-mail: davide.disanto@humanitas.it

A. Galli · M. Bussi
Department of Otolaryngology-Head and Neck Surgery, Scientific Institutes of Hospitalization and Care San Raffaele Hospital, Milan, Italy

San Raffaele Vita-Salute University, Milan, Italy

For example, if frozen sections reveal positive margins on the subglottic mucosa during an OPHL type II, the procedure will be converted to an OPHL type III, which still provides the same excellent oncological and functional outcomes.

Therefore, OPHLs provide the surgeon with an amazing tool to approach the tumor in an organ in which a few millimeters could mean everything. However, in extreme cases, if the tumor spreads to some regions (i.e., the posterior paraglottic space or both the arytenoid cartilages), the procedure can no longer be performed and must be intraoperatively converted into a total laryngectomy. The patient must be conscious and accept this eventuality.

Full comprehension and alliance between patient and surgeon are fundamental, therefore when approaching an OPHL, the surgeon should refer to a surgical plan rather than to a single procedure.

However, the great advantage of being able to tailor the procedure, even intraoperatively, to the precise extent of the disease may also hide crucial drawbacks. First, the patient may experience difficulties in understanding the complexity of the procedure and the possibility to shift from one OPHL type to another, potentially resulting in a higher complication rate, longer rehabilitation time [2], or a drastic lifestyle change in case of total laryngectomy. Second, the surgeon should specifically mention any possible intraoperative variation to the preoperatively scheduled procedure when explaining it to the patient and obtain the patient's consent to any variation, including total laryngectomy, since the procedure cannot be stopped halfway.

Providing complete and appropriate preoperative information to a patient undergoing surgery and obtaining full consent to the procedure is dictated by law and may prevent future litigations.

A unified "modular" informed consent form (ICF), in which the surgeon can specify the scheduled OPHL type and can detail any possible extension, could therefore be extremely helpful. We already presented such ICF in a previous publication [4]. In association with the ICF, an Information Form (IF), containing detailed explanations of

F. Mattioli et al. (eds.), *Atlas of Open Partial Horizontal Laryngectomy*, https://doi.org/10.1007/978-3-031-48023-2_15

laryngeal anatomy, physiology, the rationale of surgery, description of different procedures and extensions, alternatives to surgery, potential complications, and physiology of the operated larynx would be a very valuable supplement.

15.2 Essential Elements of an Appropriate Informed Consent Form

Informed consent is a legal term, defined as "voluntary authorization, by a patient or research subject, with full comprehension of the risk involved, for diagnostic or investigative procedures, and for medical and surgical treatment" (year introduced: 1973 (1971), http://www.ncbi.nlm.nih.gov/mesh/68007258?ordinalpos=1&itool=EntrezSystem2.PEntrez.Mesh_ResultsPanel.Mesh_RVDocSum) and is supported by three cornerstones: preconditions, information, and consent [5].

The *preconditions* are competence and voluntariness. Patients have the right to self-determination [6]. They must have the competence to make decisions, and they must express voluntariness, without external influence. Generally, competence is recognized by the surgeon if communication appears to be "normal." However, in a review on patient competence, Appelbaum [7] surprisingly found that the number of "incompetent" patients was higher than expected, and that doctors are unable to differentiate between competent and incompetent patients. OPHLs require a strong alliance between surgeon and patient; during the postoperative period, patient collaboration and firm compliance are essential for rehabilitation. The surgeon must be sure of the presence of these preconditions before proposing any surgical procedure and should rule out any psychiatric disorder.

Information is the second cornerstone. The 1995 WHO Declaration on the Promotion of Patients' Rights states that patient has the right to be fully informed about their health status. This includes information about their condition, proposed medical procedures, potential risks and benefits of each procedure, alternatives to the proposed procedures (including the effects of non-treatment), and the diagnosis, prognosis, and progress of treatment [8]. The surgeon should discuss with the patient a well-defined care plan and must be sure that they understood the information. Communication is fundamental; most legal cases are not due to failures in treatment, but due to failure in communication [9]. It is demonstrated that oral information is retained very poorly, and patients tend to forget crucial parts [10]. Therefore, providing the patients an IF prior to surgery can be extremely helpful. Better informed patients will have more realistic expectations and higher satisfaction and demonstrate more treatment cooperation [11].

Consent is the registration of the patient's decision and the authorization to proceed. Depending on each country's legislation, consent can be obtained orally or in writing. A consent form should be readable and written at a 12-year-old's reading level [12]. Even though it may not be mandatory, it is strongly advisable to have a written ICF.

15.3 Information Form

A booklet containing the most relevant information about the procedure should be prepared by the surgeon and provided to the patient. It should include figures to make it easier to understand. This booklet should be intended for persons without any medical knowledge, and try to explain medical terms in simple words.

It is crucial to instruct patients about the aim of the procedure, focusing on the concept of oncological safety, and describe the dynamism of OPHLs, to clarify the possibility of intraoperative variation to the scheduled plan.

Some patients prefer not being informed about the procedure and completely rely on the surgeon's decisions [13]. Even in these cases, a written IF provided in advance may be helpful to the patient whether they would need some information.

15.4 Modular Informed Consent Form

OPHLs benefit from a modular ICF that can be tailored to each patient's specific case as well as the surgical procedure.

A modular ICF does not limit itself to the registration of the patient's decision and the authorization to proceed; it represents an agreement on a tailored surgical plan. This agreement will be an insurance for both the patient, to have the best surgical procedure according to oncological safety, and for the surgeon, to perform an OPHL without any concern of extending his procedure if needed.

The consent starts with a section about the personal details of the patient and the surgeon.

To define the precise extension of the tumor, the ICF includes a multiple-choice list of all laryngeal and extra-laryngeal structures that can be involved by the neoplasm.

Extent of the disease

Dear Mr/Mrs, your tumor involves:

☐	Epiglottis		
☐	Base of tongue or glossoepiglottic folds		
☐	Mucosa of the piriform sinus		
☐	Aryepiglottic fold	☐ right	☐ left
☐	Laryngeal vestibule		
☐	Pre-epiglottic space		
☐	False vocal cord	☐ right	☐ left
☐	Laryngeal ventricule	☐ right	☐ left
☐	Vocal cord	☐ right	☐ left
☐	Anterior commissure		
☐	Arytenoid cartilage	☐ right	☐ left
☐	Thyroid cartilage		
☐	Paraglottic space	☐ right	☐ left
☐	Cricoid cartilage		
☐	Crico-arytenoid unit	☐ right	☐ left
☐	Subglottic mucosa		
☐	Crico-thyroid membrane		
☐	Prelaryngeal soft tissues		

After defining the extent of the disease, in a second multiple-choice list, the surgeon chooses the specific scheduled procedure.

Surgical Procedure

- ☐ Horizontal Supraglottic Laryngectomy (OPHL type I)
  - ☐ extended to one arytenoid cartilage (OPHL type I + ARY)
  - ☐ extended to the base of the tongue (OPHL type I + BOT)
  - ☐ extended to the piriform sinus (OPHL type I + PIR)
- ☐ Supracricoid laryngectomy with crico-hyoido-epiglottopexy (OPHL type IIa)
  - ☐ extended to one arytenoid cartilage (OPHL type IIa + ARY)
- ☐ Supracricoid laryngectomy with crico-hyoidopexy (OPHL type IIb)
  - ☐ extended to one arytenoid cartilage (OPHL type IIb + ARY)
- ☐ Supratracheal laryngectomy with tracheo-hyoido-epiglottopexy (OPHL type IIIa)
  - ☐ extended to one crico-arytenoid unit (OPHL type IIIa + CAU)
- ☐ Supratracheal laryngectomy with tracheo-hyoidopexy (OPHL type IIIb)
  - ☐ extended to one crico-arytenoid unit (OPHL type IIIb + CAU)

Finally, in a third multiple-choice list, any plausible intra-operative extension or variation to the procedure, including the conversion to a total laryngectomy, will be highlighted.

Possible Intraoperative Modulation

- ☐ Extension of a horizontal supraglottic laryngectomy (OPHL type I) to one adjacent subsite (arytenoid, base of the tongue, mucosa of the piriform sinus – OPHL type I + ARY, type I + BOT, type I + PIR respectively);
- ☐ Extension of a supracricoid laryngectomy (OPHL type II) to one arytenoid (OPHL type IIa + ARY or type IIb + ARY);
- ☐ Extension of a supratracheal laryngectomy to one crico-arytenoid unit (OPHL type IIIa + CAU or type IIIb + CAU).
- ☐ Conversion of the scheduled procedure into a:
  - ☐ Supracricoid laryngectomy with crico-hyoidopexy (OPHL type IIb), with eventual extension to one arytenoid (OPHL type IIb + ARY);
  - ☐ Supratracheal laryngectomy with tracheo-hyoido-epiglottopexy (OPHL type IIIa), with eventual extension to one crico-arytenoid unit (OPHL type IIIa + CAU);
  - ☐ Supratracheal laryngectomy with tracheo-hyoidopexy (OPHL type IIIb), with eventual extension to one crico-arytenoid unit (OPHL type IIIb + CAU);
  - ☐ Total laryngectomy.

In the last section, the declaration of consent to the procedure must be signed by both the patient and the surgeon.

It must be noted that the use of some technical terms is essential for the precise definition of the procedure. Those terms must be carefully explained by the surgeon, in order to allow the patient to understand every passage of the ICF.

It is crucial to remember that the ICF does not replace the surgeon's oral explanations to the patient. The conversation should be tailored to the patient's socio-cultural conditions, with appropriate and clear vocabulary, and the patient should be urged to ask for any further information. This conversation should take place some days before the surgery, in order to give the patient enough time to meditate. The patient is asked again for any questions the day before the procedure.

15.5 Conclusions

OPHLs can be referred to as modular surgery, being able to tailor the procedure, even intraoperatively, to a patient's specific disease. When proposing an OPHL, the surgeon should present a surgical plan rather than a single procedure. The patient must be aware of that and accept any possible intraoperative variation. Therefore, a peculiar ICF designed in a modular way can reproduce the variability of the procedure. At the same time, an IF can improve the level of patient–surgeon cooperation and avoid any possible litigation by providing full comprehension of the procedure and reaching a complete agreement on surgical planning. Both an IF and an ICF should be adopted by any surgeon performing OPHLs.

References

1. Succo G, Fantini M, Rizzotto G. Supratracheal partial laryngectomy: indications, oncologic and functional results. Curr Opin Otolaryngol Head Neck Surg. 2017;25(2):127–32. https://doi.org/10.1097/MOO.0000000000000344.
2. Rizzotto G, Crosetti E, Lucioni M, Succo G. Subtotal laryngectomy: outcomes of 469 patients and proposal of a comprehensive and simplified classification of surgical procedures. Eur Arch Otorhinolaryngol. 2012;269(6):1635–46. https://doi.org/10.1007/s00405-012-1928-4.
3. Succo G, Peretti G, Piazza C, Remacle M, Eckel HE, Chevalier D, et al. Open partial horizontal laryngectomies: a proposal for classification by the working committee on nomenclature of the European Laryngological Society. Eur Arch Otorhinolaryngol. 2014;271:2489–96. https://doi.org/10.1007/s00405-014-3024-4.
4. Giordano L, Di Santo D, Crosetti E, Bertolin A, Rizzotto G, Succo G, et al. Open partial horizontal laryngectomies: is it time to adopt a modular form of consent for the intervention? Acta Otorhinolaryngol Ital. 2016;36(5):403–7. https://doi.org/10.14639/0392-100X-769.
5. Leclercq WKG, Keulers BJ, Scheltinga MRM, Spauwen PHM, van der Wilt GJ. A review of surgical informed consent: past, present, and future. A quest to help patients make better decisions. World J Surg. 2010;34:1406–15. https://doi.org/10.1007/s00268-010-0542-0.
6. Katz J. Reflections on informed consent: 40 years after its birth. J Am Coll Surg. 1998;186:466–74. https://doi.org/10.1016/s1072-7515(98)00045-3.
7. Appelbaum PS, Clinical practice. Assessment of patients' competence to consent to treatment. N Engl J Med. 2007;357:1834–40. https://doi.org/10.1056/NEJMcp074045.
8. World Health Organization Staff. Promotion of the rights of patients in Europe. In: Proceedings of a WHO consultation; 1995.
9. Armstrong AP, Cole AA, Page RE. Informed consent: are we doing enough? Br J Plast Surg. 1997;50:637–40. https://doi.org/10.1016/s0007-1226(97)90510-5.

10. Henney S, Rakhra S. Patient information in otorhinolaryngology: a prospective audit. J R Soc Med Sh Rep. 2011;2:37. https://doi.org/10.1258/shorts.2011.011022.
11. Kessler TM, Nachbur BH, Kessler W. Patients' perception of preoperative information by interactive computer program—exemplified by cholecystectomy. Patient Educ Couns. 2005;59:135–40. https://doi.org/10.1016/j.pec.2004.10.009.
12. Paasche-Orlow MK, Taylor HA, Brancati FL. Readability standards for informed-consent forms as compared with actual readability. N Engl J Med. 2003;348:721–6. https://doi.org/10.1056/NEJMsa021212.
13. Tan LT, Jenkins H, Roberts-Harry J, et al. Should patients set the agenda for informed consent? A prospective survey of desire for information and discussion prior to routine cataract surgery. Ther Clin Risk Manag. 2008;4:1119–25. https://doi.org/10.2147/tcrm.s3706.

Information Form

1.1 The Partial Horizontal Laryngectomies

1.1.1 Anatomy and Physiology of the Larynx

The larynx is an organ located in the neck; it follows the pharynx, behind the tongue, and continues with the trachea. The larynx has several functions: first of all, serves for the passage of inspired and expired air; second, it allows the emission of sounds (phonation), but the key role of the organ is to constitute a sphincter, some kind of valve that properly directs air into the trachea during breathing and the food and drinks into the esophagus during swallowing.

The larynx is composed of some articulated cartilages with the ability to move through a series of muscles. The cartilages constitute the supporting structure of the organ. They are the thyroid cartilage, which constitutes the front portion; the epiglottis, located above, which is reversed posteriorly during swallowing, protecting the larynx; cricoid cartilage, ring-shaped, is the basis on which rests the whole organ; the arytenoid cartilages, resting on the cricoid cartilage and free to move above it. The vocal cords are two bands that lie between the arytenoid and the thyroid cartilages. A series of muscles allows the rotation of the arytenoid cartilages, opening and closing the vocal folds.

During breathing, the vocal folds are opened, allowing free passage of inspired and expired air. They are closed during phonation, and the air emitted from the lungs causes their vibration and consequent sound emission. During swallowing, the whole organ moves forward and upward, the epiglottis is reversed, and the vocal cords close, directing the food back into the esophagus.

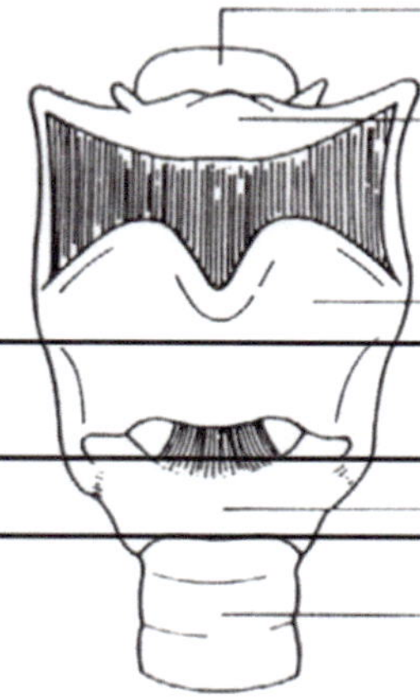

1.2 Presentation of the Surgical Procedure

Horizontal partial laryngectomies are surgical procedures reserved to the removal of laryngeal tumors. Depending on the type of surgery, different portions of the larynx can be preserved or sacrificed, and surgery may eventually be extended to other areas, beyond the organ boundaries.

According to the system of horizontal partial laryngectomies (*Open Partial Horizontal Laryngectomies - OPHL*), referring to the inferior limit of resection, we can identify the horizontal supraglottic laryngectomy (OPHL type I), the supracricoid laryngectomy (OPHL type II), and the supratracheal laryngectomy (OPHL type III).

F. Mattioli et al. (eds.), *Atlas of Open Partial Horizontal Laryngectomy*, https://doi.org/10.1007/978-3-031-48023-2

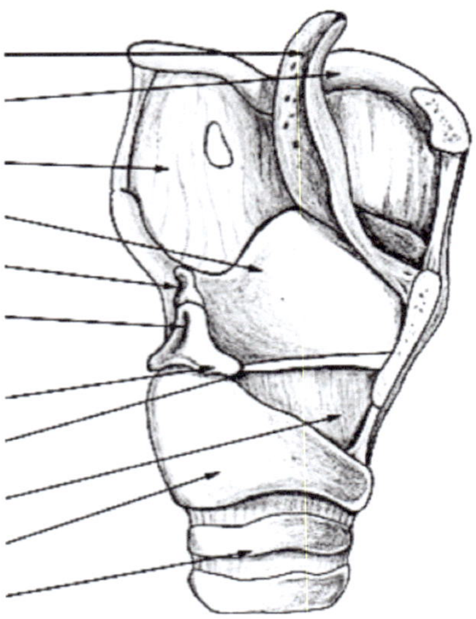

1.2.1.1 Aim of Surgery and Concept of Oncological Safety

OPHLs achieve at the same time two objectives: the complete removal of the disease and the functional preservation of the larynx.

The primary goal of a surgical procedure aiming at the removal of a neoplastic mass must always be the complete removal of the mass, that is **oncological safety**. This goal is reached by removing the mass together with a portion of healthy surrounding tissue, whose extent depends on the origin of the disease. Generally, after the removal of the tumor and a surrounding portion of macroscopically healthy tissue, the surgeon performs biopsies on the resection margins, which are sent to the pathologist for an immediate response (the so-called intraoperative consultation). Intraoperative consultation is requested to assess the need to make a further resection for clear margins. If the disease is found microscopically, the surgeon must extend the resection.

The second goal of the horizontal partial laryngectomies is to preserve laryngeal function. To maintain laryngeal function, at least one of the two crico-arytenoid units must be kept intact and functioning. The **crico-arytenoid unit** is constituted by one arytenoid cartilage together with the corresponding portion of the cricoid cartilage, on which the first rests and is free to move. This movement will recreate the larynx function after surgery.

The peculiarity of the horizontal partial laryngectomies is represented by the possibility of "modulating" the surgical procedure according to the extent of the disease. The horizontal partial laryngectomies system in fact provides for different types of intervention, each with peculiar possible extensions, and the possibility to switch from one type to another according to intraoperative findings, to guarantee oncological safety and, in most cases, also the preservation of the laryngeal function.

1.2.1.2 Types of Intervention

- The **horizontal supraglottic laryngectomy (OPHL type I)** consists of the removal of the region of the larynx above the vocal folds. Both arytenoid cartilages and both true vocal folds are spared, while epiglottis, ventricular folds, aryepiglottic folds, pre-epiglottic space (i.e., the space bounded by the cricothyroid membrane anteriorly, the hyoid bone superiorly, and the epiglottis posteriorly), superior portion of the thyroid cartilage, and hyoid bone (eventually) are removed.
  The surgery is intended for the removal of tumors arising from the supraglottic larynx, i.e., the portion above the vocal folds. In particular:
  - tumors of the laryngeal face of the epiglottis
  - tumors of the ventricular folds affecting the petiolus of the epiglottis
  - tumors extended to the anterior portion of the laryngeal ventricle, a fusiform fossa situated between the vestibular and the vocal folds, without involvement posteriorly of the arytenoids and the posterior third of the vestibular folds, anteriorly of the anterior commissure, i.e., where the two vocal folds join together, inferiorly of the floor of the ventricle
  - tumors of the suprahyoid epiglottis

  The horizontal supraglottic laryngectomy can also be extended to the resection of one adjacent subsite if affected by the disease (extension to one arytenoid - OPHL type I + ARY -, extension to the base of the tongue, located above the larynx - OPHL type I + BOT -, extension to one piriform sinus, located behind and laterally to the larynx, it constitutes the inlet to the esophagus - OPHL type I + PIR).

- The **supracricoid laryngectomy (OPHL type II)** consists of the removal of the entire thyroid cartilage, the pre-epiglottic space, and both true and false vocal folds. The cricoid cartilage is spared and it constitutes the lower limit of the resection. Arytenoid cartilages are spared too. Superiorly, according to the extent of the disease to the supraglottic larynx, the superior portion of the epiglottis can be spared or resected. Reconstruction is achieved with two different possibilities: crico-hyoido-epiglottopexy or crico-hyoidopexy.
  Supracricoid laryngectomy with crico-hyoido-epiglottopexy (OPHL type IIa) is intended for the removal of tumors arising from the true vocal folds. In particular:
  - tumors of one true vocal fold, with decreased motility of the fold
  - tumors of one vocal fold involving the anterior commissure or the laryngeal ventricle
  - tumors involving both vocal folds, if at least one of the two arytenoid cartilages appears to be spared

Supracricoid laryngectomy with crico-hyoidopexy (OPHL type IIb) is intended for the removal of tumors arising from the supraglottic larynx. In particular:

- tumors arising from the petiolus of the epiglottis, involving the false vocal folds and eventually one arytenoid cartilage with decreased vocal fold mobility
- tumors arising from the supraglottic larynx involving one or both vocal folds, if at least one of the two arytenoid cartilages appears to be spared
- tumors arising from the laryngeal ventricle, without subglottic involvement

Supracricoid horizontal laryngectomy, both if reconstruction is achieved by crico-hyoido-epiglottopexy and by crico-hyoidopexy, can also be extended to the resection of one of the two arytenoid cartilages, if affected by the disease (respectively, OPHL type IIa + ARY, OPHL type IIb + ARY).

- The **supratracheal laryngectomy (OPHL type III)** consists of the removal of the entire thyroid cartilage, the pre-epiglottic space, both true and false vocal folds, a portion of the cricoid cartilage, and the subglottic region. The organ function is guaranteed by the preservation of at least one functioning crico-arytenoid unit. First tracheal rings constitute the lower limit of the resection. Superiorly, according to the extent of the disease to the supraglottic larynx, the superior portion of the epiglottis can be spared or resected. Reconstruction is achieved with two different possibilities: tracheo-hyoido-epiglottopexy or tracheo-hyoidopexy.

  Supratracheal laryngectomy with tracheo-hyoido-epiglottopexy (OPHL type IIIa) is intended for the removal of tumors arising from the vocal folds with subglottic extension. In particular:
  - tumors arising from one vocal fold, with fixation of the vocal fold caused by involvement of the crico-arytenoid joint and/or with minimal invasion of the thyroid or cricoid cartilage
  - tumors arising from one vocal fold, which spread to the subglottic region
  - tumors of one vocal fold involving the anterior commissure, with subglottic extension and involvement of the thyroid cartilage and/or the cricothyroid membrane
  - tumors involving both vocal folds, with subglottic extension, if at least one of the two arytenoid cartilages appears to be spared

  Supratracheal laryngectomy with tracheo-hyoidopexy (OPHL type IIIb) is intended for transglottic tumors, i.e., tumors affecting supraglottic larynx and vocal folds, with subglottic extension. In particular:
  - tumors arising from the petiolus of the epiglottis or the laryngeal ventricle, extending inferiorly to involve one or both the vocal folds and the subglottic space, if at least one of the two arytenoid cartilages appears to be spared
  - tumors arising from the supraglottic larynx involving one or both the vocal folds, with the invasion of the anterior portion of the cricoid cartilage and/or the cricothyroid membrane
  - tumors arising from the supraglottic larynx, with involvement and fixation of one vocal fold caused by involvement of the crico-arytenoid joint
  - tumors of the supraglottic larynx extending to one vocal fold with minimal invasion of the thyroid or cricoid cartilage

  Supratracheal horizontal laryngectomy, both if reconstruction is achieved by tracheo-hyoido-epiglottopexy and by tracheo-hyoidopexy, can also be extended to the resection of one of the two crico-arytenoid joints, if affected by the disease (respectively, OPHL type IIIa + CAU, OPHL type IIIb + CAU).

1.2.1.3 Possibilities to "Modulate" the Surgical Procedure

The partial horizontal laryngectomy aims at preserving laryngeal function by a **"modular" surgical procedure**. It means that the surgery may change even intraoperatively, according to the intraoperative pathologic consultation, with an extension of the procedure until the maximum is reachable, such as sparing of only one functioning crico-arytenoid joint. If clear margins cannot be reached with scheduled surgery, then the procedure will be extended. As an extreme measure to achieve oncological safety, the procedure may eventually be converted to a total laryngectomy. In particular:

- **Supraglottic horizontal laryngectomy (OPHL type I)** may be extended:
  - to adjacent subsites (arytenoid, the base of the tongue, piriform sinus, respectively, OPHL Type I + ARY, type I + BOT, type I + PIR)
  - inferiorly, thus converting the procedure to a supracricoid laryngectomy with crico-hyoidopexy (OPHL type IIb), with or without the further extension to one arytenoid (OPHL type IIb + ARY)
- **Supracricoid laryngectomy with crico-hyoido-epiglottopexy (OPHL type IIa)** may be extended:
  - to one arytenoid (OPHL type IIa + ARY)
  - superiorly, thus converting the procedure to a supracricoid laryngectomy with crico-hyoidopexy (OPHL type IIb), with or without the further extension to one arytenoid (OPHL type IIb + ARY)
  - inferiorly, thus converting the procedure to a supratracheal laryngectomy with tracheo-hyoido-epiglottopexy (OPHL type IIIa), with or without the further extension to one crico-arytenoid unit (OPHL type IIIa + CAU)

- **Supracricoid laryngectomy with crico-hyoidopexy (OPHL IIb)** may be extended:
  - to one arytenoid (OPHL type IIb + ARY)
  - inferiorly, thus converting the procedure to a supratracheal laryngectomy with tracheo-hyoidopexy (OPHL type IIIb), with or without the further extension to one crico-arytenoid unit (OPHL type IIIb + CAU)
- **Supratracheal laryngectomy with tracheo-hyoido-epiglottopexy (OPHL type IIIa)** may be extended:
  - To one crico-arytenoid unit (OPHL type IIIa + CAU)
  - Superiorly, thus converting the procedure to a supratracheal laryngectomy with tracheo-hyoidopexy (OPHL type IIIb), with or without the further extension to one crico-arytenoid unit (OPHL type IIIb + CAU)
  - In case your surgeon, according to intraoperative findings, believes that supratracheal laryngectomy with tracheo-hyoido-epiglottopexy (OPHL type IIIa or type IIIa + CAU) is not adequate to achieve clear margins, the procedure may be intraoperatively converted to a total laryngectomy.
- **Supratracheal laryngectomy with tracheo-hyoidopexy (OPHL type IIIb)** may be extended:
  - To one crico-arytenoid unit (OPHL type IIIb + CAU)
  - In case your surgeon, according to intraoperative findings, believes that supratracheal laryngectomy with tracheo-hyoidopexy (OPHL type IIIb or type IIIb + CAU) is not adequate to achieve clear margins, the procedure may be intraoperatively converted to a total laryngectomy.

The extreme possibility of surgical "modulation" consists in the intraoperative conversion to a **total laryngectomy**. This eventuality becomes necessary if sparing the minimal portion of the larynx that is essential for postoperative functioning (i.e., one functioning crico-arytenoid unit) is not possible. It will happen only in rare cases, if intraoperative consultation reveals microscopic extension of the disease beyond macroscopically involved regions. Total laryngectomy entails performing a definitive tracheostomy.

Although the need for conversion to total laryngectomy is most likely for patients candidates for supratracheal laryngectomy (OPHL type III), because they are generally affected by more extended lesions or because they already need the removal of one crico-arytenoid unit, the patient should keep in mind that this possibility can never be completely excluded.

1.2.1.4 Alternatives to Surgery

For many years, total laryngectomy was the only available procedure for the removal of advanced tumors of the larynx. Since the 1970s, partial laryngectomy procedures were introduced, which at the same time aim at the complete removal of the disease and the preservation of laryngeal function. To date total laryngectomy, it is still performed for very advanced tumors.

Starting from the 1990s, new options of treatment based on non-surgical protocols have been developed, even for patients with advanced cancers of the larynx. They are the so-called organ preservation protocols, and they consist of radiation therapy or chemo-radiation therapy. Today, the best alternative to surgery is **concurrent chemo-radiation therapy**. In some studies, although performed in tertiary referral centers and in selected groups of patients, organ preservation protocols have demonstrated efficacy comparable to surgery; to date, they represent a valid alternative to surgical treatment.

Radiation therapy is the administration of radiations that damage the diseased cells, preventing their growth and causing their death. To provide at the same time, the highest possible dose of radiation to the tumor cells and the lowest dose to healthy tissues, the radiation beams are emitted from different angles. It is therefore necessary that the patient stays completely still during the treatment. For this reason, a containment mask of plastic material is realized before the treatment, which immobilizes the patient on the table where the treatment takes place. To be effective, the treatment should be administered continuatively for several days. Generally, it consists of a session of about 10 min, 5 days a week, with a duration of 6 weeks. However, radiation therapy should be individualized; further information, if required, will be provided by your radiation oncologist.

Chemotherapy is the administration of one or more drugs that inhibit and fight the development of cancer cells. These drugs are mostly directed against rapidly replicating cells, such as cancer cells, but they damage healthy cells too. The treatment is usually administered intravenously, during a day hospital, once a week. However, also chemotherapy should be individualized; further information, if required, will be provided by your oncologist.

Concomitant use of radiation and chemotherapy enhances the effects of each treatment, maximizing the chances of success. Chemotherapy would aim to sensitize cancer cells, making them more susceptible to radiation damage.

Despite no surgical procedure being required (including tracheostomy), also chemo-radiation therapy bears some risks. First, there is the risk of not being able to complete the treatment because of excessive toxicity caused by the treatment itself. Second, chemo-radiation therapy, as well as surgery, has some possible complications: dysphagia, even severe, with the need for positioning of a percutaneous gastrostomy (PEG), such as a tube passed into your stomach through the abdominal wall; poor quality of the voice; chronic penetration of small amounts of saliva in the trachea and bronchi, with consequent severe bronchopneumonia. In rare cases, the function of the larynx may be completely lost, causing persistent inhalation of saliva in the tracheobronchial tree, resulting in repeated bronchopneumonia; in such cases, a total laryngectomy may be necessary.

Also with chemo-radiation treatment, there is a risk for recurrence of the disease. If recurrence happens after a chemo-radiation, an eventual surgical procedure would present greater technical difficulties and increased risks of complications. In this case, a horizontal partial laryngectomy may not be feasible anymore.

Involvement of specific subsites of the larynx, such as anterior commissure or cartilage infiltration, may make some tumors less susceptible to chemo-radiation treatment, and they are associated with a higher rate of recurrence. If these conditions are present, your surgeon will disclose them.

The correct therapeutic approach must be individualized for each patient, taking into account their preferences, their physical and mental status, their comorbidities, their lifestyle habits, and the laryngeal function they intend to preserve. The patient, informed of any possible treatment and relative risks and benefits, will choose the preferred treatment.

If you decide not to undertake any treatment, the disease will inevitably progress over a period that could be more or less long. It will increase its dimensions in the larynx; it will cause metastases to lymph nodes (if they are still not present at diagnosis) and distant metastases to other organs, such as lung, liver, brain, bones, etc. At a certain time, the disease will not be resectable anymore with a partial horizontal laryngectomy and, subsequently, neither with a total laryngectomy, and your chances of survival will reduce considerably.

1.3 Surgical Procedure

The surgery will be performed under general anesthesia. Therefore, it is essential for a preoperative anesthesiologist evaluation. The anesthesiologist will answer all your questions about general anesthesia.

The surgery is intended for the removal of the portions of the larynx affected by the disease, and resection will follow one of the above-mentioned types of intervention, such as horizontal supraglottic laryngectomy, sopracricoid laryngectomy with crico-hyoido-epiglottopexy or with crico-hyoidopexy, and supratracheal laryngectomy with tracheo-hyoido-epiglottopexy or with tracheo-hyoidopexy.

A "U"-shaped skin incision is performed, extending from one retro auricular region to the other, going down into the anterior neck. The procedure requires the creation of a temporary opening on the trachea (tracheotomy). Tracheotomy allows respiration until postsurgical swelling will reduce and until rehabilitation of deglutition will be completed. When the tracheostomy will be closed, you will be able to speak and breathe by the natural ways. Your voice will be preserved, but a certain degree of **dysphonia** (hoarseness) will be permanent.

Partial horizontal laryngectomy may be associated with a unilateral or bilateral functional neck dissection (removal of the lymph nodes, which are small rounded organs, composed of lymphatic tissue, connected by lymphatic vessels).

During the first postoperative days, you will be fed through a **nasogastric tube** (tube passing through the nose into the stomach), which will be placed during surgery.

The duration of the procedure may vary, according to the encountered difficulties. Hospital stay and postoperative care depend on the type of intervention and they will be specified by your surgeon.

Surgery will be followed by a period of **rehabilitation** that will include a series of exercises to accelerate the recovery of swallowing and phonation functions. A speech therapist will help you during the hospital stay. Rehabilitation will continue after discharge.

Like all medical procedures (examinations, endoscopies, and interventions), even if conducted properly with expertise and experience following the current medical standards, even partial horizontal laryngectomies bear the risk of some complications. Some of these complications are more common, while others are exceptional. The incidence of complications is increased by some patient's conditions (for example, diabetes, immunodeficiency, malnutrition, etc.), as well as from previous treatments, such as prior radiation or chemo-radiation therapy on the larynx or the neck.

1.4 How the Operated Larynx Works

Partial horizontal laryngectomies exploit the redundancy of the anatomical structures of the larynx, which can be considerably reduced, maintaining the ability to efficiently carry out its functions.

After a partial horizontal laryngectomy, especially after OPHL type II and III that involve a significant reduction of the laryngeal framework including the vocal folds, anatomy and physiology are intensely modified.

In OPHL type I, glottic sphincter is preserved, and it keeps its function and compensates for the lack of the structures located above. After OPHL Type II and III instead, as already explained, the crico-arytenoid unit(s) will recreate the functional sphincter. After surgery, the organ will be called "neo-larynx," and the sphincter will be called "neo-glottis." The neo-glottis is a three-dimensional structure, which has the role of maintaining the three main functions of the larynx: respiration, phonation, and deglutition. It is composed of the tongue base and an optional residual portion of the epiglottis anteriorly (the neo-larynx is located in a superior position compared to the original one) and by at least one of the two crico-arytenoid units posteriorly.

The function of the neo-larynx will be guaranteed by the movement of the crico-arytenoid unit(s), which closes the neo-glottis anteriorly against the base of the tongue and eventually the remaining portion of the epiglottis.

Postoperative rehabilitation will be hard for the patient. Achieving recovery of the laryngeal function means learning how to coordinate the structures of the neo-glottis. A correct rehabilitation is crucial after surgery, for this reason, you will be assisted by a speech therapist. During this period, you will be instructed about a series of exercises and then you will have to perform many deglutition attempts, both together with the surgeon and/or the speech therapist, and alone. Your dedication and your resolution during this period are critical for the proper recovery.

1.5 Complications

Possible complications are as follows:

- Intra- and postoperative bleedings. Massive hemorrhages due to the rupture of large vessels of the neck may require urgent surgical treatment, although they are very rare, and they occur more often in patients who had undergone prior radiation therapy
- Infections of the surgical wound. They are generally controlled by systemic antibiotic therapy
- Hematoma (localized collection of blood) in the cervical region
- Fistulas, which may heal by conservative treatment (compression bandages and antibiotic therapy) or may require a surgical procedure if conservative treatments are ineffective;
- Aspiration pneumonia, i.e., a lung infection due to food penetration into the trachea and bronchi. It may occur especially in the immediate postoperative period or in the early stages of swallowing rehabilitation;
- Laryngocele, which is a collection of air around the larynx
- Rupture of the pexy is a very rare event, but requires an immediate surgical revision
- Malpositioning/prolapse of the remaining portion of the epiglottis or formation of the mucosal flap, resulting in breathing difficulties, which may require surgical revision
- Hypopharyngeal stenosis (narrowing of the lowest portion of the pharynx), resulting in swallowing difficulties
- Laryngeal stenosis (narrowing of the larynx), resulting in the need to maintain the tracheostomy or to undergo a revision surgery
- Tracheal stenosis (narrowing of the trachea), resulting in breathing difficulties, which may require further medical and/or surgical treatment to be able to remove the tracheostomy. Rarely, it will be necessary to permanently maintain the tracheostomy
- Difficult functional recovery of swallowing. It will be more frequent if one arytenoid or one crico-arytenoid unit must be removed (sparing of both arytenoids will produce contraction of interarytenoid muscles, providing a more valid closure of the neo-larynx and thus facilitating correct swallowing)
- Exuberant skin scarring (keloid) is generally related to a patient's congenital characteristic, or abnormal reaction following exposure to sunlight during any season period, mainly in the summer
- Mucus plugs, which may block the tracheostomy tube resulting in insufficient air passage. Mucus plugs formation is more frequent in the early postoperative days because of stagnation of the abundant catarrhal secretion, non-physiological breathing, poor humidification of inspired air, insufficient expectoration due to the local pain, and lack of physical activity. To free the airways, it will be sufficient to remove the tracheostomy tube and, if needed, to aspirate tracheal secretions; sometimes the same aspirator, stimulating the cough reflex, helps the expulsion of the plug. Death by suffocation due to the formation of a mucus plug that cannot be removed in time is a very rare event
- If the patient experiences difficulties in swallowing rehabilitation, it is possible to place a percutaneous endoscopic gastrostomy (PEG), which is the surgical positioning, under local anesthesia, of a tube passing through the abdominal wall into the stomach, which will feed the patient during the prolonged rehabilitation period
- If you refuse the PEG and if swallowing recovery is impossible, despite all rehabilitation attempts, resulting in inhalation of solids and liquids leading to aspiration pneumonia, a total laryngectomy may be necessary
- Inappropriate phonation recovery. A certain degree of dysphonia will be permanent, but the voice may not be powerful enough to be understandable. Speech therapy and surgical aids may be necessary
- Persistence of stitches from the pexy, which may cause granulomas or fistulas; they require a surgical revision for removal
- Recurrence of the disease. A regular follow-up will be necessary, according to your surgeon's indications
- Complications due to the general anesthesia, with possible very serious complications, including anaphylactic shock

Modular Informed Consent Form

1.1 Declaration of Patient's Consent to Partial Horizontal Laryngectomy

Dear Mr/Mrs,

You are affected by

....

....

According to the extent and location of your tumor, you are candidate for a partial horizontal laryngectomy.

To inform you as clearly and as completely as possible about the surgical procedure, together with this form, **an Information Form has been provided to you**, which contains any information about partial horizontal laryngectomies. You are kindly invited to carefully read both these documents. You don't have to be concerned by the information contained therein; this information is mandatory to allow you to freely and consciously decide whether to undergo or not the procedure. You can ask your surgeon for any more information at any moment.

It is crucial that you tell your surgeon, to doctors who will collect your medical history, and to the anesthesiologist, the drugs that you are taking (in particular analgesics, anti-inflammatories, painkillers, antihypertensives, anticoagulants, etc.). It is important as well to tell whether you ever experienced any allergies, especially to drugs, and if you have ever undergone general anesthesia. Finally, you should provide all your clinical documentation (laboratory, clinical and radiological examinations, etc.).

1.1.1 The Extent of the Disease

Dear Mr/Mrs, your tumor involves:

☐ Epiglottis		
☐ Base of tongue or glossoepiglottic folds		
☐ Mucosa of the piriform sinus		
☐ Aryepiglottic fold	☐ Right	☐ Left
☐ Laryngeal vestibule		
☐ Pre-epiglottic space		
☐ False vocal fold	☐ Right	☐ Left
☐ Laryngeal ventricule	☐ Right	☐ Left
☐ Vocal fold	☐ Right	☐ Left
☐ Anterior commissure		
☐ Arytenoid cartilage	☐ Right	☐ Left
☐ Thyroid cartilage		
☐ Paraglottic space	☐ Right	☐ Left
☐ Cricoid cartilage		
☐ Crico-arytenoid unit	☐ Right	☐ Left
☐ Subglottic mucosa		
☐ Crico-thyroid membrane		
☐ Prelaryngeal soft tissues		

1.1.2 Surgical Procedure

There are different types of partial horizontal laryngectomies, as already discussed in the Information Form. According to the extent of your lesion, the scheduled surgical procedure is as follows:

- ☐ Horizontal supraglottic laryngectomy (OPHL type I)
  - ☐ Extended to one arytenoid cartilage (OPHL type I + ARY)
  - ☐ Extended to the base of the tongue (OPHL type I + BOT)
  - ☐ Extended to the piriform sinus (OPHL type I + PIR)
- ☐ Supracricoid laryngectomy with crico-hyoido-epiglottopexy (OPHL type IIa)
  - ☐ Extended to one arytenoid cartilage (OPHL type IIa + ARY)
- ☐ Supracricoid laryngectomy with crico-hyoidopexy (OPHL type IIb)
  - ☐ Extended to one arytenoid cartilage (OPHL type IIb + ARY)
- ☐ Supratracheal laryngectomy with tracheo-hyoido-epiglottopexy (OPHL type IIIa)
  - ☐ Extended to one crico-arytenoid unit (OPHL type IIIa + CAU)
- ☐ Supratracheal laryngectomy with tracheo-hyoidopexy (OPHL type IIIb)
  - ☐ Extended to one crico-arytenoid unit (OPHL type IIIb + CAU)

F. Mattioli et al. (eds.), *Atlas of Open Partial Horizontal Laryngectomy*, https://doi.org/10.1007/978-3-031-48023-2

1.1.3 Possible Intraoperative Modulation

Partial horizontal laryngectomy is a "modular" surgical procedure. According to the intraoperative pathological consultation, it may be necessary to convert the surgery. In your particular case, although other options can never be completely excluded, the most plausible extensions may be:

- ☐ Extension of a horizontal supraglottic laryngectomy (OPHL type I) to one adjacent subsite (arytenoid, the base of the tongue, mucosa of the piriform sinus – OPHL type I + ARY, type I + BOT, type I + PIR, respectively)
- ☐ Extension of a supracricoid laryngectomy (OPHL type II) to one arytenoid (OPHL type IIa + ARY or type IIb + ARY)
- ☐ Extension of a supratracheal laryngectomy to one crico-arytenoid unit (OPHL type IIIa + CAU or type IIIb + CAU)
- ☐ Conversion of the scheduled procedure into a:
  - ☐ Supracricoid laryngectomy with crico-hyoido-pexy (OPHL type IIb), with eventual extension to one arytenoid (OPHL type IIb + ARY)
  - ☐ Supratracheal laryngectomy with tracheo-hyoido-epiglottopexy (OPHL type IIIa), with eventual extension to one crico-arytenoid unit (OPHL type IIIa + CAU)
  - ☐ Supratracheal laryngectomy with tracheo-hyoido-pexy (OPHL type IIIb), with eventual extension to one crico-arytenoid unit (OPHL type IIIb + CAU)
  - ☐ Total laryngectomy

Surgeon's annotation on possible extensions

....
....
....
....
....
....
....
....
....
....

Furthermore, you confirm that:

- ☐ You didn't ask for any more information;
- ☐ You asked for further information about:

....
....
....
....
....
....
....
....
....
....

Surgeon's Signature ....

Patient's Signature ....

1.2 Declaration of Consent

During oral explanations of the procedure and after reading the Information Form, I received information about:

- Anatomy and physiology of the larynx
- Horizontal partial laryngectomies: indications and aim of surgery and how it is performed
- The possibility that the scheduled surgery may be intraoperatively extended or converted according to the OPHL system, to achieve oncological safety
- How the larynx will work after surgery, and the need for a postoperative rehabilitation period with the speech therapist
- Achievable benefits of the procedure, and the possibility of obtaining them according to the results reported in the literature and to my condition; the possibility that revision surgeries may be necessary for any defects, even aesthetic, not always secondary to technical errors
- Risks of the procedure, according to the incidence reported in the literature and to my condition; the possibility that any surgical procedure may lead to unforeseeable risks
- Possible alternatives to surgery, in particular, a radiation or chemo-radiation treatment, with relative risks and benefits
- Possible complications after surgery, and how to try to avoid these complications
- **The possibility that, if necessary according to the intraoperative findings, to achieve the complete removal of the disease, the procedure may be intraoperatively converted to a total laryngectomy, without the need for additional consent. In this case, a definitive tracheostomy will be performed**

During oral explanations of the procedure and after reading the Information Form, I obtained any information I asked for.

After reading the Information Form and after oral explanation, **I received a copy of this Consent Form**, and I was asked to carefully think about the information provided by my surgeon, to ask for any further information, to reveal my doubts even about medical terms, and finally to declare my consent to the procedure.

I declare that I was informed about the risks of partial horizontal laryngectomies, that the surgeon answered all my questions that I completely understood all the information provided in the Information Form and during oral explanations, and that I had enough time to think about it. Then, today **I express/I don't express** my conscious and informed consent to the scheduled surgical procedure that will be performed by the surgical team under general anesthesia, and I authorize the specific surgical technique. I am aware that, according to oncological safety, the procedure may be intraoperatively extended or converted, even into a total laryngectomy. I am aware that, in the need to save my life from imminent and not predictable danger or to avoid serious harm to my person, any medical or surgical procedure will be attempted to prevent or limit this danger, to safely complete the surgery.

I authorize/I don't authorize the surgical team to treat any disease revealed during surgery and previously unknown, according to surgeon's knowledge and judgment, even with modification to the scheduled surgical procedure.

I authorize/I don't authorize the use of tissues and/or organs removed during surgery to obtain a pathological diagnosis, and also for eventual procedures aiming at the improvement of scientific knowledge.

Finally, **I authorize/I don't authorize** the use of images and videos taken during surgery, which may be used in scientific publications, with complete respect for my privacy.

Place, Date Patient's Signature

....

MIX
Papier aus verantwortungsvollen Quellen
Paper from responsible sources
FSC® C105338

If you have any concerns about our products,
you can contact us on
ProductSafety@springernature.com

In case Publisher is established outside the EU,
the EU authorized representative is:
Springer Nature Customer Service Center GmbH
Europaplatz 3, 69115 Heidelberg, Germany

Printed by Libri Plureos GmbH
in Hamburg, Germany